Community Pharmacy

Commissioning Editor: Ellen Green
Project Development Manager: Hannah Kenner
Project Manager: Frances Affleck
Designer: George Ajayi
Illustrator: PCA Creative

Community Pharmacy

Symptoms, Diagnosis and Treatment

Paul Rutter BPharm MRPharmS PhD

Senior Lecturer, Pharmacy Practice Division
School of Pharmacy and Biomedical Sciences
University of Portsmouth, UK

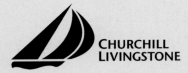

CHURCHILL LIVINGSTONE

Edinburgh   London   New York   Oxford   Philadelphia   St Louis   Sydney   Toronto 2004

CHURCHILL LIVINGSTONE
An imprint of Elsevier Limited

First published 2004

ISBN 0 4430 7362 7

British Library Cataloguing in Publication Data
A catalogue record for this book is available from the British Library

Library of Congress Cataloging in Publication Data
A catalog record for this book is available from the Library of Congress

Notice
Medical knowledge is constantly changing. Standard safety precautions must be followed, but as new research and clinical experience broaden our knowledge, changes in treatment and drug therapy may become necessary or appropriate. Readers are advised to check the most current product information provided by the manufacturer of each drug to be administered to verify the recommended dose, the method and duration of administration, and contraindications. It is the responsibility of the practitioner, relying on experience and knowledge of the patient, to determine dosages and the best treatment for each individual patient. Neither the Publisher nor the author assumes any liability for any injury and/or damage to persons or property arising from this publication.

The Publisher

The
Publisher's
policy is to use
**paper manufactured
from sustainable forests**

Printed in China

Contents

Preface

Demand on healthcare professionals to deliver high quality patient care has never been greater. A multitude of factors impinge on healthcare delivery today, including an aging population, more sophisticated medicines, high patient expectation, health service infrastructure as well as adequate and appropriate staffing levels. In primary care the medical practitioner role is pivotal in providing this care and they remain the central member of the healthcare team, but demands on their time mean other models of service delivery are being adopted in the UK and in other developed countries that utilise other healthcare professionals.

This is leading to the traditional boundaries of care between doctors, nurses, and pharmacists being broken down. In particular, certain medical practitioner responsibilities, which were once seen as their sole domain are now being performed by nurses and pharmacists, for example it is now common practice in many doctors' surgeries to have practice nurses who run specialist clinics, for example asthma and diabetes clinics, and more recently nurse and pharmacist prescribing.

Probably of greatest impact to community pharmacy practice in the UK and elsewhere is the continued de-regulation of medicines. This has included products from new therapeutic classes (e.g. anti-emetics and H_2 antagonists) allowing community pharmacists scope to manage more conditions without the need to refer patients to a medical practitioner. The global market for over-the-counter medicines is considerable, and rising. In 1991 US customers spent $10.2 billion on OTC medicines, which had risen to $19.1 billion by 2000. Similar trends have been seen in UK and European markets and this upward trend looks set to continue.

A combination of factors has fuelled this worldwide increase in OTC sales: including government healthcare policies that have encouraged self-care and self-medication; a greater emphasis on cost containment by healthcare organisations; an unprecedented rise in the number of medicines deregulated from prescription-only control to OTC status, aided by streamlined and less bureaucratic administration; and the profit interests of pharmaceutical companies, especially when ethical patents expire.

Pharmacists will have to demonstrate that they are competent practitioners to be trusted with this additional responsibility. Therefore pharmacists will require greater levels of knowledge and understanding about commonly occurring medical conditions. They will need to be able to recognise their signs and symptoms, and use an evidence-based approach to treatment.

This is the catalyst for this book. Although other books targeted for pharmacists on diagnosis are published, this book aims to give a more in-depth view of minor conditions and how to differentiate them from more sinister pathology that may present in a similar way. The book is intended for all pharmacists, from undergraduate students to experienced practitioners.

It is hoped that the information contained within the book is both informative and useful.

PR

Introduction

Community pharmacists are the most accessible healthcare professional. In the UK one report suggested that 6 million people a day visit community pharmacies. No appointment is needed to consult a pharmacist and patients can receive free, unbiased advice almost anywhere. On a typical day a pharmacist practising in an 'average' community pharmacy can realistically expect to help between 5 and 15 patients a day who present with various symptoms for which they are seeking advice, reassurance, treatment or a combination of all three. Unlike most other healthcare professionals community pharmacists do not normally have access to the patient's medical record and thus have no idea about what the person's problem is until a conversation is initiated. This presents the community pharmacist with a great challenge to correctly differentially diagnose the patient.

Communication skills

For the most part pharmacists will be totally dependent on their ability to question patients in order to arrive at a differential diagnosis. This is in stark contrast to the GP and, to a lesser extent, the nurse, who can draw on physical examination and diagnostic tests to help them arrive at a diagnosis. Opportunities for pharmacists to perform a physical examination are limited by the lack of privacy within a pharmacy and also a lack of training in correct examination technique; diagnostic testing is never employed because of the costs (which would have to be passed on to the patient) and the invasive nature of most tests (e.g. blood taking for analysis).

Having said this, a number of studies have shown that in more than three-quarters of all cases taking a patient history alone will result in the correct diagnosis. This figure rises slightly if a history is supplemented with a physical examination and yet further if laboratory investigations are also conducted.

It is vital, therefore, that pharmacists possess excellent communication skills to ensure the correct information is obtained from the patient. This will be drawn from a combination of good questioning technique, listening actively to the patient and picking up on non-verbal cues.

Approaches to differential diagnosis

Try to avoid using acronyms

Traditionally, the use of acronyms has been advocated to help pharmacists remember what questions to ask a patient. However, it is important that pharmacists do not rely solely on acronyms in trying to differentially diagnose a person's presenting complaint; acronyms are rigid, inflexible and often inappropriate. Every patient is different and therefore it is unlikely that an acronym can be fully applied and, more importantly, using acronyms can mean that you miss vital information that could shape your course of action. Some of the more commonly used acronyms are discussed briefly below.

WWHAM

This is the simplest acronym to remember but it is also the worst one to use. It gives the pharmacist very limited information from which to work and it is unlikely that a correct differential diagnosis will be made. If used at all, it should be with caution and it is probably only useful for counter assistants to use when a patient first presents, so that a general picture of the person's presenting complaint can be established.

	Meaning of the letter	Attributes of the acronym
W	Who is the patient?	**Positive points**
W	What are the symptoms?	Establishes presenting
H	How long have the symptoms been present?	complaint
A	Action taken?	**Negative points**
M	Medication being taken?	Fails to consider general appearance of patient. No social/lifestyle factors taken into account; no family history sought; not specific or in-depth enough; no history of previous symptoms

Other acronyms that have been suggested as being helpful for pharmacists in differential diagnosis are ENCORE, ASMETHOD and SIT DOWN SIR. Although these three acronyms are more comprehensive than WWHAM, they are still limited. No one acronym takes into consideration all the factors that might impinge on the differential diagnosis. All fail to establish a full history from the patient in respect to lifestyle and social factors or the relevance of a family history. They are very much designed to establish the nature and severity of the presenting complaint. This, in many instances, will be adequate but for intermittent conditions (e.g. irritable bowel syndrome, asthma, hayfever) they might well miss important information. Likewise, positive family history with certain conditions (e.g. psoriasis, eczema) provides useful clues in establishing a diagnosis.

Meaning of the letter	Attributes of the acronym
E Explore	**Positive points**
N No medication	'Observe' section suggests
C Care	taking into account the
O Observe	appearance of the patient –
R Refer	does he or she look poorly?
E Explain	
	Negative points
	Sections on 'No medication' and 'Refer' add little to the differential diagnosis process. No social/lifestyle factors taken into account; no family history sought

Meaning of the letter	Attributes of the acronym
A Age/appearance?	**Positive points**
S Self or someone else?	Establishes the nature of
M Medication?	problem and if patient has
E Extra medicines?	suffered from previous
T Time persisting?	similar episodes
H History?	
O Other symptoms?	**Negative points**
D Danger symptoms?	Exact symptoms and severity not fully established. No social/lifestyle factors taken into account; no family history sought

Meaning of the letter	Attributes of the acronym
S Site or location?	**Positive points**
I Intensity or severity?	Establishes the severity and
T Type or nature?	nature of problem and if the
D Duration?	patient has suffered from
O Onset?	previous similar episodes
W With (other symptoms)?	
N Annoyed or aggravated?	**Negative points**
S Spread or radiation?	Fails to consider general
I Incidence or frequency pattern?	appearance of patient. No social/lifestyle factors taken
R Relieved by?	into account; no family history sought

Clinical decision making

Whether we are conscious of it or not, most people will – at some level – use clinical decision making to arrive at a differential diagnosis. Diagnostic reasoning is a component of clinical decision making and involves recognition of cues and analysis of data. Very early in a clinical encounter, and based on limited information, a pharmacist will arrive at a small number of hypotheses. The pharmacist then sets about testing these hypotheses by asking the patient a series of questions. The answer to each question allows the pharmacist to narrow down the possible diagnosis either by eliminating particular conditions or confirming his or her suspicions of a particular condition. Once the questioning is over, the pharmacist should be in a position to differentially diagnose the patient's condition.

Key steps in the process

1. Formulating a diagnosis based on the patient and the initial presenting complaint

Before any questions are asked of the patient you should think about the line of questioning you are going to take:

- What is the general appearance of the patient? Does the person look well or poorly? Is the person you are about to talk to the patient or someone acting on the patient's behalf? This will shape your thinking as to the severity of the problem.
- How old is the patient? This is very useful information. Epidemiological studies for a wide range of conditions and disease states has shown that certain age groups will suffer from certain problems. For example, it is very unlikely that a child who presents with cough will have chronic bronchitis but the probability of an elderly person having chronic bronchitis is much higher.
- What sex is the patient? As with age, sex can dramatically alter the chances of suffering from certain conditions. Migraines are five times more common in women than men, yet cluster headache is nine times more common in men than women.
- What is the presenting complaint? Some conditions are much more common than others. Therefore you could form an idea of what condition the patient is likely to be suffering from based on the laws of probability. For example, if a person presents with a headache then you should already know that the most common cause of headache is tension headache,

followed by migraine and then cluster headache. Other causes of headache are rare but obviously need to be eliminated. Your line of questioning should try to confirm or refute the most likely causes of headache.

2. Asking questions

The questions you ask the patient will be specific to that patient. After establishing who the person is, how poorly he or she is and what the presenting complaint is, a number of targeted questions specific to that patient should be asked. The following scenario will illustrate this point:

A 31-year-old female asks for advice about a headache she has.

What are your initial thoughts? (1. Formulating a diagnosis based on the patient and the initial presenting complaint):

- the patient is present
- the patient is female and in her early thirties
- the patient looks and sounds OK
- epidemiology states that tension headache is most likely but females are more prone to migraine than males.

What line of questioning do you take? (2. Asking questions.) Your main aim is to differentiate between tension and migraine headache:

Nature of the pain

Tension headache usually produces a dull ache, as opposed to the throbbing nature of migraine pain:

- patient's response: dull ache
- pharmacist's thoughts: suggestive of tension headache.

Location of the pain

Tension headache is generally bilateral; migraine is often unilateral:

- patient's response: all over
- pharmacist's thoughts: suggestive of tension headache.

Severity of pain

Tension headache is not usually severe and disabling; migraine can be disabling:

- patient's response: bothersome more than stopping her doing things
- pharmacist's thoughts: suggestive of tension headache.

The answers so far are indicative of tension headache. However, further specific questions relating to lifestyle and previous and family history should be asked. It would be expected that there was no family history of migraine and there is probably some trigger factor causing the headache, for example increased stress due to work or personal pressures. The patient might therefore have had similar headaches in the past.

Finally, even though at this stage you are confident of your differential diagnosis you should still ask a couple of questions to rule out any sinister pathology. Obviously you are expecting the answers from these questions to be negative to support your differential diagnosis. Any questions that invoke the opposite response to that expected will require further investigation.

3. Confirm facts

Before making a recommendation to the patient it is always helpful to try and re-cap on the information elicited. This is especially important when you have had to ask a lot of questions. It is well known that short-term working memory is relatively small and that remembering all the pertinent facts is difficult. Summarising the information at this stage will not only help you formulate your final diagnosis but will also allow the patient to add further information or to correct you on facts that you have failed to remember correctly.

The way in which one goes about establishing what is wrong with the patient will vary from practitioner to practitioner. However, it is important that whatever method is adopted it must be sufficiently robust to be of benefit to the patient. Using a clinical decision-making approach to differential diagnosis allows you to build a fuller picture of the patient's presenting complaint. It is both flexible and specific to each individual, unlike acronyms.

How to use this book

This book is divided into ten chapters. The first nine are systems based and structured in the format shown in Fig. 1. The final chapter is product based and has a slightly different format. A list of abbreviations and a glossary are included at the end of the book.

Key features of each chapter

At the beginning of each chapter a short section addressing basic anatomy and history taking specific to that body system is presented. A basic understanding of the anatomical location of major structures is useful when attempting to diagnose/exclude conditions from a patient's presenting complaint. It would be almost impossible to know whether to treat or refer a patient who presented with symptoms suggestive of renal colic if one doesn't know where the kidneys are. However, this book is not intended to replace an anatomy text and the reader is referred to the list of further reading for anatomy texts.

Self-assessment questions

Twenty multiple choice and two case-study questions are presented at the end of each chapter. These are designed

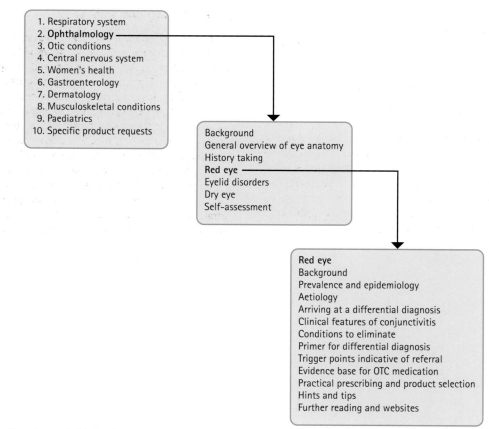

Figure 1   Structure of this book

to test factual recall and applied knowledge. The multiple choice questions are constructed to mimic those set in the pre-registration examination. They start with simple traditional multiple choice questions in which the right answer has to be picked from a series of five possible answers, and work up to more complex, interrelated questions.

The case studies challenge you with 'real-life' situations. All are drawn from practice and have been encountered by practising pharmacists, but have been modified for inclusion in the book. They all begin with an initial presenting complaint followed by a series of questions that guide you through the case.

For all questions, a set of answers are provided to allow self-reflection.

Elements included under each condition

The same structure has been adopted for every condition. This is intended to help the reader approach differential diagnosis from the position of clinical decision making. To help summarise the information, tables and algorithms are included for many of the conditions.

Arriving at a differential diagnosis

A table summarising the key questions that should be asked for each condition is included. The relevance (i.e. the rationale for asking the question) is given for each question. This will allow pharmacists to determine what questions to ask of every patient to enable a differential diagnosis.

Primer for differential diagnosis

A 'primer for differential diagnosis' is available for a number of the conditions covered. This algorithmic approach to differential diagnosis is geared towards nearly or recently qualified pharmacists. They are not intended to be solely relied upon in making a differential diagnosis but to act as an aide memoire. It is anticipated that the primers will be used in conjunction with the text, thus allowing a broader understanding of the differential diagnosis of the condition being considered.

Trigger points indicative of referral

A summary box of trigger factors when it would be prudent to refer the patient to a medical practitioner is presented for each condition.

Evidence-based OTC medication and Practical prescribing and product selection

These two sections present the reader, first, with an evaluation of the current literature on whether over-the-counter medicine works and, second, with a quick reference to the dose of the medicine and when it cannot be prescribed. This does not replace standard textbooks such as *Stockley's drug interactions* or Briggs' *Drugs in pregnancy and lactation* but it does allow the user to find basic data in one text without having to reach for three or four other texts to answer simple questions.

Hints and tips boxes

A summary box of useful information is provided near the end of each condition. This contains information that does not fall readily into any of the other sections but is none the less useful. For example, some of the hints and tips boxes give advice on how to administer eye drops, suppositories and other forms of medicines that are not taken via the oral route.

Further reading and web sites

To supplement the text, at the end of each condition a list of selected references and reading is provided for those who wish to seek further information on the subject. Web sites are also provided, as many people now have internet access. All the sites have been checked and were active and relevant at the time of writing (summer 2003).

Finally, all information presented in the book is accurate and factual as far as the author is aware. It is acknowledged that guidelines change, products become discontinued and new information becomes available over the life-time of a book. Therefore, if any information in the book is not current or valid, the author would be grateful of any feedback; positive or negative to ensure that the next edition is as up-to-date as possible.

Acknowledgements

Every chapter has been reviewed by a GP with a particular speciality in that area, or by another expert in that field.

Chapter 1 (Respiratory system) and Chapter 4 (The central nervous system)
Dr Nick Dunn MB DM MRCGP MSc
Senior Lecturer in Primary Medical Care, Southampton
Dr Dunn teaches at Southampton University medical school and works in general practice part time.

Chapter 2 (Ophthalmology) and Chapter 3 (Otic conditions)
Dr David Raw MBBS FRCCP MA
General Practitioner, Sunnyside Surgery, Portsmouth
Dr Raw specialises in education for primary healthcare professionals from GP registrars to clerical staff.

Chapter 5 (Women's health)
Dr Charlotte Day MBBS BSc (Hons) MRCGP MFFP DRCOG
Principal General Practitioner, Baffin's Road Surgery, Portsmouth
Dr Day specialises in contraceptive and sexual health services.

Chapter 6 (Gastroenterology)
Dr Patrick Craig-McFeely MA MBBS MRCGP DCH DRCOG Dip Ther
General Practitioner, The Surgery, High Street, Hindon, Wiltshire
Dr Craig-McFeely specialises in therapeutics and medical education and has an interest in rheumatology.

Chapter 7 (Dermatology)
Dr A R Tollast BM DRCOG DPD MRCGP
General Practitioner, Sunnyside Surgery, Portsmouth
Dr Tollast lectures in primary care dermatology and is a clinical assistant at the Portsmouth Skin Centre.

Chapter 8 (Musculoskeletal conditions)
Mr Keith Waldon
Vice-chair of the Society of Sports Therapists

Chapter 9 (Paediatrics)
Mrs Amanda Bevan MRPharmS
Southampton General Hospital, Directorate Pharmacist specialising in Paediatrics

Chapter 10 (Specific product requests)
Dr John Purvis MRPharmS PhD CertVetPharm ILT
Associate Dean for teaching and learning and Senior Lecturer in clinical pharmacy, University of Bradford
Dr Purvis specialises in pathophysiology and differential diagnosis.

Respiratory system

In this chapter

Background

Diseases of the respiratory tract are among the most common reasons for consulting a GP; the average GP sees 700–1000 patients each year with respiratory disease. Although respiratory disease can cause significant morbidity and mortality, the vast majority of conditions are minor and self-limiting.

Community pharmacists are often the first health professional the patient seeks advice from and, as such, provide a filtering mechanism whereby minor self-limiting conditions can be treated appropriately with the correct medication and patients with more sinister pathology referred on to the GP for further investigation.

General overview of the anatomy of the respiratory tract

The basic requirement for all living cells to function and survive is a continuous supply of oxygen. However, a by-product of cell activity is carbon dioxide, which if it is not removed, poisons and kills the cells of the body. The principal function of the respiratory system is therefore the exchange of carbon dioxide and oxygen between the blood and atmospheric air. This exchange takes place in the lungs, where pulmonary capillaries are in intimate contact with the linings of the air spaces in the lung: the alveoli. All other structures associated with the respiratory tract serve to facilitate this gaseous exchange.

The respiratory tract is divided arbitrarily into the upper and lower respiratory tracts. In addition to these structures, the respiratory system also includes the oral cavity, rib cage and diaphragm.

Upper respiratory tract

The upper respiratory tract comprises those structures located outside the thorax: the nasal cavity, the pharynx and the larynx.

Nasal cavity

The internal portion of the nose is known as the nasal cavity. The nasal cavity is connected to the pharynx through two openings called the internal nares. Besides receiving olfactory stimuli (smell), the nasal cavity plays an important part in respiration because it filters out large dust particles and warms and moistens incoming air.

Pharynx

The pharynx is divided into three sections:

- nasopharynx, which exchanges air with the nasal cavity and moves particulate matter towards the mouth
- oropharynx and laryngopharynx, which serve as a common passageway for air and food
- laryngopharynx, which connects with the oesophagus and the larynx and, like the oropharynx, serves as a common pathway for the respiratory and digestive systems.

Larynx (voice box)

The larynx is a short passageway that connects the pharynx with the trachea. The glottis and epiglottis are located here and act like 'trap doors' to ensure that liquids and food are rooted into the oesophagus and not the trachea.

Lower respiratory tract

The lower respiratory tract is located almost entirely within the thorax and comprises the trachea, bronchial tree and lungs.

Trachea and bronchi

The trachea connects the larynx with the bronchi. The bronchi divide and subdivide into bronchioles and these in turn divide to form terminal bronchioles, which give rise to the alveoli where gaseous exchange takes place. The epithelial lining of the bronchial tree acts as a defence mechanism and is known as the mucociliary escalator. Cilia on the surface of cells beat upwards in organised waves of contraction, thus expelling foreign bodies.

Lungs

The lungs are cone shaped and lie in the thoracic cavity. Enclosing and protecting the lungs are the pleural membranes; the inner membrane covers the lungs and the outer membrane is attached to the thoracic cavity. Between the membranes is the pleural cavity, which contains fluid and prevents friction between the membranes during breathing.

History taking and physical exam

Cough, cold, sore throat and rhinitis often coexist and an accurate history is therefore essential to differentially diagnose a patient who presents with symptoms of respiratory disease. A number of similar questions must be asked for each symptom, although symptom specific questions are also needed (these are discussed under each heading, below). Currently, examination of the respiratory tract is outside the remit of the community pharmacist.

Cough

Background

The main function of coughing is airway clearance. Particles are cleared from the lungs by a combination of coughing and the mucociliary escalator. Cough is the most common respiratory symptom and one of the few ways by which abnormalities of the respiratory tract manifest themselves.

Coughs can be described as either productive (chesty) or non-productive (dry, tight, tickly). However, many patients will say that they are not producing sputum, although they go on to say that they 'can feel it on their chest'. In these cases the cough is probably productive in nature and should be treated as such.

Coughs can be either acute or chronic. Any cough of less than 3 weeks duration is said to be acute; any cough lasting longer than 3 weeks is classed as chronic.

Prevalence and epidemiology

Conditions that present with cough are among the most common reasons why patients seek care. They are most often associated with viral infection, for example the common cold, and are therefore extremely prevalent. Additionally, acute bronchitis is one of the major causes of cough and consistently ranks among the top ten reasons to visit a GP.

Aetiology

A five-part cough reflex is responsible for cough production. Receptors located mainly in the pharynx, larynx, trachea and bifurcations of the large bronchi are stimulated via mechanical, irritant or thermal mechanisms. Neural impulses are then carried along afferent pathways of the vagal and superior laryngeal nerves, which terminate at the cough centre in the medulla. Efferent fibres of the vagus and spinal nerves carry neural activity to the muscles of the diaphragm, chest wall and abdomen. These muscles contract, followed by the sudden opening of the glottis that creates the cough.

Arriving at a differential diagnosis

The most common causes of an acute cough are infection, allergies and postnasal drip. Viral infections are the most common cause of an acute cough at all ages. Recurrent viral bronchitis is most prevalent in preschool and young school-aged children and is the most common cause of persistent cough in children of all ages. It is the pharmacist's responsibility to differentiate other causes of cough from viral causes and also to refer those cases of cough that might have more serious pathology. Asking symptom-specific questions will help the pharmacist to determine if referral is needed (Table 1.1).

Clinical features of acute viral cough

Viral coughs typically present with sudden onset and associated fever. Sputum production is minimal and symptoms are often worse in the evening. Associated cold symptoms are also often present; these usually last between 7 and 10 days. Duration of longer than 14 days might indicate a bacterial secondary infection but this is clinically difficult to establish without analysing sputum samples.

Table 1.1
Specific questions to ask the patient: Cough

Question	Relevance
Sputum colour	<ul><li>Mucoid (clear and white) is normally of little consequence and suggests that no infection is present</li><li>Yellow, green or brown sputum normally indicates infection. However, mucopurulent sputum is probably caused by a viral infection and does not require automatic referral</li><li>Haemoptysis can be rust coloured (pneumonia), pink tinged (left ventricular failure) or dark red (carcinoma)</li></ul>
Nature of sputum	<ul><li>Thin and frothy suggests left ventricular failure</li><li>Thick, mucoid to yellow can suggest asthma</li><li>Offensive, foul-smelling sputum suggests either bronchiectasis or lung abscess</li></ul>
Onset of cough	<ul><li>A cough that is worse in the morning suggests postnasal drip, bronchiectasis or chronic bronchitis</li></ul>
Duration of cough	<ul><li>Coughs lasting longer than 3 weeks should be viewed with caution because they might indicate a more sinister pathology</li><li>The longer the cough is present, the more likely serious underlying pathology is responsible. E.g. the most likely diagnosis of a cough of 3 days duration will be an upper respiratory tract infection but at 3 weeks duration acute or chronic bronchitis are more likely; at 3 months duration conditions such as chronic bronchitis, tuberculosis and carcinoma become more likely</li></ul>
Periodicity	<ul><li>Adult patients with recurrent cough might have chronic bronchitis, especially if they smoke</li><li>Care should be exercised in children who present with recurrent cough and have a family history of eczema, asthma or hayfever. This might suggest asthma and referral would be required for further investigation and pulmonary function tests (e.g. peak expiratory flow assessment)</li></ul>
Age	<ul><li>Children will most likely be suffering from an upper respiratory tract infection but asthma, especially if the cough is non-productive and at night, should be considered</li><li>With increasing age conditions such as bronchitis, pneumonia and carcinoma become more prevalent</li></ul>
Smoking history	<ul><li>Patients who smoke are more prone to chronic and recurrent cough. Over time this might develop into chronic bronchitis and emphysema</li></ul>

Conditions to eliminate

Acute cough

Laryngotracheobronchitis (croup)
One of the less common causes of acute cough is croup. This is viral in origin and typically affects infants aged between 9 and 18 months old; it is said to be more common in boys. The cough is described as having a barking quality and the child usually has a preceding history of an upper respiratory tract infection. Attacks typically occur in the middle of the night and subside within a few hours, although they can recur. Steam inhalation is recommended but in severe cases referral to the GP or casualty should be the first line of action.

Postnasal drip
Postnasal drip is characterised by a sinus or nasal discharge that flows behind the nose and in to the throat. Patients should be asked if they are swallowing mucous or notice that they are clearing their throat more than usual, as these features are commonly seen in patients with postnasal drip.

Allergy-related cough
Coughs caused by allergies are often non-productive and worse at night. However, there are usually other associated symptoms, such as sneezing, nasal discharge/blockage, conjunctivitis and itching oral cavity. Cough of allergic origin might show seasonal variation, for example hayfever.

Chronic cough

Chronic bronchitis
Chronic bronchitis (CB) is the most common cause of chronic cough in adults. Patients often present with a longstanding history of recurrent acute bronchitis in which episodes become increasingly severe and persist for increasing duration until the cough becomes continual. CB has been defined as coughing up sputum on most days for three or more consecutive months over

the previous 2 years. A history of smoking is the single most important factor in the aetiology of CB. In non-smokers the likely cause of CB is postnasal drip, asthma or **gastro-oesophageal reflux**. One study has shown that 99% of non-smokers with CB and a normal chest X-ray suffered from one of these three conditions.

CB starts with a non-productive cough that later becomes productive. The patient should be questioned regarding smoking habit. If the patient is a smoker the cough will usually be worse on waking. Pharmacists have an important role to play in identifying smokers with CB as this provides an excellent opportunity for health promotion advice and assessing the patient's willingness to quit smoking.

Asthma

Estimates of asthma prevalence suggest that up to 5% of the UK and US populations suffer from asthma. It is a chronic inflammatory condition of the airways characterised by coughing, wheeze, chest tightness and shortness of breath. However, asthma can present solely as a non-productive cough. This is especially true in young children, in whom the cough is often worst at night. Over time, other symptoms such as wheeze, **dyspnoea** and a productive cough can develop. Diagnosis should be made by a combination of a medical history, symptoms and lung function tests.

Rare causes of cough

Cough can be a symptom of many other conditions, although the majority will be rarely encountered in community pharmacy. However, it is important to be aware of these rare causes of cough to ensure that appropriate referrals are made.

Productive coughs

Heart failure

Heart failure is a condition of the elderly. The prevalence of heart failure rises with increasing age; 3 to 5% of people aged over 65 are affected and this increases to approximately 10% of patients aged 80 and over. Heart failure is characterised by insidious progression and diagnosing early mild heart failure is extremely difficult because the symptoms are not pronounced. Often, the first symptoms patients experience are shortness of breath and dyspnoea at night. As the condition progresses from mild/moderate to severe heart failure patients might complain of a productive, frothy cough, which may have pink-tinged sputum.

Bronchiectasis

Bronchiectasis is caused by irreversible dilation of the bronchi. Characteristically, the patient has a chronic cough of very long duration, which produces copious amounts of mucopurulent sputum (green–yellow in colour) that is usually foul smelling. The cough tends to

be worse in the morning and evening. In longstanding cases the sputum is said to display characteristic layering, with the top being frothy, the middle clear and the bottom dense with **purulent** particles.

Tuberculosis

Tuberculosis (TB) is a bacterial infection caused by *Mycobacterium tuberculosis* and is transmitted primarily by inhalation. After many decades of decline, the number of new TB cases occurring in industrialised countries is now starting to increase. Each year there are more than 6000 new cases of TB notified in the UK, and over 500 deaths. The incidence is higher in inner city areas, and among the elderly and immigrants from developing countries. TB is characterised by its slow onset and initial mild symptoms. The cough is chronic in nature and sputum production can vary from mild to severe with associated **haemoptysis**. Other symptoms of the condition are **malaise**, fever, night sweats and weight loss. However, not all patients will experience all symptoms. A patient with a productive cough for more than 3 weeks and exhibiting one or more of the associated symptoms should be referred for further investigation, especially if they fall into one of the groups listed above. Chest X-rays and sputum smear tests can be performed to confirm the diagnosis.

Pneumonia

Bacterial infection is usually responsible for pneumonia, which can be caused by *Klebsiella*, *Staphylococcus* or *Mycoplasma* bacteria. Initially, the cough is non-productive and painful but it rapidly becomes productive, with the sputum being stained red. The intensity of the redness varies depending on the causative organism. The cough tends to be worst at night. The patient will be unwell, with a high fever, malaise, chills and headache, and will experience pleuritic pain (inflammation of pleural membranes, manifested as pain to the sides) that worsens on inspiration.

Carcinoma of the lung

A number of studies have shown that between 20 and 90% of patients will develop a cough at some point during the progression of carcinoma of the lung. The possibility of carcinoma increases in long-term cigarette smokers who have had a cough for a number of months or who develop a marked change in the character of their cough. The cough produces small amounts of sputum that might be blood streaked. Other symptoms that can be associated with the cough are dyspnoea, weight loss and fatigue.

Nocardiosis

Nocardiosis is an extremely rare bacterial infection caused by *Nocardia asteroides*; it is transmitted primarily by inhalation. It is very unlikely that a pharmacist will ever encounter this condition and it is included in this text only for the sake of completeness. It has a higher incidence in the elderly population, especially men. The sputum is purulent, thick and possibly blood tinged. Fever is prominent and night sweats, **pleurisy**, weight loss and fatigue might also be present.

Non-productive coughs

Gastro-oesophageal reflux disease

Gastro-oesophageal reflux disease (GORD) does not usually present with cough but patients with this condition might cough when recumbent (lying down). It should always be considered in all cases of unexplained chronic cough.

Lung abscess

A typical presentation is of a non-productive cough with pleuritic pain and dyspnoea. Signs of infection such as malaise and fever can also be present. Later the cough produces large amounts of purulent and often foul-smelling sputum.

Medicine-induced cough or wheeze

A number of medicines can cause bronchoconstriction, which presents as cough or wheeze. Angiotensin converting enzyme (ACE) inhibitors are most commonly associated with cough and can affect up to one in five patients. Other medicines associated with cough or wheeze are non-steroidal anti-inflammatories (NSAIDs) and beta-blockers.

Spontaneous pneumothorax (collapsed lung)

Rupture of the bullae (the small air or fluid filled sacs in the lung) can cause spontaneous pneumothorax, although there is normally no underlying cause. Spontaneous pneumothorax affects approximately 1 out of 10 000 people, usually tall, thin men aged between 20 and 40 years. Cigarette smoking and a family history of pneumo-thorax are contributing risk factors. This can be a life-threatening disorder causing a non-productive cough and severe respiratory distress. The patient experiences sudden sharp chest pain that worsens on chest movement. The symptoms often begin suddenly and can occur during rest or sleep.

Figure 1.1 will aid the differentiation between serious and non-serious conditions of cough in adults.

Evidence base for over-the-counter medication

There is a plethora of over-the-counter (OTC) medication to treat cough. Any member of the public will find the choice overwhelming. The pharmacist must ensure that the most appropriate medication is selected for the patient and this must be done using an evidence-based approach.

> **❗ TRIGGER POINTS indicative of referral: Cough**
> - Chest pain
> - Cough that recurs on a regular basis
> - Duration longer than 3 weeks
> - Haemoptysis
> - Pain on inspiration
> - Persistent nocturnal cough in children
> - Wheeze and/or shortness of breath

All the active ingredients to treat cough were brought to the market many years ago when clinical trials suffered from flaws in study design compared to today's standards, thus their clinical efficacy is difficult to establish.

Expectorants

A number of active ingredients have been formulated to help expectoration, including guaifenesin (guaiphenesin), ammonium salts, ipecacuanha, creosote and squill. The majority of products marketed in the UK for productive cough contain guaifenesin, although products containing squill (Buttercup syrup Traditional), ipecacuanha (Galloway's cough syrup) and ammonium salts (Histalix syrup) are available. The clinical evidence available for any active ingredient is limited. Older ingredients such as ammonium salts, ipecacuanha and squill were traditionally used to induce vomiting as it was believed that at subemetic doses they would cause gastric irritation, triggering reflex expectoration. This has never been proven and belongs in the annals of folklore. At best they offer a placebo effect but should not be recommended. Guaifenesin is the only active ingredient that has any evidence of effectiveness. It is the only substance that has been approved by the United States Food and Drug Administration (FDA) as being effective, although some trials have shown it to be ineffective.

Summary

Based on evidence, guaifenesin should be recommended as first-line treatment for productive cough. However, as all products to treat productive cough are probably no more than placebos, if the patient has confidence in a product's efficacy then their use should not be discouraged.

Cough suppressants (antitussives)

The effectiveness of antitussives has been investigated in acute and chronic cough as well as citric-acid-induced cough. Although trials on healthy volunteers – in whom coughing was induced by citric acid – allowed repro-ducible conditions to assess the activity of antitussives, they are of little value because they do not represent physiological cough. Of greatest relevance to OTC medication are trials investigating acute cough, because patients suffering from chronic cough should be referred to the GP.

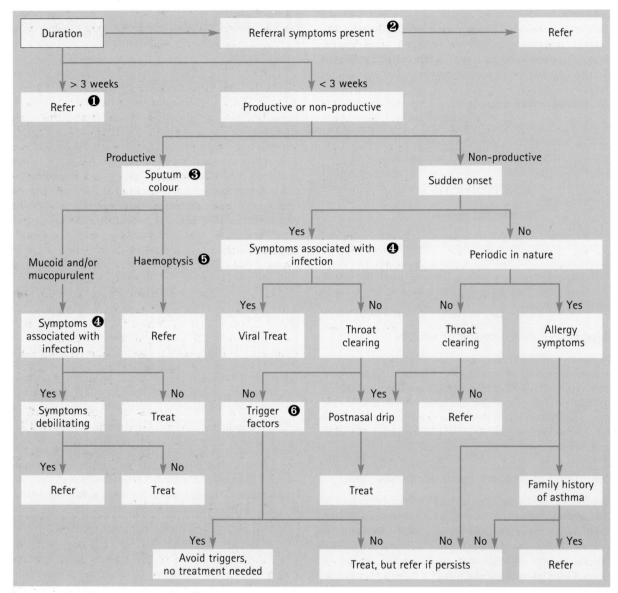

Fig. 1.1 Primer for differential diagnosis of cough in adult

❶ **Duration of cough**
Coughs lasting longer than 3 weeks are considered chronic in nature. Most acute, self-limiting coughs usually resolve within 3 weeks; conditions with sinister pathology are more likely the longer the cough has been present. However, not all coughs that have lasted 3 weeks have to be referred automatically. Postnasal drip and seasonal allergies (e.g. hayfever) can persist for weeks and be managed by community pharmacists.

❷ **Referral symptoms**
Certain symptoms warrant direct referral to the GP or even casualty. For example, shortness of breath, breathlessness (possible asthma), chest pain (possible cardiovascular cause) or pain on inspiration (pleurisy or pneumothorax).

❸ **Sputum colour**
Sputum colour can be helpful in deciding when to refer. However, there is a common misconception that patients who present with green-yellow or brown sputum have a bacterial infection; this is

not normally the case. If the cough has persisted for more than 7 to 10 days it is possible that an initial viral infection has become secondarily infected with a bacterial infection. This could indicate referral, especially if the symptoms are debilitating or if the patient is elderly.

❹ **Symptoms associated with infection**
The patient might have associated symptoms of fever, rhinorrhoea and sore throat.

❺ **Haemoptysis**
Blood in the sputum requires further investigation, especially if the person has had the symptoms for a period of time.

❻ **Trigger factors**
Certain atmospheric factors can trigger cough. These factors include air temperature changes, pollution (e.g. cigarette smoke) and dry atmospheres (e.g. air conditioning).

Codeine

Codeine is generally accepted as a standard or bench-mark antitussive against which all others are judged. A review by Eddy et al showed codeine to be an effective antitussive in animal models, and cough-induced studies in humans have also shown codeine to be effective. However, these findings appear to be less reproducible in acute and pathological chronic cough. More recent studies have failed to demonstrate a significant clinical effect of codeine compared with placebo in patients suffering with acute cough. Greater voluntary control of the cough reflex by patients has been suggested for the apparent lack of effect codeine has on acute cough.

Pholcodine

Pholcodine, like codeine, has been subject to limited clinical trials, with the majority being either animal models or citric-acid-induced cough studies in man. These studies have shown pholcodine to have antitussive activity. A review by Findlay (1988) concluded that, on balance, pholcodine appears to possess antitussive activity but advocates the need for better, well-controlled studies.

Dextromethorphan

Trial data for dextromethorphan, like that for codeine and pholcodine, is limited. It has been shown to be effective in citric-acid-induced cough and chronic cough but studies assessing the efficacy of dextromethorphan in acute cough have shown it to be no better than placebo. It appears to have limited abuse potential and fewer side-effects than codeine.

Antihistamines

Antihistamines have been included in cough remedies for decades. Their mechanism of action is thought to be through the anticholinergic-like drying action on the mucous membranes and not via histamine. There are numerous clinical trials involving antihistamines for the relief of cough and cold symptoms, most notably with diphenhydramine.

Citric-acid-induced cough studies have demonstrated significant antitussive activity compared with placebo and results from chronic cough trials support an antitussive activity for diphenhydramine. However, trials that showed a significant reduction in cough frequency suffered from having small patient numbers, thus limiting their usefulness. Additionally, poor methodological design of trials investigating the antitussive activity of diphenhydramine in acute cough makes assessment of its effectiveness difficult.

Demulcents

Demulcents, such as simple linctus, are pharmacologically inert and are used on the theoretical basis that they reduce irritation by coating the pharynx and so prevent coughing. There is no evidence for their efficacy and they are used mainly for their placebo effect. They are a suitable recommendation for very young children who cannot take other cough suppressants.

Summary

Antitussives have traditionally been evaluated for efficacy in animal or cough-induced models on healthy volunteers. This presents serious problems in assessing their effectiveness because support for their antitussive activity does not come from patients with acute cough associated with upper respiratory tract infection. Indeed, a recent systematic review of trial data of any cough medication for acute cough in adults concluded that evidence of efficacy was lacking. Furthermore, there appear to be no comparative studies of sound study design to allow judgements to be made on their comparable efficacy. Compounding these problems is the self-limiting nature of acute cough, which further hinders differentiation between clinical efficacy and normal symptom resolution.

Antitussives therefore probably have a limited role in the treatment of acute non-productive cough. Patients should be encouraged to drink more fluid and told that their symptoms will resolve in time on their own. If medication is required then any active ingredient could be recommended; side-effect profile and abuse tendency rather than clinical efficacy will drive choice. On this basis, pholcodine and dextromethorphan would be first-line therapy and codeine, because of its greater side-effect profile and tendency to be abused, should be reserved for second-line treatment. Antihistamines should not be used routinely, unless night-time sedation is perceived as an additional benefit to help the patient sleep.

Cough medication for children

Very few well-designed studies have been conducted in children. A review published in the *Drug and Therapeutics Bulletin* identified just five trials of sound methodological design. However, of these five trials, one study used illogical drug combinations (expectorant combined with suppressant) and a further three used combination products that are not available on the UK market. This left one study, involving Dimotapp elixir, that could be evaluated. The results from this study showed no significant differences between the active ingredients, placebo and no medication. It therefore appears, from the limited data available, that cough medication for children is no better than placebo. However, many parents will insist on treatment for their children and in such cases, as long as no contraindications are present, supplying a suitable 'theoretical' cough medication would not be unjustified because adverse events from cough medication are rare.

Practical prescribing and product selection

Prescribing information relating to the cough medicines reviewed in the section 'Evidence base for over-the-

Table 1.2
Practical prescribing: Summary of cough medicines

Medicine	Use in children	Likely side-effects	Drug interactions of note	Patients in whom care should be exercised	Pregnancy
Cough expectorants					
Guaifenesin	>1 year	None	None	None	OK
Cough suppressants					
Codeine	> 1 year	Sedation, constipation	Increased sedation with alcohol, opioid analgesics, anxiolytics, hypnotics and antidepressants	Asthmatics	Best avoided in the third trimester
Pholcodine	> 1 year	Possible sedation			
Dextromethorphan	> 1 year				
Antihistamines					
Brompheniramine	> 3 years	Dry mouth, sedation and constipation	Increased sedation with alcohol, opioid analgesics, anxiolytics, hypnotics and antidepressants	Glaucoma, prostate enlargement	*BNF* states OK but some manufacturers advise avoidance
Chlorphenaramine (chlorphenamine)	> 1 year				
Diphenhydramine	> 6 years*				
Promethazine	> 1 year**				
Triprolidine	> 1 year				
Demulcents					
Simple linctus	> 3 months (paediatric version)	None	None	None	OK

* most products are licensed for children over 6, however Benylin Children's Night Coughs can be used from 1 year.
** Not normally recommended below 2 years of age.

HINTS AND TIPS BOX 1.1: COUGH

Insulin-dependent diabetics	People with insulin-dependent diabetes should be asked to monitor their blood glucose more frequently because insulin requirements increase during acute infections
Avoid theophylline	Theophylline is available in OTC products but it is best avoided because patients requiring medication to help with shortness of breath or wheeze are best referred
Alternative delivery routes	Dextromethorphan is available as a lozenge (Strepsils Cough Lozenges). This is a useful alternative for those patients who find carrying a bottle of liquid around with them difficult
Avoid illogical combinations	Very few cough remedies now have illogical medicine combinations. However, there are still a few on the market and these are best avoided. For example, combinations of expectorants and suppressants (e.g. Famel Original and Pulmo Bailley) and expectorant antihistamine combinations (e.g. Bronalin Expectorant and Histalix)

counter medication' is discussed and summarised in Table 1.2 and useful tips relating to patients presenting with cough are given in Hints and Tips Box 1.1.

Cough expectorants

Guaifenesin
A number of manufacturers include guaifenesin in their cough product ranges, including Benylin, Robitussin and Vicks. It can be given to children over 1 year old (e.g. Benylin Children's Chesty Coughs 50 mg (5 mL) four times a day); children aged between 6 and 12 years should take 100 mg four times a day and the dose for adults – if it is going to work – must be 200 mg four times a day. Some products deliver suboptimal doses or the quantity taken in a single dose would be so large that the product would last only 2 or 3 days. It is therefore advisable to check the label of any branded guaifenesin

product before recommendation to ensure the patient is receiving appropriate treatment. Guaifenesin-based products have no cautions in their use and no side-effects; they are also free from clinically significant drug interactions and so can be given safely with prescribed medication. Sugar-free versions (e.g. Robitussin range) are available for diabetic patients.

Cough suppressants (codeine, pholcodine, dextromethorphan)

Codeine, pholcodine and dextromethorphan are all opiate derivatives and therefore – broadly – have the same interactions, cautions in use and side-effect profile. They do interact with prescription-only medications (POMs) and also with OTC medications, especially those that cross the blood–brain barrier. Their combined effect is to potentiate sedation and it is important to warn the patient of this, although short-term use of cough suppressants with the interacting medication is unlikely to warrant dosage modification. Care should be exercised when giving cough suppressants to asthmatics because, in theory, cough suppressants can cause respiratory depression. However, in practice this is very rarely observed and does not preclude the use of cough suppressants in asthmatic patients. However, other side-effects can occur (e.g. constipation), especially with codeine. If a cough suppressant is unsuitable, for example in late pregnancy and children, then a demulcent can be offered.

Codeine

Children from 1 year upwards can be treated with codeine linctus (e.g. codeine linctus paediatric BP, 5 mL (3 mg) three or four times a day), although codeine is generally not recommended for children under 5 years of age. The adult dose is 5 mL (15 mg) three or four times a day, and half the adult dose is suitable for children aged between 5 and 12 years of age. The maximum dose should not exceed 5 mL because doses higher than this change the legal status of codeine to a POM. Codeine is still available in a number of proprietary brands, for example Dimotane Co, but the majority of pharmacies restrict sales due to the abuse potential of codeine. Sugar-free versions are available for diabetic patients (e.g. the Galen range).

Pholcodine

Pholcodine can also be recommended for children aged over 1 year old (e.g. Tixylix Daytime 2.5 mL (2 mg) four times a day or Benylin Children's Dry Cough 5 mL (2 mg) three times a day) but, like codeine, treatment of children less that 5 years of age is generally not recommended. The adult dose is 5 to 10 mL (5 to 10 mg) three or four times a day, and half the adult dose for children between 5 and 12 years of age. Sugar-free versions are available for diabetic patients (e.g. Pavacol-D).

Dextromethorphan

Dextromethorphan can also be given in children older than 1 year of age (e.g. Benylin Children's Coughs and Colds Medicine 2.5 mL (2.5 mg) three or four times a day) but, like other opiate derivatives, dextromethorphan is generally not recommended for children less than 5 years old. The adult dose is 10 mL (15 mg) four times a day (e.g. Covonia Bronchial Balsam and Benylin Dry Cough Non-drowsy), and half the adult dose is suitable for children aged between 5 and 12 years old.

Antihistamines

Routine use of antihistamines is unjustified in treating non-productive cough. However, the sedative side-effects from antihistamines can, on occasion, be useful to allow patients an uninterrupted night's sleep.

All antihistamines included in cough remedies are first-generation antihistamines and associated with sedation. They interact with other sedating medication, resulting in potentiation of the sedative properties of the interacting medicines. They also possess antimuscarinic side-effects, which commonly result in dry mouth and possibly constipation. It is these antimuscarinic properties that mean that patients with glaucoma and prostate enlargement should ideally avoid their use, because it could lead to increased intraocular pressure and precipitation of urinary retention. The vast majority of products that contain an antihistamine are combination products, usually with a cough suppressant.

Demulcents

Demulcents, for example simple linctus, provide a safe alternative for at-risk patient groups such as the elderly, pregnant women, young children and those taking multiple medication. They can act as useful placebos when the patient insists on a cough mixture and will not take no for an answer. If recommended they should be given three or four times a day.

Further reading

[Anonymous] 1999 Cough medications in children. Drug and Therapeutics Bulletin 37:19–21

Eddy N B, Friebel H, Hahn K J et al 1970 Codeine and its alternatives for pain and cough relief. World Health Organization, Geneva, pp 1–253

Findlay J W A 1988 Review articles: pholcodine. Journal of Clinical and Pharmacological Therapy 13:5–17

Schroeder K, Fahey T 2002 Systematic review of randomised controlled trials over the counter cough medicines for acute cough in adults. British Medical Journal 324:1–6

Web sites

Action on Smoking and Health (ASH): www.ash.org.uk
British Lung Foundation: www.britishlungfoundation.com
National Asthma Campaign: www.asthma.org.uk

The common cold

Background

Colds, along with coughs, represent the largest caseload for primary healthcare workers. Because the condition has no specific cure and is self-limiting in nature it would be easy to dismiss the differential diagnosis as unimportant. However, because of the very high number of cases seen it is essential that pharmacists have a thorough understanding of the condition so that severe symptoms or symptoms suggestive of influenza are identified.

Prevalence and epidemiology

The common cold is extremely prevalent. Upper respiratory tract infections are the most common affliction that affects the general population, with people on average suffering between 3 and 12 colds per year, depending on their age. Children aged between 4 and 8 years are most likely to contract a cold and it can appear to a child's parents that one cold follows another with no respite. By the age of 10 the number of colds contracted is half that observed in preschool children.

Aetiology

A number of different virus types can produce symptoms of the common cold, including rhinoviruses, adenoviruses and the influenza virus – rhinoviruses account for almost half of all cases. Transmission is primarily by the virus coming into contact with the hands, which then touch the nose, mouth and eyes (direct contact transmission) and not by droplet transmission (e.g. sneezing), which is a secondary mechanism. The virus then invades the nasal and bronchial epithelia, attaching to specific receptors and causing damage to the ciliated cells. This results in the release of inflammatory mediators, which in turn leads to inflammation of the tissues lining the nose. Permeability of capillary cell walls increases, resulting in oedema, which is experienced by the patient as nasal congestion and sneezing. Fluid might drip down the back of the throat, spreading the virus to the throat and upper chest and causing cough and sore throat.

Arriving at a differential diagnosis

Viral infection will account for the vast majority of cases. The pharmacist must try to differentiate between viral infection and conditions that present with similar symptoms (e.g. influenza and allergic and chronic rhinitis), as well as complications associated with the common cold. Asking symptom-specific questions will help the pharmacist to determine whether the patient should be referred to a GP (Table 1.3).

Clinical features of the common cold

The symptoms of the common cold are well known. However, the nature and severity of symptoms will be influenced by factors such as the causative agent and the patient's age and underlying medical condition. Following an incubation period of between 1 and 3 days the patient develops a sore throat and sneezing, followed by profuse nasal discharge and congestion. Cough and postnasal drip commonly follow. In addition headache, fever (< 102°F, 38.9°C) and general malaise might be present. It is not unusual for a common cold to last for 14 days or more.

Conditions to eliminate

Influenza

Patients often use the word 'flu' when describing a common cold. However, subtle differences in symptoms between the two conditions should allow differentiation.

Table 1.3
Specific questions to ask the patient: Cold

Question	Relevance
Onset of symptoms	● Peak incidence of flu is in the winter months; the common cold occurs any time throughout the year ● Flu symptoms tend to have a more abrupt onset than the common cold – a matter of hours rather than 1 or 2 days ● Summer colds are common but they must be differentiated from seasonal allergic rhinitis (hayfever)
Nature of symptoms	● Marked myalgia, chills and malaise are more prominent in flu than the common cold. Loss of appetite is also common with flu
Aggravating factors	● Headache/pain that is worsened by sneezing, coughing and bending over suggests sinus complications. If ear pain is present, especially in children, middle ear involvement is likely

It is helpful to remember that the 'flu' season tends to be between December and March, whereas the common cold can strike at any time. The onset of influenza is sudden and the typical symptoms are shivering, chills, malaise, marked aching of the limbs, insomnia, a non-productive cough (cough in the common cold is usually productive) and loss of appetite. Influenza is therefore normally debilitating and a person with flu is much more likely to send a third party to the pharmacy for medication than present in person.

Rhinitis

A blocked or stuffy nose, whether acute or chronic in nature, is a common complaint. Rhinitis is covered in more detail on page 19 and the reader is referred to this section for differential diagnosis of rhinitis from the common cold.

Acute sinusitis

Complications can arise from the common cold, for example sinusitis. Anatomically the sinuses are described in four pairs: frontal, ethmoid, maxillary and sphenoid (Fig. 1.2). All are air-filled spaces that drain in to the nasal cavity.

Following a cold, sinus air spaces can become filled with nasal secretions, which stagnate because of a reduction in ciliary function of the cells lining the sinuses. Bacteria – commonly *Streptococcus* and *Haemophilus* – can then secondarily infect these stagnant secretions. The pain in the early stages tends to be relatively localised, usually unilateral and dull, but becomes bilateral and more severe the longer the condition persists. Bending down, moving the eyes from side to side, coughing or sneezing often exacerbates the pain. If the ethmoid sinuses are involved, retro-orbital pain (behind the eye) is often experienced. Oral or nasal sympathomimetics can be tried to remove the nasal secretions but if this fails then referral is needed because appropriate antibiotic therapy will probably be needed.

Otitis media

This is commonly seen in children following a common cold and results from the virus spreading to the middle ear via the Eustachian tube. The overriding symptom is pain due to an accumulation of pus within the middle ear or inflammation of the tympanic membrane (eardrum). Rupture of the eardrum causes purulent discharge and relieves the pain. Referral to the GP would be appropriate for **auroscopical examination**. GPs tend to prescribe antibiotic treatment, although the importance of antibiotics in speeding the resolution of otitis media has not been definitively established. The pharmacist should offer symptomatic relief of pain.

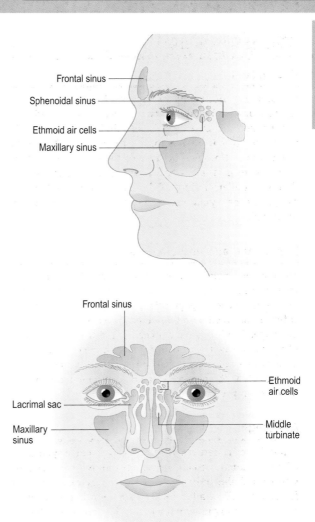

Fig. 1.2 Location of the sinuses

> ❗ **TRIGGER POINTS indicative of referral: The common cold**
>
> - Acute sinus involvement
> - Ear pain originating from the middle ear
> - Patients with symptoms indicative of flu
> - Vulnerable patient groups, such as the very elderly

Evidence base for over-the-counter medication

Many of the active ingredients found in cold remedies are also constituents of cough products. In many cases they are combined and marketed as cough and cold or flu remedies. For information relating to cough ingredients the reader is referred to the sections on OTC medication for coughs (page 5).

Antihistamines

A review article published in the *Journal of the American Medical Association* on OTC cold medications illustrates the lack of high quality methodological studies. Only four trials involving chlorphenamine and one trial each of diphenhydramine and triprolidine met the inclusion criteria for the article. Three of the trials for chlorphenamine showed a reduction in sneezing and decreased symptom scores, whereas the other showed no benefit. Both trials involving diphenhydramine and triprolidine showed them to be no better than placebo.

Systemic and topical sympathomimetics

Sympathomimetics help to clear nasal passages and are clinically effective, although only pseudoephedrine and oxymetazoline appear to have trial data to support their efficacy.

Multi-ingredient preparations

There is no shortage of cold and flu remedies marketed. Many combine three or more ingredients. In the majority of cases either the patient will not require all the active ingredients to treat symptoms or the 'drug cocktail' administered will not contain active ingredients that have proven efficacy. A more sensible approach to medicine management would be to match symptoms with active ingredients with known evidence of efficacy. In many cases this can be achieved by providing the patient with monotherapy or a product containing two active ingredients. Preparations with multiple ingredients therefore have a very limited role to play in the management of coughs and colds. However, patients might perceive an 'all in one' medicine as better value for money and, potentially, compliance with such preparations might be improved.

Alternative therapies

Many products are advocated to help treat cold symptoms. Three products in particular have received much attention and are widely used.

Zinc lozenges

The argument for zinc as a plausible treatment in ameliorating symptoms of the common cold can be traced back to 1984. A number of studies have investigated whether zinc lozenges can decrease the severity and duration of the common cold. A meta-analysis conducted in 2000 concluded that there was insufficient evidence to establish efficacy and that any benefit would probably be modest. A further trial by Prasad et al (2000), which was published after the meta-analysis, did show zinc lozenges to significantly decrease the duration and severity of the common cold, although numbers in the study were low. This latter study provides important additional evidence that zinc lozenges might have a beneficial effect. Larger studies are needed to establish the role of zinc in the common cold but if patients wanted to try a zinc supplement then it would not seem unreasonable.

Vitamin C

Vitamin C has been widely recommended as a 'cure' for the common cold by many sources – both medical and non-medical. However, controversy still remains as to whether it is an effective weapon in combating the common cold. A large number of clinical trials have investigated the effect of vitamin C on the prevention and treatment of the common cold. A review of trial data conducted in 2000 concluded that prophylactic use of vitamin C does not prevent colds. However, vitamin C appears to reduce the duration of cold symptoms when ingested in high doses (up to 1 g daily) although the response is variable.

Echinacea

The herbal remedy echinacea is marketed as a treatment for upper respiratory tract infections, including the common cold. Current evidence suggests that some echinacea preparations might be better than placebo at decreasing the duration of the common cold. A review by Melchart et al, conducted in 2000, stated that echinacea products differ greatly and no strong evidence was found to recommend a specific echinacea product, its dose or times when to use it.

Vapour inhalation

Steam inhalation has long been advocated to aid symptoms of the common cold, usually with the addition of menthol crystals. Current trial data supports the use of vapour inhalation in relieving the symptoms of the common cold although it appears that steam is the key to symptom resolution, and not any additional ingredient that is added to the water.

Practical prescribing and product selection

Prescribing information relating to the cold medicines reviewed in the section 'Evidence base for over-the-counter medication' is discussed and summarised in Table 1.4 and useful tips relating to patients presenting with a cold are given in Hints and Tips Box 1.2.

Antihistamines

First-generation antihistamines do have some evidence of efficacy in reducing cold symptoms in adolescents and adults. It is therefore reasonable to select cold remedies that contain an antihistamine. Further information on antihistamines can be found on page 9.

Sympathomimetics

Sympathomimetics constrict dilated blood vessels and swollen nasal mucosa, easing congestion and helping

Table 1.4
Practical prescribing: Summary of cold medicines

Medicine	Use in children	Likely side-effects	Drug interactions of note	Patients in whom care should be exercised	Pregnancy
Antihistamines					
Brompheniramine	> 3 years	Dry mouth, sedation and constipation	Increased sedation with alcohol, opioid analgesics, anxiolytics, hypnotics and antidepressants	Glaucoma, prostate enlargement	BNF states OK but some manufacturers advise avoidance
Chlorphenamine	> 1 year				
Diphenhydramine	> 6 years*				
Promethazine	> 1 year**				
Triprolidine	> 1 year				
Systemic sympathomimetics					
Phenylpropanolamine	> 2 years	At OTC doses insomnia is most likely. Possibly causes tachycardia	Avoid concomitant use with MAOIs and moclobemide because of risk of hypertensive crisis. Avoid in patients taking beta-blockers and TCAs	CSM advice is that patients with high blood pressure, heart disease or hyperthyroidism should avoid. Control of hypertension and diabetes might be affected but a short treatment course is unlikely to be clinically important	OK but best avoided in first trimester because mild fetal malformations have been reported
Phenylephrine	> 2 years				
Pseudoephedrine	> 2 years				
Topical sympathomimetics					
Oxymetazoline	> 5 years	Possible local irritation in ~5% of patients	Avoid concomitant use with MAOIs and moclobemide because of risk of hypertensive crisis	None	OK
Xylometazoline	> 2 years				

* Most products licensed for children over 6, however Benylin Children's Night Coughs can be used from 1 year.
** Not normally recommended under 2 years of age.
CSM, Committee of Safety of Medicines; MAOI, monoamine oxidase inhibitor; OTC, over-the-counter; TCA, tricyclic antidepressant.

HINTS AND TIPS BOX 1.2: THE COMMON COLD

Stuffy noses in babies	Saline nose drops can be used from birth to help with congestion. This would be a more suitable and safer alternative than a topical sympathomimetic
General Sales List cold remedies	Products such as the Lemsip and Beechams ranges contain paracetamol. It is important to ensure patients are not taking excessive doses of analgesia unknowingly. Also, many products contain subtherapeutic doses of sympathomimetics. If a sympathomimetic is needed then these products are generally best avoided
Administration of nasal drops	The best way to administer nose drops is to have the head in the downwards position, facing the floor. Tilting the head backwards and towards the ceiling is incorrect because it facilitates swallowing the drops. However, most patients will find the latter way of putting drops into the nose much easier than the former

breathing. However, they interact with monoamine oxidase inhibitors (MAOIs) (e.g. phenelzine, isocarboxazid, tranylcypromine and moclobemide), which can result in a fatal hypertensive crisis. The danger of the interaction persists for up to 2 weeks after treatment with MAOIs is discontinued. In addition, systemic sympathomimetics can also increase blood pressure, which might, although unlikely with short courses of treatment, alter control of blood pressure in hypertensive patients and disturb blood glucose control in diabetics. However, coadministration of medicines such as beta-blockers is probably clinically unimportant and does not preclude patients on beta-blockers taking a sympathomimetic. However, a topical sympathomimetic could be given to such patients to negate this potential interaction. The most likely side-effects of sympathomimetics are insomnia, restlessness and tachycardia. Patients should therefore be advised not to take a dose just before bed-time because their mild stimulant action can disturb sleep.

Systemic sympathomimetics

Phenylephrine

Phenylephrine is available in a number of proprietary cold remedies, for example Lemsip and Beechams, in doses ranging between 5 and 20 mg three or four times a day. Most products are not licensed for use in children, although phenylephrine is one of the ingredients in Beechams Powders capsules, which can be given to children over 6 years of age.

Pseudoephedrine

Pseudoephedrine is widely available as either a single ingredient (e.g. Sudafed Tablets) or in multi-ingredient products in cold and cough remedies (e.g. Benylin Four Flu Tablets or some of the Dimotane, Expulin, Actifed cough range). The standard adult dose is 60 mg four times a day and half the adult dose is suitable for children between 6 and 12 years of age. It can be given to children older than 1 year of age (e.g. Tixycolds Syrup, 2.5 ml (11.25 mg) every 6 hours).

Phenylpropanolamine

Following the recent safety concerns over phenylpropanolamine and the possible increased risk of haemorrhagic stroke, the Committee for Safety of Medicines (CSM) has stated that the maximum daily dose of phenylpropanolamine should not exceed 100 mg. Consequently, it appears that all manufacturers have either reformulated their products and replaced phenylpropanolamine with pseudoephedrine. (e.g. Mucron Tablets is now called Otrivine Mucron and Contact 400 is called Contact 12-hour Relief) or discontinued their products (e.g. Eskornade).

Topical sympathomimetics

Topical administration of sympathomimetics represents the safest route of administration. They can be given to most patient groups, including children over 2 years of age, pregnant women after the first trimester and patients with pre-existing heart disease, diabetes, hypertension and hyperthyroidism. However, a degree of systemic absorption is possible, especially when using drops, as a small quantity might be swallowed, and they should therefore be avoided in patients taking MAOIs. No topical decongestant should be used for longer than 7 days because rhinitis medicamentosa (rebound congestion) can occur.

Ephedrine and phenylephrine

Both are short acting and need to be administered four times a day. Ephedrine can be given to babies from 3 months but phenylephrine (e.g. Fenox Nasal Spray) is licensed only for children over 5 years old.

Oxymetazoline and xylometazoline

These agents are longer acting than ephedrine and phenylephrine and require only twice-daily dosing. They are made by a number of manufacturers (e.g. Afrazine Nasal Spray, Otrivine range and Sudafed Decongestant Nasal Spray). Within the Otrivine range is a paediatric drop that can be given to children over 2 years of age.

Further reading

Damoiseaux R A, van Balen F A, Hoes AW et al 1998 Antibiotic treatment of acute otitis media in children under two years of age: evidence based? British Journal of General Practice 48:1861–1864

Douglas R M, Chalker E B, Treacy B 2000 Vitamin C for preventing and treating the common cold. Cochrane Database Systems Review 2:CD000980

Marshall I 2000 Zinc for the common cold. Cochrane Database Systems Review 2:CD001364

Melchart D, Linde K, Fischer P et al 2000 Echinacea for preventing and treating the common cold. Cochrane Database Systems Review 2:CD000530

Monto A S 1994 The common cold. Cold water on hot news. Journal of the American Medical Association 271:1122–1124

Mossad S B 1998 Treatment of the common cold. British Medical Journal 317:33–36

Prasad A S, Fitzgerald J T, Bao B et al 2000 Duration of symptoms and plasma cytokine levels in patients with the common cold treated with zinc acetate. A randomized, double-blind, placebo-controlled trial. Annals of Internal Medicine 133:245–252

Singh M 2000 Heated, humidified air for the common cold. Cochrane Database Systems Review 2:CD001728

Smith M B, Feldman W 1993 Over-the-counter cold medications. A critical review of clinical trials between 1950 and 1991. Journal of the American Medical Association 269:2258–2263

Thibodeau G A, Patton K T 2003 Anatomy and physiology. Mosby, St Louis

Web sites

Common Cold Centre: www.cf.ac.uk/biosi/associates/cold/
Commoncold, Inc: www.commoncold.org
The National Institute for Health: www.nih.gov/health/

Sore throat

Background

Throat pain generally refers to discomfort of any part of the pharynx. Symptoms can range from scratchiness to severe pain. It has been reported that viruses account for between 70 and 90% of all cases. Bacterial infection (streptococcal sore throat), glandular fever, herpes simplex, candidiasis and varicella normally account for the remaining cases.

Prevalence and epidemiology

Sore throats are often associated with the common cold and therefore the prevalence of sore throat is extremely common. The average adult experiences two or three sore throats each year. Streptococcal sore throat is more commonly associated with people under the age of 30, particularly those of school age (5 to 15). Other causes of sore throat such as candidiasis (oral thrush) and herpes simplex are more common in children, and glandular fever is most prevalent in adolescents and young adults.

Aetiology

Most sore throats will be caused by viral and, to a lesser extent, bacterial infection and result from the body's response to invading pathogens. A fuller account of the aetiology of viral and bacterial pathogens that affect the upper respiratory tract appears on page 19.

Arriving at a differential diagnosis

Pharmacists must try to differentiate between viral infection and other causes of sore throat. Unfortunately, differentiation between viral and bacterial causes of sore throat is extremely difficult. A number of marker symptoms that might point to sore throat of bacterial origin can be identified, but these are by no means fool proof. Asking symptom-specific questions will help the pharmacist to determine the cause and whether referral is needed (Table 1.5). After questioning, the pharmacist should inspect the mouth and cervical glands (located just below the angle of the jaw) to substantiate the

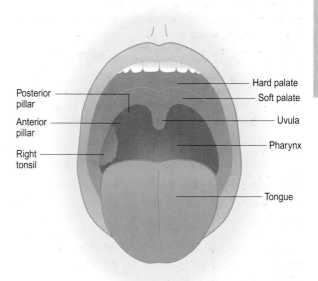

Fig. 1.3 Major structures of the mouth

differential diagnosis (Fig. 1.3). When examining the mouth, pay particular attention to the fauces and tonsils – are they red and swollen? Is any exudate present? Is there any sign of ulceration?

Clinical features of viral sore throat

Unlike streptococcal infections, there is no particular distribution with regard to age or time of year when a person can contract a viral infection. Symptoms obviously include sore throat but there might be more marked systemic symptoms than with streptococcal infection, such as malaise, fever, headache and cough. Symptoms resolve spontaneously after about 7 to 10 days.

Table 1.5
Specific questions to ask the patient: Sore throat

Question	Relevance
Age	• The likely cause of sore throat is influenced by the age of the patient. Although viral causes are the most common cause, *Streptococcal* infections are more prevalent in school-aged children • Viral causes are the most common cause of sore throat in adults • Glandular fever is most prevalent in adolescents • Oral thrush affects the very young and very old
Tender cervical glands	• On examination, patients suffering from glandular fever and streptococcal sore throat often have markedly swollen glands. This is less so in viral sore throat
Presence of tonsillar exudate	• Marked tonsillar exudate is more suggestive of a bacterial cause than a viral cause
Ulceration	• Herpetiform and herpes simplex ulcers can also cause soreness in the mouth, especially in the posterior part of the mouth. For further information see Chapter 6, page 99.

Conditions to eliminate

Streptococcal sore throat

Differentiating between bacterial and viral sore throat is plagued with difficulty. However, the probability that the sore throat is bacterial in origin rises if the patient has marked tonsillar exudate, tender cervical glands, a fever over 101°F (39.4°C), no cough and the sore throat has persisted for more than a week.

Glandular fever (infectious mononucleosis)

Glandular fever is caused by the Epstein–Barr virus and is often called the 'kissing disease' because transmission occurs primarily via saliva. It has a peak incidence in adolescents and young adults. The signs and symptoms of glandular fever often mimic those of streptococcal sore throat. It is characterised by pharyngitis (occasionally with exudate), fever, **cervical lymphadenopathy** and fatigue. The person can also suffer from general malaise prior to the start of the other symptoms.

Trauma-related sore throat

Occasionally patients develop a sore throat from direct irritation of the pharynx. This can be due to substances such as cigarette smoke, a lodged foreign body or from acid reflux.

Medicine-induced sore throat

A rare complication associated with certain medication is **agranulocytosis**, which can manifest as a sore throat. The patient will also probably present with signs of infection, including fever and chills. Medicines known to cause this adverse event are listed in Table 1.6.

Table 1.6 Examples of medication known to cause agranulocytosis
Captopril
Carbimazole
Cytotoxics
Neuroleptics, e.g clozapine
Penicillamine
Sulfasalazine
Sulfur-containing antibiotics

Laryngeal and tonsillar carcinoma

Both these cancers have a strong link with smoking and excessive alcohol intake, and are more common in men than women. Sore throat and dysphagia are the common presenting symptoms. In addition, patients with tonsillar cancer often develop referred ear pain. Any person, regardless of age, who presents with dysphagia should be referred.

Figure 1.4 will help in the differentiation of serious and non-serious conditions in which sore throat is a major presenting compliant.

TRIGGER POINTS indicative of referral: Sore throat

- Adverse drug reaction
- Associated skin rash
- Duration of more than 2 weeks
- Dysphagia
- Marked tonsillar exudate accompanied with a high temperature and swollen glands

Evidence base for over-the-counter medication

The majority of sore throats are viral in origin and self-limiting. Medication therefore aims to relieve symptoms and discomfort while the infection runs its course. Lozenge and spray formulations incorporating anti-bacterials and anaesthetics provide the mainstay of treatment, and there is no shortage of these on the market. In addition, systemic analgesics will help reduce the pain associated with sore throat.

Local anaesthetics

Lidocaine and benzocaine are the two local anaesthetics included in a number of marketed products. Very few published clinical trials involving products marketed for sore throat have been conducted yet local anaesthetics have proven efficacy. It therefore appears that manufacturers are using trial data on local anaesthetic efficacy for conditions other than sore throats to substantiate their effect.

Antibacterial and antifungal agents

Antibacterial agents include chlorhexidine, tyrothricin, dequalinium chloride and benzalkonium chloride. In vitro testing has shown that many of the proprietary products do have antibacterial activity, and some inhibit the growth of *Candida albicans*. In vivo tests have also shown antibacterial effects. The use of antibacterial and antifungal agents should not be routinely recommended because the vast majority of sore throats are caused by viral infections, against which these agents have no action. As adverse effects are rare and stimulation of saliva from sucking the lozenge can confer symptomatic relief, the use of such products may be justified.

Anti-inflammatories

Benzydamine is available as a spray or mouthwash and has proven efficacy in relieving pain associated with sore throat.

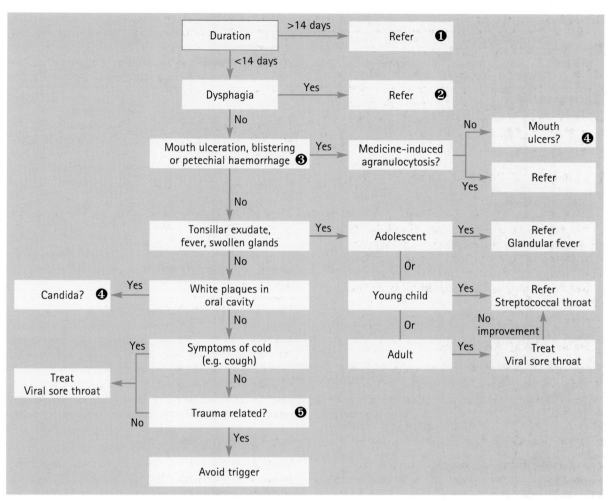

Fig. 1.4 Primer for differential diagnosis of sore throat

❶ **Duration longer than 2 weeks**
The overwhelming majority of cases resolve spontaneously in this time; it is therefore prudent to refer these cases for further investigation.

❷ **Dysphagia**
True difficulty in swallowing (i.e. not just caused by pain but by a mechanical blockage) should be referred. Most patients with sore throat will find it less easy to swallow but this has to be differentiated from actual difficulty in swallowing. Severe inflammation of the throat can cause restriction of the airways and thus hinder breathing. Additionally, rare causes of sore throat also have associated dysphagia symptoms, such as peritonsillar abscess, thyroiditis and oesophageal carcinoma.

❸ **Signs of agranulocytosis**
A severe reduction in the number of white blood cells can result in neutropenia, which is manifested as fever, sore throat, ulceration and small haemorrhages under the skin.

❹ **Mouth ulceration and Candida (oral thrush) primers**
See Chapter 6 and Figs 6.6 & 6.7 for further differentiation of these conditions.

❺ **Trauma related**
Simple acts of drinking fluids that are too hot can give rise to ulceration of the pharynx. It is worth asking whether any such factors could have triggered the sore throat.

Analgesia

There is good evidence to show that simple systemic analgesia, for example paracetamol, aspirin and ibuprofen, is effective in reducing the pain associated with sore throat. In addition, flurbiprofen lozenges have shown to be significantly more effective than placebo in reducing pain associated with sore throat; these have recently become available in the UK.

Practical prescribing and product selection

Prescribing information relating to the sore throat medicines reviewed in the section 'Evidence base for over-the-counter medication' is discussed and summarised in Table 1.7 and useful tips relating to patients presenting with a sore throat are given in Hints and Tips Box 1.3.

Table 1.7
Practical prescribing: Summary of sore throat medicines

Medicine	Use in children	Likely side-effects	Drug interactions of note	Patients in whom care should be exercised	Pregnancy
Local anaesthetics					
Lidocaine	> 12 years	Can cause sensitisation reactions	None	None	Neonatal respiratory depression in large doses
Benzocaine					
lozenge	> 3 years				Avoid in the third trimester
spray	> 6 years				
Anti-inflammatories					
Benzydamine		Oral rinse may cause stinging	None	None	OK
rinse	> 12 years				
spray	> 6 years				
Flurbiprofen	> 12 years	None reported	None	Pregnancy and breast feeding	Avoid in third trimester

---

HINTS AND TIPS BOX 1.3: SORE THROAT

Stimulation of saliva production	Sucking a lozenge or pastille promotes saliva production, which will lubricate the throat and thus exert a soothing action
Gargles or lozenges?	Gargles have very short contact time with inflamed mucosa and therefore any effect will be short lived. A lozenge or a pastille is preferable, as contact time will be longer

---

Local anaesthetics (lidocaine, benzocaine)

All local anaesthetics have a short duration of action and frequent dosing is required to maintain the anaesthetic effect, whether formulated as a lozenge or spray. They appear to be free from any drug interactions, have minimal side-effects and can be given to most patients, although they should be avoided in the third trimester of pregnancy. A small number of patients might experience a hypersensitivity reaction with either ingredient; this appears to be more common with benzocaine. Because of differences in their chemical structure, cross-sensitivity is unusual and therefore if a patient experiences side-effects with one, then the other can be tried. Most products contain a sugar base but the amount of sugar is too small to affect blood glucose control and the products can therefore be recommended to diabetic patients.

Lidocaine

Lidocaine is available as a spray (Covonia throat spray 0.05%, Dequaspray 2% or Strepsils Pain Relief Spray). Lidocaine is licensed only for adults and is best taken on a when-needed basis. Patients should be told that a maximum of six sprays of Dequaspray and ten sprays of Covonia throat spray are allowed in any 24 h.

Benzocaine

Unlike lidocaine, benzocaine can be given to children. Lozenges are available and can be given from aged 3 and over (Tyrozets 1 lozenge (5 mg) every 3 h when needed, maximum six in 24 h). Additionally, children over the age of 6 can also use a spray formulation (Ultra Chloraseptic or AAA Spray). Lozenges for adults contain 10 mg of benzocaine (e.g. Merocaine, Dequacaine) and a maximum of eight in 24 h can be taken.

Anti-inflammatories (Benzydamine, Difflam)

Benzydamine should be used every 1½ to 3 h for maximum benefit. It has no drug interactions of note, can be used by all patient groups and only occasionally does the rinse cause stinging, in which case it can be diluted with water. The manufacturers advise that the product should be stored in the box away from direct sunlight, however, the stability of the product is not known to be affected by sunlight. Benzydamine is probably the treatment of choice for adults and children over the age of 6 years who wish to use a non-systemic treatment. However, it is expensive and many patients may prefer to purchase a cheaper alternative.

Flurbiprofen (Strefen)

Strefen lozenges (7.5 mg flurbiprofen) can only be given

to adults and children over the age of 12. The dose is one lozenge to be sucked every 3 to 6 h with a maximum of five lozenges in 24 h. They are contraindicated in patients with peptic ulceration and those patients allergic to flurbiprofen, and must be used with caution in pregnant and breast-feeding women.

Further reading
Komaroff A L, Pass T M, Aronson M D et al 1986 The prediction of streptococcal pharyngitis in adults. Journal of General and Internal Medicine 1:1–7
Middleton D B 1996 Pharyngitis. Primary Care 23:719–739
Thomas M, Del Mar C, Glasziou P 2000 How effective are treatments other than antibiotics for acute sore throat? British Journal of General Practice 50:817–820
Watson N, Nimmo W S, Christian J et al 2000 Relief of sore throat with the anti-inflammatory throat lozenge flurbiprofen 8.75 mg: a randomised, double-blind, placebo-controlled study of efficacy and safety. International Journal of Clinical Practice 54:490–496

Web sites
Sinus Care Center: www.sinuscarecenter.com

Rhinitis

Background

Rhinitis is simply inflammation of the nasal lining. It is characterised by **rhinorrhoea**, nasal congestion, sneezing and itching. The majority of cases that present in a community pharmacy will be either viral infection (see page 10), colds or allergic rhinitis, which can either be seasonal (hayfever) or year round (perennial rhinitis).

Prevalence and epidemiology

The prevalence of allergic rhinitis has dramatically increased since the 1970s, with studies confirming a doubling of prevalence over this time. Hayfever affects roughly 16% of people in the Western world. However, this might be an underestimate because many people do not consult their doctor and choose to self-medicate; it has been suggested that the figure might be nearer to 40%. Hayfever commonly affects young people, with 10 to 30% of the adolescent population suffering from the condition. In addition, a person is more likely to suffer from allergic rhinitis if there is a family history of asthma, eczema or hayfever. It has also been reported that patients with concurrent asthma have up to an 80% chance of developing allergic rhinitis.

Aetiology

Initially, the patient must come into contact with an allergen; for hayfever this is pollen. The pollen season can last from early spring (tree pollen), through the summer months (grass, peaking in June and July) and finish in the autumn (fungal spores). Pollen lodges within the mucous blanket lining the nasal membranes and activates immunoglobulin E (IgE) antibodies (formed from previous pollen exposure) on the surface of mast cells. Potent chemical mediators – primarily histamine, but also leukotrienes, kinins and prostaglandins – are released, which exert their action via neural and vascular mechanisms. Nasal itch, rhinorrhoea and sneeze are neural in origin whereas nasal congestion arises from **vascular engorgement**. The house-dust mite is the allergen most responsible for perennial allergic rhinitis, although animal dander, particularly from cats, can also give rise to symptoms.

Also of importance is the phenomenon of nasal priming. After a period of continuous allergen exposure, patients can find that they experience the same level of severity in symptoms with lower levels of allergen exposure. Similarly, symptoms will be worse than previously experienced when levels of the allergen are the same. This explains why patients complain of worsening hayfever symptoms the longer the season goes on.

Arriving at a differential diagnosis

Rhinitis is not difficult to diagnose. Within the community pharmacy setting the majority of patients who present with rhinitis will be suffering from a cold or hayfever. Diagnosis is largely dependent upon the patient having a family history of **atopy**, clinical symptoms and worsening symptoms at a particular time of year. Asking symptom-specific questions will help the pharmacist to determine the cause and whether referral is needed (Table 1.8).

Clinical features of hayfever

The patient will experience a combination or all four of the classical rhinitis symptoms of nasal itch, sneeze, rhinorrhoea and nasal congestion. However, in addition the patient might also suffer from ocular irritation, giving rise to allergic conjunctivitis. The symptoms should occur intermittently (i.e. times of pollen exposure) and tend to be worse in the morning and evening as pollen levels peak at this time, as they do when the weather is hot and humid.

Conditions to eliminate

Perennial allergic rhinitis

Perennial allergic rhinitis is 10 times less common than hayfever. As its name suggests, the problem tends to be persistent and does not exhibit seasonality. However, it must be remembered that patients suffering from

Table 1.8
Specific questions to ask the patient: Rhinitis

Question	Relevance
Seasonal variation	● Symptoms in the summer months suggest hayfever; year-round symptoms suggest perennial rhinitis
History of asthma, eczema or hayfever in the family	● If a first-degree relative suffers from atopy then hayfever is the most likely cause of rhinitis
Triggers	● Pollen is the main allergen in hayfever, therefore symptoms are worse when pollen counts are high ● Infective rhinitis will be unaffected by pollen count; patients with perennial rhinitis might suffer from worsening symptoms but symptoms should persist when indoors, unlike hayfever sufferers who usually see improvement of symptoms when away from pollen

perennial allergic rhinitis might also be allergic to pollen and experience worsening symptoms in the summer months. Besides not having a seasonal cause, there are a number of other clues to look out for that aid differentiation. Nasal congestion is much more common, which often leads to hyposmia (poor sense of smell) and ocular symptoms are uncommon. Additionally, perennial allergic rhinitis sufferers also tend to sneeze less frequently and experience more episodes of chronic sinusitis. In the UK, the house-dust mite and animal dander are the main allergens. It is therefore prudent to ask about pets in the home when trying to establish the cause.

Infective rhinitis

This is normally viral in origin and associated with the common cold. Nasal discharge tends to be more mucopurulent than allergic rhinitis and nasal itching is uncommon. Sneezing tends not to occur in paroxysms and the condition resolves more quickly, whereas allergic rhinitis lasts for as long as the person is exposed to the allergen. Other symptoms, such as cough and sore throat, are much more prominent in infective rhinitis than allergic rhinitis.

Vasomotor rhinitis (intrinsic rhinitis)

The symptoms are very similar to allergic rhinitis yet an allergy test will be negative. Itching and sneezing are less common and patients might experience worsening nasal symptoms in response to climatic factors, such as a sudden change in temperature.

Rhinitis of pregnancy

This occurs as a result of hormonal changes; it resolves spontaneously after childbirth.

Rhinitis medicamentosa

Prolonged use of topical decongestants (more than 7 to 10 days) causes rebound **vasodilatation** of the nasal

arterioles leading to further nasal congestion. Patients should always be questioned about the use of topical nasal decongestants.

Nasal blockage

In the absence of rhinorrhoea, nasal itch and sneezing it is possible that the problem is mechanical or anatomical. Continuous and unilateral blockage might relate to a deviated nasal septum in adults. This might develop or be a result of trauma. Referral is needed and surgery is recommended. If the obstruction is bilateral this could relate to nasal polyps in adults. Nasal obstruction is progressive and is often accompanied by hyposmia. Referral is needed for corticosteroids or surgery.

Nasal foreign body

A trapped foreign body in a nostril commonly occurs in young children, often without the parents' knowledge. Within a matter of days of the foreign body being lodged the patient experiences an offensive nasal discharge. Any unilateral discharge, particularly in a child, should be referred for nasal examination because it is highly likely that a foreign body is responsible.

Figure 1.5 will aid in differentiating the different types of rhinitis.

 TRIGGER POINTS indicative of referral: Rhinitis

● Failed medication
● Medicine-induced rhinitis
● Nasal obstruction that fails to clear
● Unilateral discharge, especially in children

Evidence base for over-the-counter medication

Before medication is started it is important to try and identify the causative allergen. If this can be achieved then measures to limit the exposure to the allergen will help to reduce the symptoms experienced by the patient. This is more easily accomplished in perennial allergic rhinitis than in hayfever.

Allergen avoidance

Avoiding pollen is almost impossible but if the patient obeys a few simple rules then exposure to pollen can be diminished. Patients can choose to stay indoors when pollen counts are high. Windows should be closed (both when in the house and when travelling in cars) and 'wrap around' sunglasses worn. Patients should avoid walking in areas with the potential for high pollen exposure (grassy fields, parks and gardens) as well as areas such as city centres, because many hayfever sufferers will have increased sensitivity to other irritants such as car exhaust fumes and cigarette smoke.

The two main causative agents of perennial allergic rhinitis – house dust mite and animal dander – can be avoided more easily. The offending pet can be banished from certain parts of the house, such as living areas and bedrooms. Using allergen-impermeable bed linen and acaricidal sprays can reduce house-dust mite. Replacing carpeted rooms with wooden flooring will also help reduce both animal dander and house-dust mite.

Medication

Pharmacists now possess a wide range of therapeutic options to treat both hayfever and perennial rhinitis. A number of deregulated POM products enable the vast majority of sufferers to be managed appropriately without the need for referral to the GP. However, for many patients the cost of treatment will be too prohibitive to self-medicate for the entire period for which they suffer, and they will seek a prescription. Management of allergic rhinitis falls broadly in to two categories: systemic and topical.

Systemic therapy: antihistamines

Both sedating and non-sedating antihistamines are clinically effective in reducing the symptoms associated with allergic rhinitis. However, sedating antihistamines should not be recommended routinely because of their sedative effects when compared to second-generation, non-sedating antihistamines.

Of the second-generation antihistamines, the community pharmacist has a choice between acrivastine, cetirizine and loratadine. All are equally effective and are considered to be non-sedating. However, they are not truly non-sedating and cause different levels of sedation. Loratadine has been shown to have the lowest affinity for histamine receptors in the brain and a paper published in the *British Medical Journal* in 2000, reviewing reported sedation with second-generation antihistamines, showed loratadine to be least sedating of the non-sedating anti-histamines. In comparison cetirizine was 3.5 times more likely to cause sedation and acrivastine 2.5 times more likely to cause sedation than loratadine. On this basis, loratadine would be the antihistamine of choice.

Topical therapy

A range of topically administered medication is available to combat nasal congestion and ocular symptoms, including antihistamines, corticosteroids, mast cell stabilisers and decongestants. All can be administered intranasally but corticosteroids cannot be administered intraocularly.

Intranasal medication

Corticosteroids Corticosteroids are the medicine of choice for nasal congestion and have been recommended by the World Health Organization (WHO) as first-line therapy for allergic rhinitis because a number of clinical trials have confirmed their efficacy. Additionally, a recent meta-analysis demonstrated superiority to antihistamines in the treatment of allergic rhinitis for all nasal symptoms. However, patients should be advised that maximum clinical efficacy will take a number of weeks to develop and that regular prophylactic use is necessary to maintain symptom control. Patients who regularly suffer from nasal congestion associated with allergic rhinitis should be advised to start therapy before exposure to the allergen to ensure symptom control.

Antihistamines Two nasally administered antihistamines are currently available OTC: azelastine and levocabastine. Clinical trials have proved their efficacy and a recent review paper concluded that azelastine was well tolerated and provided an effective alternative to other anti-histamine agents because it had a rapid onset of action. This finding seems to be equally applicable to levo-cabastine and studies show comparable efficacy to oral antihistamines.

Mast cell stabilisers Like corticosteroids, sodium cromo-glicate is a prophylactic agent. However, the effect of sodium cromoglicate is only partial – it is less effective than corticosteroids, although it is not clear why. A further drawback with nasal cromoglicate is the frequency of administration; between four and six times a day. Although no data is available for the compliance with such a regimen it is likely to be poor and result in inadequate symptom control. Their place in nasal symptoms of allergic rhinitis is therefore limited.

Decongestants Topical decongestants are clinically effective in the treatment of nasal congestion. They are associated with rebound congestion (rhinitis medica-mentosa) when used for prolonged periods of time. Their place in therapy is probably best reserved for when nasal congestion needs to be treated quickly and can provide symptom relief while corticosteroid therapy is initiated, allowing it time to begin to exert its action.

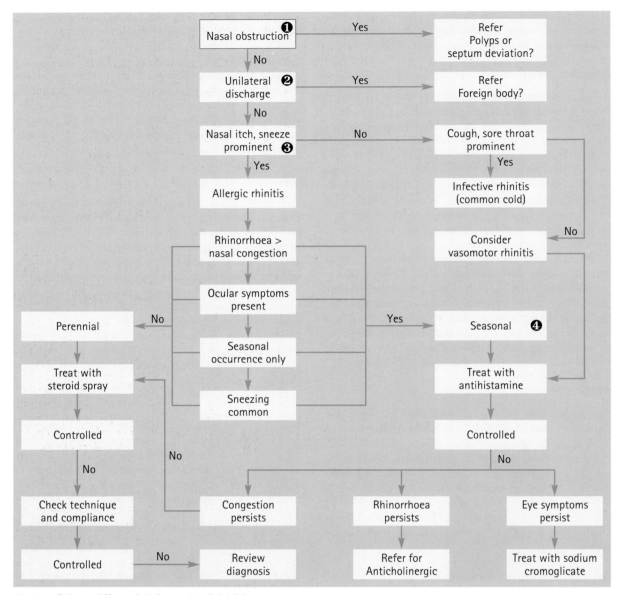

Fig. 1.5 Primer differential diagnosis of rhinitis

❶ Nasal obstruction
Nasal obstruction differs from nasal congestion in that obstruction refers to a physical blockage of the nasal passage and is normally due to an anatomical fault, whereas congestion refers to the nasal passages being temporarily blocked by nasal secretions that can easily be cleared by nose blowing. Obstruction therefore warrants referral.

❷ Unilateral discharge
Any one-sided nasal discharge must be viewed with suspicion. Accidental lodging of a foreign body by young children is the usual cause.

❸ Nasal itch and sneeze prominent
Nasal itching and sneezing are classically associated with hayfever, although these symptoms are also associated with perennial rhinitis, but to a lesser extent. Sneezing is often said to occur in multiple bouts, which is unlike infective rhinitis. Coughing can occur but is infrequent.

❹ Treatment of vasomotor rhinitis
Because symptoms are similar to hayfever then it is reasonable to assume that first-line therapy for vasomotor rhinitis would be a systemic antihistamine.

Intraocular medication

Mast cell stabilisers Sodium cromoglicate has proven efficacy and is significantly better than placebo. However, it does require four-times-a-day dosing and compliance might be a problem.

Antihistamines (levocabastine, antazoline) Trial data have shown levocabastine to be an effective and well-tolerated treatment in controlling ocular symptoms. Comparative trials have shown it to be significantly better than placebo and at least as effective as sodium cromoglicate.

Antazoline is available in combination with xylometazoline. There appears to be little trial data in the public domain regarding decongestant/antihistamine combinations, although one small trial involving 25 patients concluded that a combination of the two drugs was superior to either alone. At best it should be used short term to avoid possible rebound conjunctivitis caused by xylometazoline.

Sympathomimetics OTC ocular sympathomimetics are commonly used to control ocular redness and discomfort. There appears to be no significant differences between ocular decongestants on the basis of their vasoconstrictive effectiveness. They should be restricted to short-term use to avoid rebound effects.

Summary

Loratadine should be recommended as first-line therapy if the patient suffers from general symptoms such as nasal itching, sneezing, rhinorrhoea and associated ocular symptoms. If this fails to control all symptoms then a topical eye drop (antihistamine or mast cell stabiliser) or nasal spray (corticosteroid) should be added in to the regimen. If nasal congestion predominates then regular topical nasal corticosteroids are recommended as first line treatment.

Practical prescribing and product selection

Prescribing information relating to the rhinitis medicines reviewed in the section 'Evidence base for over-the-counter medication' is discussed and summarised in Table 1.9 and useful tips relating to patients presenting with rhinitis are given in Hints and Tips Box 1.4.

Systemic antihistamines (acrivastine, cetirizine and loratadine)

Systemic antihistamines selectively inhibit histamine H_1 receptors and suppress many of the vascular effects of histamine. They possess very few side-effects and can be given safely with other prescribed medication. They can also be prescribed to all patient groups, although manufacturers advise against prescribing to the elderly. Studies in pregnancy with second-generation antihistamines have shown no sign of teratogenicity, although manufacturers advise avoidance.

Acrivastine (Benadryl Allergy Relief)

Acrivastine is recommended for adults and children over 12 years of age. The dose is one capsule (8 mg) as necessary, up to three times a day. Acrivastine can also be purchased as a combination product (Benadryl Plus), which contains a sympathomimetic (pseudoephedrine). However, if nasal congestion is a problem, corticosteroids should be used in preference to the addition of a decongestant.

Cetirizine (Zirtek Allergy, Benadryl One-a-Day, Benadryl Allergy Oral Solution, Piriteze Allergy)

Cetirizine is available as either tablets or solution. The solution can be given to children aged over 2 (5 mL once daily or 2.5 mL twice daily). The dose for adults and children 6 years and over is one tablet (10 mg) daily.

Loratadine (Clarityn Allergy)

Loratadine is available as either a tablet or syrup. The dose for people aged over 6 years is one tablet (10 mg) each day. The syrup (1 mg/mL) can be given to children aged between 2 and 5 years old at a dose of 5 mg each day.

Nasal corticosteroids (beclometasone, fluticasone)

Currently, only beclometasone (beclomethasone) and fluticasone are available for sale to the public. In addition, flunisolide, budesonide and triamcinolone possess pharmacy status but the manufacturers have not produced an OTC product.

Beclometasone (Beconase)

This is licensed for adults and children over 18 years old, although it can be given to children over the age of 6 on prescription. The recommended dose is two sprays into each nostril twice daily (400 µg/day). Once symptoms have improved it might be possible to decrease the dose to one spray twice daily. However, should symptoms recur, patients should revert to the standard dosage.

Fluticasone (Flixonase)

In common with beclometasone, fluticasone is licensed for adults and children over 18 years old. The dose is two sprays into each nostril once daily (200 mcg/day). If symptoms are not controlled, the dose can be increased to twice daily.

Antihistamines

Azelastine (Rhinolast Hayfever Nasal Spray, Aller-eze Nasal Spray)

Azelastine can be given to adults and children over 5 years of age. The dose is one application (0.14 mL) in each nostril twice daily (0.56 mg of azelastine hydrochloride). It should not be recommended to elderly patients. It appears to have no drug interactions and can be used safely in pregnancy.

Ocular and nasal levocabastine (Livostin Direct)

Levocabastine is only recommended for adults and children over the age of 12. The usual dose is one drop in each eye or two sprays per nostril, twice daily. The dose for eye drops can be increased to three to four times daily, if necessary. When using the eye drops, if no improvement is seen in 3 days, treatment should be discontinued. Levocabastine is safe to use in pregnancy.

Table 1.9
Practical prescribing: Summary of rhinitis medicines

Medicine	Use in children	Likely side-effects	Drug interactions of note	Patients in whom care should be exercised	Pregnancy
Systemic antihistamines					
Acrivastine	> 12 years	Sedation but least likely with loratadine	None	None	OK but all manufacturers advise avoidance
Cetirizine	> 6 years				
Loratadine	> 2 years				
Ocular antihistamines					
Antazoline*	> 5 years	Local irritation, bitter taste	Avoid concomitant use with MAOIs and moclobemide due to risk of hypertensive crisis	Avoid in glaucoma	OK
Levocabastine	> 12 years	Local irritation, blurred vision	None	None	
Nasal antihistamines					
Azelastine	> 5 years	Nasal irritation (5%), bitter taste (3%)	None	None	OK
Levocabastine	> 12 years	Nasal irritation, headache		Severe renal impairment	
Nasal corticosteroids					
Beclometasone	> 18 years	Nasal irritation, bitter taste, nosebleeds	None	Avoid in glaucoma	OK
Fluticasone					
Ocular and nasal mast cell stabilisers					
Sodium cromoglicate ocular	> 12 years	Local irritation, blurred vision	None	None	OK
Sodium cromoglicate nasal	> 5 years	Rare wheezing and shortness of breath			
Ocular sympathomimetics					
Naphazoline	> 12 years	Local irritation	Avoid concomitant use with MAOIs and moclobemide because of risk of hypertensive crisis	None	OK

*only available in combination with naphazoline.
MAOI, monoamine oxidase inhibitor.

HINTS AND TIPS BOX 1.4: RHINITIS

Livostin Direct Eye Drops and Nasal Spray	These are microsuspensions and the bottle should be shaken before each application
Corticosteroid nasal sprays	Regular usage is essential for full therapeutic benefit. It should also be explained that maximum relief might not be obtained for several days
Breakthrough symptoms with one-a-day antihistamines	Patients who suffer breakthrough symptoms using a once-daily preparation (loratadine, cetirizine) might benefit from changing to acrivastine, because three-times-a-day dosing may confer better symptom control

Mast cell stabilisers

Ocular and nasal sodium cromoglicate

Sodium cromoglicate can be given intranasally (Rynacrom) or intraocularly (e.g. Opticrom Allergy). It is not known to be teratogenic or to have any drug interactions, and it can be given to all patient groups. The dose for the eye drops is four times a day and the nasal spray four to six times a day. Sodium cromoglicate is a prophylactic agent and therefore has to be given continuously whilst exposed to the allergen.

Sympathomimetics

For general information about sympathomimetics and product information on nasally administered products, see page 12.

Ocular sympathomimetics

Ocular products either contain a combination of sympathomimetic and antihistamine (Otrivine Antistin) or sympathomimetic alone (e.g. Naphazoline 0.01%). They are useful in reducing redness in the eye but will not treat the underlying cause that is causing the eye to be red. They should be limited to short-term use to avoid rebound effects. Like all sympathomimetics they can interact with monoamine oxidase inhibitors and should not be used by patients receiving such treatment or within 14 days of ceasing therapy. They are safe to use in pregnancy.

Otrivine Antistin Adults and children over 5 years old should administer Otrivine Antistin two or three times a day. Patients with glaucoma should avoid this product because of the potential of the antihistamine component to increase intraocular pressure. Local transient irritation and a bitter taste after application have been reported.

Naphazoline (Murine, Eye Dew and Optrex Clear Eyes). The use of products containing naphazoline is restricted to adults and children over the age of 12 years old. One to two drops should be administered into the eye four times a day.

Further reading

[Anonymous] 1995 Hayfever. MeReC Bulletin 6:13–16

Demichiei M E, Nelson L 1988 Allergic rhinitis. American Family Physician 37:251–263

Fleming D M, Crombie L D 1987 Prevalence of hayfever in England and Wales. British Medical Journal 294:279–283

Jones N 2001 Management of allergic rhinitis in primary care. Prescriber 12:81–96

Jones N S, Carney A S, Davis A 1998 The prevalence of allergic rhinosinusitis: a review. Journal of Laryngology and Otolaryngology 112:1019–1030

Mann R D, Pearce G L, Dunn N et al 2000 Sedation with 'non-sedating' antihistamines: four prescription-event monitoring studies in general practice. British Medical Journal 320:1184–1186

McNeely W, Wiseman L R 1998 Intranasal azelastine. A review of its efficacy in the management of allergic rhinitis. Drugs 56:91–114

Slater J W, Zechnich A D, Haxby D G 1999 Second-generation antihistamines: a comparative review. Drugs 57:31–47

Soparkar C N S, Wilhelmus K R, Douglas D et al 1997 Acute and chronic conjunctivitis due to over-the-counter ophthalmic decongestants. Archives of Ophthalmology 115:34–38

Self-assessment questions

The following questions are intended to supplement the text. Two levels of questions are provided; multiple choice questions and case studies. The multiple choice questions are designed to test factual recall and the case studies allow knowledge to be applied to a practice setting.

Multiple choice questions

1.1. Which respiratory condition is characterised by shortness of breath and bronchoconstriction?

    a. Acute bronchitis
    b. Heart failure
    c. Asthma
    d. Chronic bronchitis
    e. Pneumonia

1.2. What course of action would be most appropriate if a baby was suffering with croup-like symptoms?

    a. Take the infant to casualty
    b. Put the infant into a steamy room
    c. Give the infant paracetamol
    d. Give the infant a cough suppressant
    e. Give the infant an antihistamine

1.3. Which patient group is most at risk of pneumothorax?

    a. Elderly women
    b. Young men
    c. Young women
    d. Elderly men
    e. None of the above

1.4. Which one of the following medicines can cause rebound congestion with over use?

    a. Pseudoephedrine tablets
    b. Guaifenesin cough mixture
    c. Oxymetazoline nasal spray
    d. Chlorphenamine tablets
    e. Codeine linctus

1.5. Which medicine is drug of choice for nasal congestion caused by allergic rhinitis?

    a. Loratadine
    b. Nasal sodium cromoglicate
    c. Nasal levocabastine
    d. Nasal beclometasone
    e. Chlorphenamine

1.6. Which patient group is most likely to suffer from infectious mononucleosis?

    a. Infants
    b. Children
    c. Adolescents
    d. Adults
    e. The elderly

1.7. What symptoms are commonly associated with acute sinusitis?

    a. Dull, localised unilateral pain that is often worse on bending down
    b. Dull, localised unilateral pain that often eases on bending down
    c. Dull, diffuse bilateral pain that is often worse on bending down
    d. Dull, diffuse bilateral pain that often eases on bending down
    e. Sharp, localised bilateral pain that often eases on bending down

1.8. The most likely cause of acute cough in children is:

    a. Bacterial infection
    b. Viral infection
    c. Postnasal drip
    d. Croup
    e. Asthma

Questions 1.9 to 1.11 concern the following conditions:

A. Tuberculosis
B. Left ventricular failure
C. Chronic bronchitis
D. Pneumonia
E. Acute bronchitis

Select in which of the above conditions (A to E):

1.9. Is shortness of breath often the main presenting symptom

1.10. Is cigarette smoking the main cause of the condition

1.11. A higher prevalence is seen in ethnic groups

Questions 1.12 to 1.14 concern the following medicines:

A. Codeine
B. Phenylpropanolamine
C. Pholcodine
D. Beclometasone
E. Benzydamine

Select, from A to E, which of the above medicines:

1.12. Should be avoided by patients taking beta-blockers

1.13. Can be abused by patients

1.14. Has been linked to causing stroke

Questions 1.15 to 1.17: for each of these questions *one* or *more* of the responses is (are) correct. Decide which of the responses is (are) correct. Then choose:

A. If a, b and c are correct
B. If a and b only are correct
C. If b and c only are correct
D. If a only is correct
E. If c only is correct

Directions summarised

A	B	C	D	E
a, b and c	a and b only	b and c only	a only	c only

1.15. Which of the following symptoms are associated with sinusitis:

a. Localised pain
b. Pain is worsened on bending over
c. Pain is described as throbbing

1.16. A pharmacist should refer patients when the following symptoms are associated with the common cold:

a. Duration of more than 5–7 days
b. If fever is present
c. If middle ear involvement is suspected

1.17. Which of the following precautions should a patient take if he or she suffers from perennial rhinitis:

a. Avoid contact with animals, especially household pets
b. Reduce house-dust mite by regular cleaning of carpets
c. Close the windows when in the house

Questions 1.18 to 1.20: these questions consist of a statement in the left-hand column followed by a statement in the right-hand column. You need to:

● decide whether the first statement is true or false
● decide whether the second statement is true or false

Then choose:

A. If both statements are true and the second statement is a correct explanation of the first statement
B. If both statements are true but the second statement is NOT a correct explanation of the first statement
C. If the first statement is true but the second statement is false
D. If the first statement is false but the second statement is true
E. If both statements are false

Directions summarised

	First statement	Second statement	
A	True	True	Second explanation is a correct explanation of the first
B	True	True	Second statement is *not* a correct explanation of the first
C	True	False	
D	False	True	
E	False	False	

	First statement	*Second statement*
18.	Carbimazole can cause a sore throat	Carbimazole is used to treat hypothyroidism
19.	Conjunctivitis is a common symptom in hayfever sufferers	The redness is concentrated in the fornices of the eyes
20.	Pholcodine is an antitussive	It blocks nerve conduction to the medulla

Case study

Mr RT has asked to speak to the pharmacist because he has a troublesome cough.

a. Discuss the appropriately worded questions you will need to ask Mr RT to determine the seriousness of the cough and to establish whether he can be treated or must be referred. Explain your rationale for each question.

   Questions should fall broadly into two groups:

   - *Those that relate to the presenting complaint, for example: nature, duration, onset, periodicity, sputum colour (if applicable), associated symptoms, aggravating/alleviating symptoms.*
   - *Those that look at the medical, family and social history of the patient: current medication regimen (recent changes to medication or dosage adjustment), self-medication, general well-being of patient, smoking status.*

Discussion with Mr RT indicates he has a productive cough that appeared a few days ago and that the sputum is white. His nose is 'a bit blocked'. He has a headache and he does not have any chest pain. Before you can make a recommendation for the symptoms you identify he is taking the following medication:

- Manerix 150 mg bd – he has taken this for over 6 months.
- Trusopt tds – he has used this for 2 years.
- Paracetamol 2 qd prn – for lower back pain.

b. Compare and contrast the different products available to treat Mr RT's symptoms and indicate which you consider would be the most beneficial to him and which are contraindicated.

Information related to products to treat a productive cough with nasal congestion should be sought. This involves expectorant medication and sympathomimetics. Mr RT's current drug regimen will have to be taken into consideration and checks for interactions and suitability made. For example, Mr RT is taking Manerix, therefore sympathomimetics should be avoided.

A few weeks later Mr RT returns to the pharmacy complaining that he is still having trouble clearing his blocked nose. A friend at work recommended Otrivine Nasal Spray and he has been using it 2 to 3 times a day for about 10 days.

c. The use of local decongestants is associated with the phenomenon known as rhinitis medicamentosa. Explain what this is and what advice you would give to Mr RT to remedy this?

Rhinitis medicamentosa relates to the problem of overly long use of topical sympathomimetics. Prolonged use (normally more than 7 to 10 days continuous use) results in vascular engorgement of the nose on withdrawal of the medication. Patients often believe mistakenly that symptoms have returned and begin to use the medication again, and thus perpetuate the problem. This cycle of overuse has to be broken and the pharmacist will need to explain to Mr RT why he has continued nasal congestion. Strategies to relieve the problem are, if appropriate, a switch to systemically administered decongestants or, if this is not appropriate, then to withdraw the medication. If the latter course is adopted the patient will need to be counselled that the symptoms will initially worsen and then gradually resolve.

CASE STUDY 1.2

Mr SJ, a 26–year–old man, comes into the pharmacy asking for something for flu. He has tried Beechams capsules and the odd Lemsip. He looks visibly well.

a. What questions do you need to ask to determine whether the patient has flu?

   Duration and onset of symptoms:

   - *Exactly what are his symptoms?*
   - *What medication, if any, does he take from the GP?*
   - *Foreign travel in last 12 months?*

Further details you obtain from him are:

- He has had the symptoms for 5 to 7 days.
- He has a productive cough but this is not bothering him too much.
- He aches a little and has hot and cold spells.
- He takes salbutamol on a when-needed basis but has been using it a little more than normal.
- He has recently come back from holiday in India.

b. What do you think is wrong with Mr SJ?

   The most probable differential diagnosis is a common cold that might have become secondarily infected by a bacterium. Possible, but very unlikely, is malaria.

c. What course of action are you going to take?

   Analgesia for aches and pains and advice to drink more fluid. Zinc supplements could be tried if he wished. Reassurance that he has probably just got a bad cold but that if the symptoms fail to respond to treatment, or deteriorate, then he should see the GP.

Answers to multiple choice questions
1.1 = c   1.2 = b   1.3 = b   1.4 = c   1.5 = d   1.6 = c   1.7 = a   1.8 = b   1.9 = b   1.10 = c,
1.11 = a   1.12 = b   1.13 = a   1.14 = b   1.15 = b   1.16 = e   1.17 = b   1.18 = c   1.19 = b   1.20 = a.

Ophthalmology

Background

The eye is one of the most important and complex organs of the body. Vision is taken for granted and only when our sight is threatened do we truly appreciate what we have. Because of its complicated and intricate anatomy, many things can and do go wrong with the eye, and these manifest as ocular symptoms to the patient.

It is the pharmacist's role to differentiate between minor self-limiting and serious sight-threatening conditions. For pharmacists to undertake this role they need to be familiar with the gross anatomy of the eye, be able to take an eye history and perform a simple eye examination.

In addition, pharmacists can play a major role in health promotion towards eye care. Patients who present with repeat medication for degenerative conditions, such as glaucoma, could have regular contact with the pharmacist, who could check patient concordance, ability to administer eye drops and ointments correctly and, potentially, discover any deterioration of the patient's condition.

General overview of eye anatomy

A basic understanding of the main eye structures is useful to help pharmacists assess the nature and severity of the presenting complaint. Figure 2.1 (overleaf) highlights the principal eye structures.

The eyelids

The eyelids consist mainly of voluntary muscle with a border of thick connective tissue, known as the tarsal plate. This plate is felt as a ridge when everting the eyelid to remove a foreign body. Covering the inner aspect of the eyelids is the conjunctiva, which continues over the surface of the eye.

The sclera and cornea

The sclera encircles the eye, apart from a small 'window' at the very front of the eye where the cornea is located. The sclera is often referred to as the 'white of the eye'. The transparent cornea allows light to enter the eye and helps to converge light on to the retina.

The iris, pupil and ciliary body

The iris is the coloured part of the eye. It is an incomplete circle, with a hole in the middle of the iris, which forms the pupil. The iris attaches to the ciliary body, which serves to hold the lens in place. The ciliary body produces the aqueous, a watery solution that bathes the lens. This is manufactured behind the iris, travels through the posterior chamber and the pupil before draining at the anterior chamber angle (where the iris meets the cornea). If this exit becomes blocked then the intraocular pressure of the eye becomes elevated.

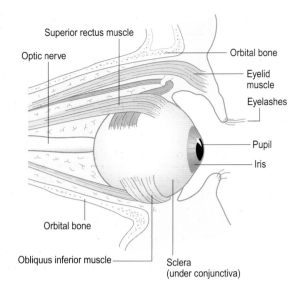

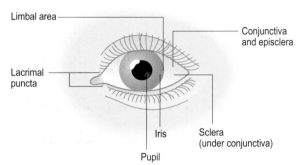

Fig. 2.1 Anatomy of the eye. Above: side view; below: front view

The lens

The lens is responsible for 'fine focusing' light onto the retina. It possesses the ability to vary its focusing power. However, this variable focus power is lost with increasing age as the lens grows harder and less elastic. This is the reason many people require reading glasses as they get older.

The retina

The retina is the light-sensitive layer of the eye; it is reason for the presence of all the other eye structures. The functioning of the retina can be compromised by many factors, such as underlying disease states, and foreign bodies causing retinal damage and detachment.

History taking and the eye exam

A detailed history should be sought from the patient when attempting to decide on the presenting complaint. Pay attention to vision, the severity and nature of dis-

comfort and the presence of discharge. Do not forget to ask about any family history of eye disease (e.g. glaucoma) and the person's previous eye and medication history. Answers to these various questions should enable the pharmacist to build up a picture of the problem and arrive at a tentative differential diagnosis.

The history gained should then be supplemented by performing an eye exam. A great deal of information can be learned from a close inspection of the eye. For example, you can check the size of the pupils, their comparative size and reaction to light, the colour of the sclera, the nature of any discharge and if there is any eye lid involvement. It is impossible to agree with a patient's self-diagnosis or for you to differentially diagnose any form of conjunctivitis from behind a counter, however intently you peer at the patient's eye! Pharmacists owe it to their patients to perform a simple eye exam.

The eye can only be examined in good light. This might mean asking the patient to move to an area within the pharmacy where this can be performed.

- First, wash your hands.
- Next, ask the patient to look straight ahead. This allows you to view the pupil, cornea and sclera.
- Then, gently pull down the lower lid and ask the patient to look upwards and to both the left and the right. This enables you to examine the conjunctiva.
- Now ask the patient to look directly in to a near light and then back at you. This is best performed using a pen-torch. This enables you to examine the reaction of the pupils to light. Any abnormal pupil reaction in the presence of ocular symptoms should always be treated seriously.

You should also endeavour to assess the **visual acuity** of the patient. Snellen charts (standard charts used to assess visual acuity) will not be available in a community pharmacy, however, you can ask a patient to read small print with the affected eye.

Red eye

Background

Redness of the eye and inflammation of the conjunctiva has been reported as being the most common ophthalmic problem encountered in the Western world. As conjunctivitis (bacterial, viral and allergic forms) is the most common ocular condition encountered by community pharmacists, this section concentrates on recognising the different types of conjunctivitis and differentially diagnosing these from more serious ocular disorders.

Prevalence and epidemiology

The exact prevalence of conjunctivitis is not known, although the prevalence of seasonal allergic conjunctivitis (hayfever) in the UK is increasing. Conjunctivitis seems to affect the sexes equally and can present in any age of patient. All three types of conjunctivitis are essentially self-limiting, although viral conjunctivitis can be recurrent and persist for many weeks.

Aetiology

Conjunctivitis can result from either an infection (viral or bacterial) or an allergen. *Staphylococcus* or *Haemophilus* bacteria most frequently cause bacterial conjunctivitis. The adenovirus is most commonly implicated in causing viral conjunctivitis and pollen usually causes seasonal allergic conjunctivitis.

Arriving at a differential diagnosis

Red eye is a presenting complaint of both serious and non-serious causes of eye pathology. Community pharmacists must be able to differentiate between those conditions that can be managed and those that need referral.

Redness of the eye can occur alone or present with accompanying symptoms of pain, discomfort, discharge and loss of visual acuity. A number of eye specific questions should always be asked of the patient to aid in diagnosis (Table 2.1).

Clinical features of conjunctivitis

The overwhelming majority of patients presenting to the pharmacy with red eye will have some form of conjunctivitis. Each of the three types of conjunctivitis has similar but varying symptoms. Each present with the three main symptoms of redness, discharge and discomfort. Table 2.2 and Figures 2.2, 2.3 and 2.4 highlight the similarities and differences in the classic presentations of the three conditions.

Table 2.1
Specific questions to ask the patient: Red eye

Question	Relevance
Discharge present	● Most commonly seen in conjunctivitis. Can vary from watery to mucopurulent, depending on the form
Associated rhinitis	● Signs and symptoms of an upper respiratory tract infection point towards a viral cause of conjunctivitis
Visual changes	● Any loss of vision or haloes around objects should be viewed with extreme caution, especially if scleral redness is also present
Pain/discomfort/itch	● True pain is generally associated with conditions requiring referral, e.g. scleritis, keratitis and acute glaucoma. Pain associated with conjunctivitis is often described as a gritty/foreign-body-type pain
Location of redness	● Redness concentrated near or around the coloured part of the eye can indicate sinister pathology, for example uveitis. Generalised redness and redness toward the fornices (corners of the eyes) is more indicative of conjunctivitis. Localised scleral redness can indicate scleritis or episcleritis
Duration	● Minor eye problems are usually self-limiting and resolve within a few days. Any ocular redness, apart from subconjunctival haemorrhage, and allergic conjunctivitis that lasts more than 1 week requires referral

Table 2.2
Symptoms that help to distinguish between the different types of conjunctivitis

	Bacterial	Viral	Allergic
Eyes affected	Both, but one eye affected a day or so before the other	Both	Both
Discharge	Purulent	Watery	Watery
Pain	Gritty feeling	Gritty feeling	Itching
Distribution of redness	Generalised and diffuse	Generalised	Generalised but greatest in fornices
Associated symptoms	None commonly	Cough and cold symptoms	Rhinitis (might also have family history of atopy)

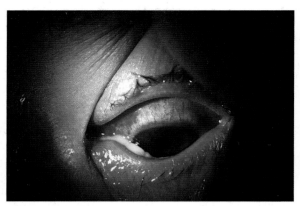

Fig. 2.2 Bacterial conjunctivitis. Reproduced from *Handbook of Ocular Disease Management* by Joseph W Sowka OD, Andrew S Gurwood OD and Alan Kabat OD, Jobson Publishing, with permission

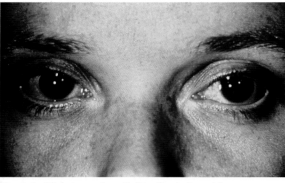

Fig. 2.4 Allergic conjunctivitis. Reproduced from *Handbook of Ocular Disease Management* by Joseph W Sowka OD, Andrew S Gurwood OD and Alan Kabat OD, Jobson Publishing, with permission

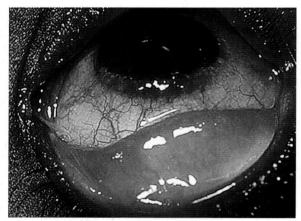

Fig. 2.3 Viral conjunctivitis. Reproduced from *Handbook of Ocular Disease Management* by Joseph W Sowka OD, Andrew S Gurwood OD and Alan Kabat OD, Jobson Publishing, with permission

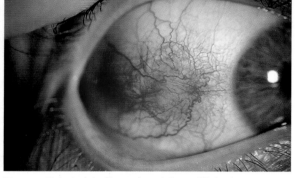

Fig. 2.5 Episcleritis. Reproduced from *Clinical Ophthalmology*, 2003, by J Kanski, Butterworth-Heinemann, with permission

Conditions to eliminate

Episcleritis

The episclera lies just beneath the conjunctiva and adjacent to the sclera. If this becomes inflamed the eye appears red, which is segmental affecting only part of the eye (Fig. 2.5). The condition is usually painless or a dull ache might be present. It is most commonly seen in young women and is usually self-limiting, but it could take 6 to 8 weeks before symptoms resolve.

Scleritis

Inflammation of the sclera is much less common than episcleritis. It is often associated with autoimmune diseases, for example rheumatoid arthritis. It presents similarly to episcleritis but is much more painful. Discharge is rare or absent in both episcleritis and scleritis.

Keratitis (corneal ulcer)

Inflammation of the cornea often results from recent trauma (e.g. eye abrasion) or administration of long-term steroid drops. Overuse of soft contact lenses has also been implicated in causing keratitis. Pain, which can be very severe, is a prominent feature. The patient usually complains of **photophobia** accompanied with a watery discharge. Redness of the eye tends to be worse around the iris.

Uveitis

Uveitis describes inflammation involving the uveal tract (iris, ciliary body and choroid). The likely cause is an antigen–antibody reaction, which can occur as part of a systemic disease such as rheumatoid arthritis or ulcerative colitis. Photophobia is a prominent feature and pain is moderate to severe and might keep the person awake. Usually, only one eye is affected and the redness is often localised to the **limbal area** (known as the ciliary flush). On examination, the pupil will appear irregular shaped

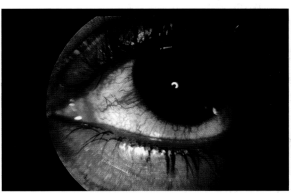

Fig. 2.6 Uveitis. Reproduced from *Handbook of Ocular Disease Management* by Joseph W Sowka OD, Andrew S Gurwood OD and Alan Kabat OD, Jobson Publishing, with permission

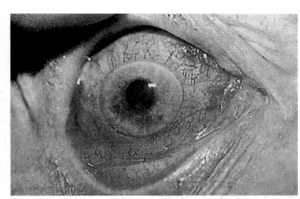

Fig. 2.8 Acute angle glaucoma. Reproduced from *ABC of Eyes*, 1999, by P Khaw and A Elkington, with permission of BMJ Books

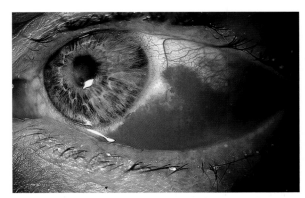

Fig. 2.7 Subconjunctival haemorrhage. Reproduced from *Clinical Ophthalmology*, 2003, by J Kanski, Butterworth-Heinemann, with permission

and constricted (Fig. 2.6). The patient might also complain of impaired reading vision.

Subconjunctival haemorrhage

The rupture of a blood vessel under the conjunctiva causes subconjunctival haemorrhage. A segment, or even the whole eye will appear bright red (Fig. 2.7). It occurs spontaneously but can be precipitated by coughing, straining or lifting. There is no pain and the patient should be reassured that symptoms will resolve in 10 to 14 days without treatment. However, a patient with a history of trauma should be referred to exclude ocular injury.

Acute closed-angle glaucoma

There are two main types of glaucoma:

● chronic open-angle glaucoma, which does not cause pain
● acute closed-angle glaucoma, which can present with a painful red eye.

The latter requires immediate referral to the GP or even casualty. It is the result of inadequate drainage of aqueous fluid from the anterior chamber of the eye, which results in an increase in intraocular pressure. The onset can be very quick and characteristically occurs in the evening. The eye appears red and may be cloudy (Fig. 2.8). Vision is blurred and the patient might also notice haloes around lights. Vomiting is often experienced because of the rapid rise in intraocular pressure. As it is such a painful condition, patients are unlikely to present to the community pharmacist.

Figure 2.9 can be used to help differentiation between serious and non-serious red eye conditions.

> ❗ **TRIGGER POINTS indicative of referral: Red eye**
>
> ● Associated vomiting
> ● Clouding of the cornea
> ● Distortion of vision
> ● Irregular shaped pupil
> ● Photophobia
> ● Redness caused by a foreign body
> ● Redness localised around the pupil
> ● True eye pain

Evidence base for over-the-counter medication

Viral conjunctivitis

Currently, there are no OTC preparations available to treat viral conjunctivitis. The condition is highly contagious and the pharmacist should instruct the patient to follow strict hygiene measures (e.g. washing hands frequently and not sharing towels), which will help to control the spread of the virus. Antibacterial preparations, if used, will only prevent secondary infection.

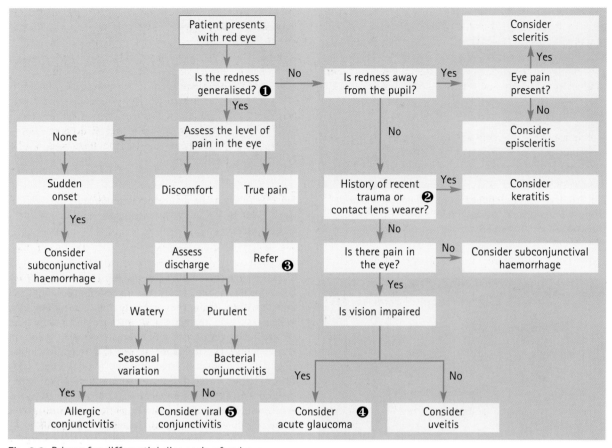

Fig. 2.9 Primer for differential diagnosis of red eye

❶ **Generalised redness**
Most episodes of conjunctivitis will show generalised redness, although the intensity of redness tends to be worse towards the corners of the eye or away from the pupil. Occasionally, severe conjunctivitis can have marked redness throughout the eye; these cases are best referred.

❷ **Contact lens wearers**
Contact lens wearers are more predisposed to keratitis because the space between the contact lens and cornea can act as an incubator for bacteria and enhance mechanical abrasion. This is especially true if patients sleep with their lenses in, because contact time for abrasion to occur is prolonged.

❸ **True pain**
It is important to distinguish true pain from ocular irritation. Red eye caused by conjunctivitis causes discomfort, often described as

gritty or a 'foreign body' sensation. It does not normally cause true eye pain. True pain would indicate more serious ocular pathology, such as scleritis, uveitis or keratitis. It is important to encourage the patient to describe the sensation carefully to enable an accurate assessment of the type of pain experienced.

❹ **Glaucoma**
This is more common in people aged over 50 years and longsighted people. Dim light can precipitate an attack. It is a medical emergency and immediate referral is needed.

❺ **Viral conjunctivitis**
Associated symptoms of an upper respiratory tract infection might be present (e.g. cough and cold). Viral conjunctivitis often occurs in epidemics and it is not unusual to see a number of cases in a very short space of time.

Bacterial conjunctivitis

Symptoms usually resolve without the need for treatment of any kind and the use of an antibacterial will hasten recovery by only a day or so. However, if treatment is instigated then dibromopropamidine isetionate and propamidine are available. Both compounds are active against a wide range of organisms, including those responsible for bacterial conjunctivitis. However, clinical trials are lacking to substantiate their effectiveness in treating bacterial conjunctivitis. The lack of trials might,

in part, be due to the self-limiting nature of the condition. A further possible limitation of these products is the licensed dosage regimen of four times a day for drops, which has been reported to be too infrequent to achieve sufficient concentrations to kill or stop the growth of the infecting pathogen.

Chloramphenicol remains the most frequently prescribed ocular antibiotic in the UK. Community pharmacists have expressed a desire to see deregulation of chloramphenicol to Pharmacy-only status to treat bacterial conjunctivitis.

However, although chloramphenicol has proven efficacy, it has also been associated with reports of aplastic anaemia following topical use. It therefore seems unlikely that chloramphenicol will be deregulated to Pharmacy-only status in the near future, despite more recent studies challenging its association with aplastic anaemia.

Allergic conjunctivitis

Avoidance of the allergen will, in theory, result in control of symptoms. However total avoidance is almost impossible and the use of prophylactic medication is usually advocated.

The evidence base for mast cell stabilisers, antihistamines and sympathomimetics is discussed in Chapter 1 (page 21).

Practical prescribing and product selection

Prescribing information relating to medication for red eye reviewed in the section 'Evidence base for over-the-counter medication' is discussed and summarised in Table 2.3 and useful tips relating to treatment are given in Hints and Tips Box 2.1.

Products for bacterial conjunctivitis

Propamidine (Brolene and Golden Eye drops) and dibromopropamidine isetionate (Brolene and Golden Eye ointment)

Propamidine and dibromopropamidine isetionate are licensed only for adults and children over the age of 12.

The dose for eye drops is one or two drops up to four times daily, whereas the ointment should be applied once or twice daily. If there has been no significant improvement after 2 days the person should be referred to a GP. Blurring of vision on instillation can occur but is transient. The manufacturers state that use in pregnancy has not been established but there do not appear to be any reports of teratogenic effects and therefore these products could be used in pregnancy if deemed appropriate. They are free from drug interactions and can be given to all patient groups.

Products for allergic conjunctivitis

Antihistamines (levocabastine)

Levocabastine (Livostin Direct) is recommended only for adults and children over the age of 12. The usual dose is one drop in each eye twice daily. The dose can be increased to three or four times a day if necessary. If no improvement is seen in 3 days, treatment should be discontinued because it is unlikely that levocabastine is going to help. It can be given to all patient groups, has no interactions and can be given in pregnancy. Instillation of the drops can cause a transient blurring of vision.

Mast cell stabilisers (sodium cromoglicate)

Intraocular sodium cromoglicate (e.g. Opticrom Allergy) is a prophylactic agent and therefore has to be given continuously when the person is exposed to the allergen. One or two drops should be administered in each eye four times a day. It is not known to be teratogenic or have any

Table 2.3
Practical prescribing: Summary of medicines for red eye

Medicine	Use in children	Likely side-effects	Drug interactions of note	Patients in whom care should be exercised	Pregnancy
Drugs for allergic conjunctivitis					
Mast cell stabilisers sodium cromoglicate	> 12 years.	Local irritation, blurred vision	None	None	OK
Sympathomimetic					
Naphazoline	> 12 years.	Local irritation	Avoid concomitant use with MAOIs and moclobemide due to risk of hypertensive crisis	None	
Antihistamines					
Antazoline	> 5 years.	Local irritation, bitter taste		Avoid in glaucoma	
Levocabastine	> 12 years.	Local irritation, blurred vision	None	None	
Drugs for bacterial conjunctivitis					
Propamidine and dibromopropamidine isetionate	> 12 years.	Blurred vision	None	None	OK

HINTS AND TIPS BOX 2.1: EYE DROPS

Contact lens wearers	Patients who wear soft contact lenses should be advised to stop wearing them while treatment continues, and for 48 h afterwards. This is because preservatives in eye drops can damage the lenses
Brolene and Golden Eye drops	If the patient is instructed to use the drops every 2 h rather than four times a day then the drops will probably be more efficacious
Administration of eye drops	1. Wash your hands 2. Tilt your head backwards, until you can see the ceiling 3. Pull down the lower eyelid by pinching outwards to form a small pocket, and look upwards 4. With the dropper in the other hand, hold it as near as possible to the eyelid without touching it 5. Place one drop inside the lower eyelid then close your eye 6. Wipe away any excess drops from the eyelid and lashes with the clean tissue 7. Repeat steps 2 to 6 if more than one drop needs to be administered
Administration of eye ointment	1. Repeat eye drop steps 1 and 2 2. Pull down the lower eyelid 3. Place a thin line of ointment along the inside of the lower eyelid 4. Close your eye, and move the eyeball from side to side 5. Wipe away any excess ointment from the eyelids and lashes using clean tissue 6. After using the ointment, vision may be blurred, but will soon be cleared by blinking

drug interactions and can be given to all patient groups. Instillation of the drops can cause a transient blurring of vision.

Sympathomimetics

These agents can be used to reduce redness of the eye. Products either contain a combination of sympathomimetic and antihistamine (Otrivine Antistin) or sympathomimetic alone (e.g. Naphazoline 0.01%, Murine, Eye Dew and Optrex Clear Eyes).

They should be limited to short-term use because prolonged use leads to rebound effects. Like all sympathomimetics they interact with MAOIs and should not be used by patients receiving such treatment, or within 14 days of ceasing therapy.

Otrivine Antistin

Adults and children over 5 years old should administer Otrivine Antistin twice or three times a day. Patients with glaucoma should avoid this product because of the potential of the antihistamine component to increase intraocular pressure. Local transient irritation and a bitter taste after application have been reported.

Naphazoline

The use of products containing naphazoline is restricted to adults and children over the age of 12 years old. One to two drops should be administered into the eye four times a day.

Further reading

Bond C M, Sinclair H K, Winfield A J et al. 1993 Community pharmacists' attitudes to their advice-giving role and to the deregulation of medicines. International Journal of Pharmacy Practice 2:26–30.

Cassel G H, Billig M D, Randall H G 1998 The eye book: a complete guide to eye disorders and health. The Johns Hopkins University Press, Baltimore

Khaw P T, Elkington A R 1999 ABC of eyes. BMJ Publishing Group, London

Laporte J R, Vidal X, Ballarin E et al 1998 Possible association between ocular chloramphenicol and aplastic anaemia – the absolute risk is very low. British Journal of Clinical Pharmacology 46:181–184

Titcomb L 2000 Over-the-counter ophthalmic preparations. Pharmaceutical Journal 264:212–218.

Vaughan D, Asbury T 1980 General ophthalmology. Lange Medical Publications, California

Web sites

International Glaucoma Association: www.iga.org.uk
Uveitis Information Group: www.uveitis.net

Eyelid disorders

Background

A number of disorders can afflict the eyelids, ranging from mild dermatitis to malignant tumours. In the context of community pharmacy consultations, the most common presenting conditions will be blepharitis, hordeola (styes) and chalazion.

Prevalence and epidemiology

There seems to be no data published on the incidence or prevalence of eyelid disorders. However, clinical practice would suggest that all three conditions are encountered frequently.

Aetiology

Blepharitis

Blepharitis is characterised by a dysfunction of lipid secretions and is caused by either **meibomianitis** (increased production of sebum from the sebaceous glands located at the base of the eyelids) or staphylo-coccal infection.

Hordeola (styes)

Styes are caused by bacterial infection and can either be internal or external. External styes occur on the outside surface of the eyelid and are due to an infected meibo-mian gland. Internal styes occur on the inner surface of the eyelid and are due to an infection of the ciliary glands (the **glands of Zeiss and Moll**). Occasionally, internal styes can evolve into a chalazion, a granulo-matous inflammation that develops into a painless lump.

Arriving at a differential diagnosis

Blepharitis and hordeola should be relatively straight-forward to recognise, so long as a careful history, eye exam and appropriate questioning are undertaken (Table 2.4).

Clinical features of blepharitis

Typically, blepharitis is bilateral with symptoms ranging from irritation, itching, burning, excessive tearing and crusty debris or skin flakes around the eyelashes

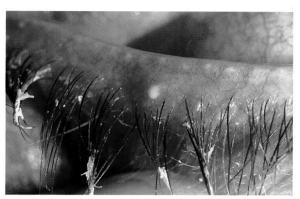

Fig. 2.10 Blepharitis. Reproduced from *Clinical Ophthalmology*, 2003, by J Kanski, Butterworth-Heinemann, with permission

(Fig. 2.10). Accompanying ocular symptoms include redness on the eyelid margins, madarosis (missing lashes) and trichiasis (inturned lash). This latter symptom can lead to further local irritation and result in conjunctivitis. Blepharitis can be acute or chronic and generally responds to therapy.

Clinical features of styes

Patients will present with a swollen upper or lower lid, which will be painful and sensitive to touch; there might be associated conjunctivitis (Fig. 2.11). Styes are usually self-limiting and often resolve spontaneously.

Conditions to eliminate for blepharitis and styes

Contact or irritant dermatitis

Many products – especially cosmetics – can be sensitis-ing and result in itching and flaking skin that mimics blepharitis. The patient should be questioned about recent use of such products to allow dermatitis to be eliminated. For further information on dermatitis, see page 155.

?	Table 2.4 **Specific questions to ask the patient: The eye lid**	
Question	**Relevance**	
Duration	● A long standing history of sore eyes is indicative of blepharitis, a chronic, persistent condition, although it can be intermittent with periods of remission	
Lid involvement	● If the majority of the lid margin is inflamed and red then this suggests blepharitis. Hordeola tend to show localised lid involvement	
Eye involvement	● Conjunctivitis is a common complication in blepharitis	
Other coexisting conditions	● Patients who suffer from blepharitis often have a coexisting hyperproliferative skin condition such as psoriasis or dandruff	

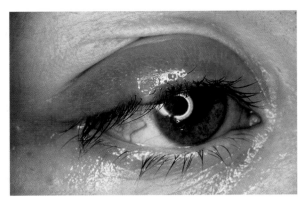

Fig. 2.11 External stye. Reproduced from *Clinical Ophthalmology*, 2003, by J Kanski, Butterworth-Heinemann, with permission

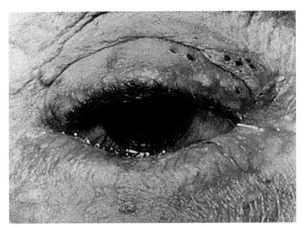

Fig. 2.12 Entropion. Reproduced from *Handbook of Ocular Disease Management* by Joseph W Sowka OD, Andrew S Gurwood OD and Alan Kabat OD, Jobson Publishing, with permission

Blepharitis unresponsive to therapy

If the patient fails to respond to OTC treatment, or if the condition recurs, then it is possible that herpes simplex, fungal infection or rosacea could be responsible for the condition. If OTC treatment has failed then the patient should be referred to the GP.

Orbital cellulitis

Inflammation of the skin surrounding the orbit of the eye is usually a complication from a sinus infection. The patient will present with unilateral swollen eyelids. The patient will be unwell and might show restricted eye movements. This has to be referred immediately because blindness is a potential complication.

Chalazion

A chalazion can be confused with a stye. Styes often have a 'head' of pus at the lid margin and will be tender and sore, whereas a chalazion presents as a painless lump. This should be clearly visible if the eyelid is everted. A chalazion is self-limiting, although it might take a few weeks to resolve completely. No treatment is needed unless the patient complains that it is particularly bothersome and is affecting vision. In these circumstances referral is recommended.

Entropion

Entropion is defined as inversion of the eyelid margin. It can occur unilaterally or bilaterally, and the lower eyelid is more frequently affected. The in-turning of the eyelid causes the eyelashes to be pushed against the cornea, resulting in ocular irritation and conjunctival redness (Fig. 2.12). Referral is needed for surgical repair to correct the problem. Taping down the lower lid to draw the eyelid margin away from the eye is sometimes employed as a temporary solution.

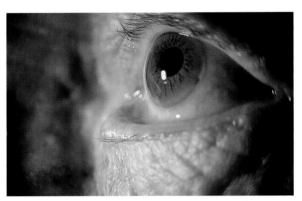

Fig. 2.13 Ectropion. Reproduced from *Clinical Ophthalmology*, 2003, by J Kanski, Butterworth-Heinemann, with permission

Ectropion

Ectropion is the converse to entropion. The eyelid turns outward exposing the conjunctiva and cornea to the atmosphere (Fig. 2.13). Patients will often present complaining of a continually watering eye. Paradoxically, this can lead to dryness of the eye, as the eye is not receiving adequate lubrication.

Basal cell carcinoma

This is the most common form of eyelid malignancy and accounts for over 90% of cases. The lesion is usually nodular with a reddish hue (due to permanent capillary dilation) and most frequently affects the lower lid margin. No pain or discomfort is present and the patient will generally have a history of prolonged exposure to the sun.

> **! TRIGGER POINTS indicative of referral: Blepharitis and styes**
>
> - Chalazion that becomes bothersome to the patient
> - Inward- or outward-turning lower eyelid
> - Middle aged/elderly patient with painless nodular lesion on or near eyelid
> - Patient with swollen eyelids and associated feelings of being unwell

Evidence base for over-the-counter medication

OTC medication is generally not required for blepharitis or styes. No specific products are available and both can respond well to conservative treatment, such as warm compresses.

Practical prescribing and product selection

Blepharitis

The mainstay of treatment for blepharitis is improved lid hygiene. A mild shampoo, such as baby shampoo, is advocated. A cotton bud can be used to apply the shampoo. A downward motion is applied to the upper eyelid and, conversely, an upward motion for the lower lid. Additionally, a warm compress applied for 10 to 20 min twice a day may be beneficial. Antidandruff shampoos can also be tried but there is no evidence to support their efficacy. Failure to respond to hygiene measures necessitates referral to the GP for possible antimicrobial therapy.

Styes

Although styes are caused by bacterial pathogens, the use of antibiotic therapy is not usually needed. Topical application of ocular antibiotics does not result in speedier symptom resolution. A warm compress applied three or four times a day might bring to a head an external stye and, once burst, the pain will subside and the symptoms resolve.

The use of dibromopropamidine has been advocated in the treatment of styes but is of unproven benefit.

> **Further reading**
> Hara J H 1996 The red eye: diagnosis and treatment. American Family Physician 54:2423–2430
> Shields S R 2000 Managing eye disease in primary care. Postgraduate Medicine 108:83–86, 91–96
>
> **Web sites**
> Handbook of Ocular Disease Management: www.revoptom.com/handbook/hbhome.htm

Dry eye

Background

Patients often complain of having dry eyes; the condition is chronic with no cure. A number of conditions can cause dry eye and keratoconjunctivitis sicca (KCS) accounts for the vast majority of cases.

Prevalence and epidemiology

The prevalence of dry eye is not known, however it is a condition associated with increasing age, especially in women. It has been hypothesised that this might be due to age-related hormonal changes.

Aetiology

Essentially, a reduction in tear volume or alteration in tear composition causes dry eyes. Underproduction of tears can be the result of increased evaporation from the eye, increased tear drainage and a decrease in tear production by the lacrimal gland. Tear composition is complex; the tear film is made up from three distinct layers:

- innermost mucin layer, which allows tears to adhere to the conjunctival surface
- middle aqueous layer, containing 90% of the tear thickness
- outermost, lipid layer, which helps to slow evaporation from the aqueous layer.

A reduction in any of these layers can lead to dryness but frequently, the mucin layer is affected due to a reduction in the mucin producing globlet cells.

Arriving at a differential diagnosis

Pharmacists receive many requests from patients wanting to buy artificial tears. Good practice would dictate that the pharmacist enquires whether the patient has been instructed from their GP or optician to buy these products or whether this is a self-diagnosis. It is important that underlying pathological causes of dry eye are eliminated. The pharmacist must ask a number of eye-specific questions to determine if a self-diagnosis is correct (Table 2.5).

Clinical features of dry eye

Symptoms frequently reported are eyes that burn, feel tired, itchy, irritated or gritty. Decreased tear production results in irritation and burning. Over time the patient experiences a chronic gritty sensation.

Table 2.5
Specific questions to ask the patient: Dry eye

Question	Relevance
Duration	● Patients suffering from dry eye usually have a longstanding history of ocular irritation
Associated symptoms	● Normally no other symptoms are present in dry eye. If the patient complains of a dry mouth, check for medication that can cause dry mouth. If medication is not implicated then this could be due to an autoimmune disease
Amount of tears produced	● If the patient complains of watery eyes but states that the eyes are dry and sore, check for ectropion

Conditions to eliminate

Sjögren's syndrome

This syndrome has unknown aetiology but is associated with rheumatic conditions. It occurs in the same patient population as KCS, although the patient does not have a history of chronic dry eyes but experiences periods of exacerbation and remission. It is also associated with dryness of other mucous membranes, such as the mouth.

Bell's palsy

Bell's palsy is characterised by unilateral facial paralysis, often with sudden onset. A complication of Bell's palsy is that the patient might be unable to close one eye or blink, resulting in a decreased tear film and dry eye.

Medicine-induced dry eye

A number of medicines can exacerbate or produce side-effects of dry eyes (Table 2.6). If medication could be causing dry eyes then the pharmacist should contact the GP to discuss possible alternative therapies to alleviate the problem.

Ectropion

Sometimes the lower eyelid turns outward. This over exposes the conjunctiva to the atmosphere leading to eye dryness (see page 40).

TRIGGER POINTS indicative of referral: Dry eye

- Associated dryness of mouth
- Outward turning lower eyelid

Evidence base for over-the-counter medication

Dry eyes are managed by the instillation of artificial tears and lubricating ointments. Products in the UK consist of hypromellose (0.3 to 1.0%), polyvinyl alcohol (1.0 to 1.4%), carbomer 940 and wool fats.

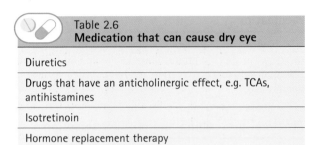

Table 2.6
Medication that can cause dry eye

Diuretics
Drugs that have an anticholinergic effect, e.g. TCAs, antihistamines
Isotretinoin
Hormone replacement therapy

Despite a lack of published trial data, hypromellose products have been in use for over half a century. They possess film-forming and emollient properties but unfortunately do not have ideal wetting characteristics, which results in up to hourly administration to provide adequate relief.

This disadvantage of frequent instillation has led to the development of other products. Polyvinyl alcohol in a concentration of 1.4% (all UK products except Hypotears (1%)) acts as a viscosity enhancer. At this concentration the products have the same surface tension as normal tears, lending them optimal wetting characteristics and hence less frequent dosing, typically four times a day. Similarly to hypromellose there is a lack of published data confirming their efficacy.

More recently, a polyacrylic polymer known as carbomer 940 has been introduced. (Viscotears and GelTears). Carbomer 940 has been shown to be more efficacious than placebo and as safe as, but better tolerated, than polyvinyl alcohol. In a comparison study between Viscotears and GelTears, both were found to be equally effective although neither was significantly better than the other.

Summary

Despite hypromellose lacking trial evidence, its place in the management of dry eye is well established. In addition, it is very cheap and should therefore be recommended as a first-line treatment. However, other newer products, which possess better wetting characteristics, provide useful alternatives to hypromellose because they can be administered less frequently; however, these products are more expensive.

Table 2.7
Practical prescribing: Summary of medicines for dry eye

Medicine	Use in children	Likely side-effects	Drug interactions of note	Patients in whom care should be exercised	Pregnancy
Hypromellose Polyvinyl alcohol Carbomer 940	Can be given but dry eye in children is rare. Patients should be referred	Transient stinging and/or burning reported. Blurred vision after instillation of carbomer	None	None	Manufacturers state to avoid as safety has not been established
Wool fats		None known			OK

Practical prescribing and product selection

Prescribing information relating to the medication for dry eye that is reviewed in the section 'Evidence base for over-the-counter medication' is discussed and summarised in Table 2.7.

The dosage of all products marketed for dry eye is largely dependent on the patient's need for lubrication, and is therefore given on a when-required basis. None of these products is known to interact with any medicine, they cause minimal and transient side-effects and are suitable for all patient groups.

Hypromellose

Hypromellose is widely available as a non-proprietary medicine in a strength of 0.3%; it is also available at 0.5% (Isopto Plain) and 1% (Isopto Alkaline). Hypromellose is pharmacologically inert and all patient groups should be able to use it safely, including pregnant women. However, because of a lack of data, manufacturers err on the side of caution and recommend that it should be avoided in pregnancy.

Polyvinyl alcohol

A number of products contain polyvinyl alcohol: Hyoptears (1%), Liquifilm Tears (1.4%) and Sno Tears (1.4%).

Carbomer 940 (Viscotears, Liposic and GelTears)

Manufacturers recommend that adults and the elderly use one drop three or four times a day or as required, depending upon patient need. Because of its viscosity, carbomer 940 should be used last if other eye drops need to be instilled.

Wool fats (Simple Eye Ointments, Lacri-Lube and Lubri-Tears)

These products contain a mixture of white soft paraffin, liquid paraffin and wool fat. They are often prescribed to help relieve ocular dryness when prolonged contact time is needed, for example at night. They are pharmacologically inert but, unlike other ocular lubricants, the manufacturers state that they can be used in pregnancy.

Further reading

Brodwall J, Alme G, Gedde-Dahl S et al 1997 A comparative study of polyacrylic acid (Viscotears) liquid gel versus polyvinylalcohol in the treatment of dry eyes. Acta Ophthalmologica Scandinavica 75:457–461

Bron A J, Daubas P, Siou-Mermet R et al 1998 Comparison of the efficacy and safety of two eye gels in the treatment of dry eyes: Lacrinorm and Viscotears. Eye 12:839–847

Gilbard J P 1999 Dry eye, blepharitis and chronic eye irritation: divide and conquer. Journal of Ophthalmic Nursing Technology 18(3):109–115

Sullivan L J, McCurrach F, Lee S et al 1997 Efficacy and safety of 0.3% carbomer gel compared to placebo in patients with moderate to severe dry eye syndrome. Ophthalmology 104:1402–1408

Web sites

Specific Eye Conditions Organisation: www.eyeconditions.org.uk/

The Schepens Eye Research Institute: www.eri.harvard.edu/htmlfiles/dryeye.html

Self-assessment questions

The following questions are intended to supplement the text. Two levels of question are provided; multiple choice questions and case studies. The multiple choice questions are designed to test factual recall and the case studies allow knowledge to be applied to a practice setting.

Multiple choice questions

2.1. Which of the following would be the *most* appropriate course of action for a patient with a chalazion?

    a. Instillation of Brolene eye drops four times a day
    b. Bathing with salt water three times a day
    c. Application of Golden Eye ointment twice a day
    d. No treatment
    e. Referral to the GP

2.2. Basal cell carcinoma usually affects?

    a. The upper eye lid
    b. The lower lid margin
    c. Upper and lower eyelids equally
    d. The lower lid margin and eye itself
    e. The eye only

2.3. How can visual acuity be assessed in the community pharmacy?

    a. By checking the reaction of the pupils to light
    b. Getting the patient to walk in a straight line
    c. Getting the patient to read print from a book
    d. Getting the patient to read distant print
    e. None of the above

2.4. Which one of the following medicines can cause dry eyes?

    a. Pseudoephedrine
    b. Atenolol
    c. Codeine
    d. Isotretinoin
    e. Pantoprazole

2.5. Sympathomimetic eye drops should be limited to how many days treatment?

    a. 3
    b. 5
    c. 7
    d. 14
    e. 21

2.6. In which of the following conditions is severe eye pain experienced?

    a. Subconjunctival haemorrhage
    b. Episcleritis
    c. Keratitis
    d. Ectropion
    e. Viral conjunctivitis

2.7. What viral pathogen is responsible for the majority of viral conjunctivitis cases?

    a. The rhinovirus
    b. The Epstein–Barr virus
    c. The adenovirus
    d. The Norwalk-like virus
    e. The rotavirus

2.8. Subconjunctival haemorrhage is associated with?

    a. A segment or whole eye appearing bright red and no pain
    b. A segment or whole eye appearing bright red and with pain
    c. A segment of the eye only that appears pale red and no pain
    d. A segment of the eye only that appears bright red and with pain
    e. None of the above

Questions 2.9 to 2.11 concern the following symptoms:

A. A clear, watery discharge
B. Haloes seen around bright lights
C. Soreness of the surface of the eye
D. A small, hard lump under the skin of the upper lid
E. Grittiness and burning of the eyes in an elderly patient

Select, from A to E, which of the above statements relate to the following conditions:

2.9. Acute closed-angle glaucoma

2.10. Chalazion

2.11. Allergic conjunctivitis

Questions 2.12 to 2.14 concern the following OTC medications:

A. Hypromellose
B. Naphalazine
C. Carbomer 940
D. Dibromopropamide isetionate
E. Levocabastine

Select, from A to E, which of the above medicines:

2.12. Is used to treat allergic conjunctivitis

2.13. Can cause rebound conjunctivitis

2.14. May require hourly administration

Questions 2.15 to 2.17: for each of the questions below, *one* or *more* of the responses is (are) correct. Decide which of the responses is (are) correct. Then choose:

A. If a, b and c are correct
B. If a and b only are correct
C. If b and c only are correct
D. If a only is correct
E. If c only is correct

Directions summarised

A	B	C	D	E
a, b and c	a and b only	b and c only	a only	c only

2.15. Which condition(s) are associated with autoimmune disease?

   a. Scleritis
   b. Keratitis
   c. Glaucoma

2.16. Subconjunctival haemorrhage is characterised by:

   a. An eye that is red and bloodshot
   b. No pain
   c. Sudden onset

2.17. Patients with dry eye syndrome usually present with:

   a. Itchy/sore eyes
   b. Associated red eye
   c. A long-standing history of dry eye

Questions 2.18 to 2.20: these questions consist of a statement in the left-hand column followed by a statement in the right-hand column. You need to:

- decide whether the first statement is true or false
- decide whether the second statement is true or false

Then choose:

A. If both statements are true and the second statement is a correct explanation of the first statement
B. If both statements are true but the second statement is not a correct explanation of the first statement
C. If the first statement is true but the second statement is false
D. If the first statement is false but the second statement is true
E. If both statements are false

Directions summarised

	First statement	Second statement	
A	True	True	Second explanation is a correct explanation of the first
B	True	True	Second statement is not a correct explanation of the first
C	True	False	
D	False	True	
E	False	False	

	First statement	Second statement
1.18.	Conjunctivitis is caused by infection only	Inflammation of the conjunctiva tends to be away from the pupil
1.19.	Ectropion should be referred	It requires surgical intervention
1.20.	Blepharitis can cause red eye	Skin flaking results in direct conjunctival irritation

Case study

CASE STUDY 2.1

Mrs JR, a 32-year-old women, asks you for something to treat her 'sore eyes'. She doesn't wear contact lenses.

a. What questions would you ask Mrs JR and what observations would you make of her eyes to help you to diagnose her eye condition?

Questions should fall broadly into two groups:

- *General questions: duration, onset, medication and family history.*
- *More specific questions: degree of discomfort, whether there is any discharge, if there have been any changes to vision, if the patient has experienced previous episodes.*

- *You perform a physical examination.*

b. What signs or symptoms would cause you to refer Mrs JR, rather than recommend OTC treatment?

Symptoms that would need referral are:

- *True eye pain.*
- *Sudden distortion of vision.*

- *Photophobia.*
- *Associated vomiting.*
- *Clouding of the cornea.*
- *Irregular-shaped pupil.*
- *Redness localised around the pupil.*
- *Redness caused by a foreign body.*
- *Swollen eyelids and associated feelings of being unwell.*
- *Inward- or outward-turning lower eyelid.*

You decide that Mrs JR appears to be suffering from allergic conjunctivitis.

c. What OTC preparations are available to treat allergic conjunctivitis?

- *First line: Topical mast-cell stabilisers, antihistamines.*
- *Second line: Systemic antihistamines.*

CASE STUDY 2.2

Mrs AY asks for your advice for her 14–year–old daughter. Emma has a sore and red eye.

a. What are the most likely conditions Emma will be suffering from based on epidemiological data alone?

One of the three forms of conjunctivitis or subconjunctival haemorrhage.

Questioning reveals that:

- Emma has had the symptoms for 2 to 3 days.
- The redness is located away from the coloured part of the eye.
- There is a slight discharge, although Emma has not noticed much colour in the discharge.
- Her eye feels slightly gritty.
- Her other eye is a little red but not as red as the problem eye.

- She is complaining of slight headaches around her eyes.
- She has taken nothing for the problem and only takes erythromycin for acne from the GP.
- She has not had these type of symptoms before.

b. What do you think is wrong with Emma?

Differential diagnosis of bacterial or viral conjunctivitis.

c. What action are you going to take?

Instigate antibacterial eye drops every 2 h and give advice about hygiene measures. If eye drops fail to resolve symptoms after 48 h then refer for further evaluation. In this instance the patient has been appropriately treated for bacterial conjunctivitis and hygiene measures will hopefully help if it were viral conjunctivitis.

Answers to multiple choice questions

2.1 = d   2.2 = b   2.3 = c   2.4 = d   2.5 = c   2.6 = c   2.7 = c   2.8 = a   2.9 = b   2.10 = d,
2.11 = a   2.12 = e   2.13 = b   2.14 = a   2.15 = d   2.16 = a   2.17 = a   2.18 = d   2.19 = a   2.20 = a.

Otic conditions

Background

Currently, community pharmacists can only offer help to patients with conditions that affect the external ear and this chapter therefore concentrates on external ear problems. However, in time, and with appropriate training, it is not unrealistic to extend the community pharmacist's role to include middle ear problems.

General overview of ear anatomy

The external ear consists of the pinna (Fig. 3.1) and the external auditory meatus (ear canal). Their function is to collect and transmit sound to the tympanic membrane (eardrum).

The pinna consists chiefly of cartilage and has a firm elastic consistency. The external auditory meatus (EAM) opens behind the tragus and curves inward for approximately 3 cm; the inner two-thirds is bony and the outer third cartilaginous. The skin lining the cartilaginous outer portion has a well-developed subcutaneous layer that contains hair follicles, ceruminous and sebaceous glands.

The two portions of the meatus have slightly different directions; the outer cartilaginous portion is upward and backward whereas the inner bony portion is forward and downward. This is important to know when examining the ear.

History taking and physical exam

The pharmacist is dependent on the patient's ability to accurately describe their symptoms because only a limited examination of the ear is possible in a commu-

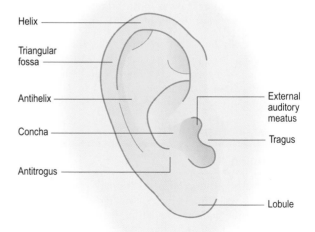

Helix
Triangular fossa
Antihelix
Concha
Antitrogus
External auditory meatus
Tragus
Lobule

Fig. 3.1 The pinna

Table 3.1
Ear symptoms and the affected ear structures

Symptom	External ear	Middle ear	Inner ear
Itch	✓		
Pain	✓	✓	
Discharge	✓	✓	
Deafness	✓	✓	✓
Dizziness			✓
Tinnitus			✓

Source: Acomb C, Pharmaceutical Journal, Aug 1991. Adapted with permission

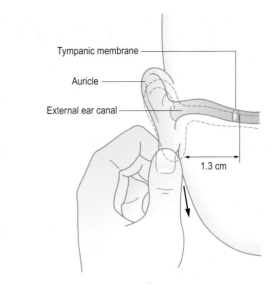

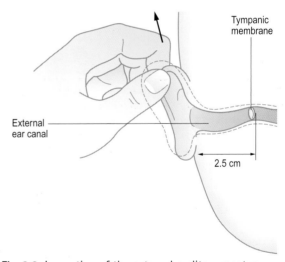

Fig. 3.2 Inspection of the external auditory meatus. Above: in children; below: in adults

nity pharmacy. This necessitates that a thorough and accurate history is taken from the patient. Certain symptoms can help decide what structure of the ear the problem originates from (Table 3.1).

After taking a history of the presenting complaint, the ear should be examined. Initially, inspect the external ear for redness, swelling and discharge. Then apply pressure to the mastoid area (directly behind the pinna). If the area is tender this suggests mastoiditis, a rare complication of otitis media. Also move the pinna up and down and manipulate the tragus. If either is tender on movement then this suggests external ear involvement. Finally, examine the EAM. Within the confines of the community pharmacy the external ear can be examined using a pen torch. Because of the shape of the EAM, when performing an examination the pinna needs to be manipulated to obtain the best view of the ear canal (Fig. 3.2). This should provide some clues as to the origin of the problem (Table 3.2). To inspect the EAM of an:

- Adult, gently but firmly hold the helix and pull it *up* and *back*.
- Infant or young child, gently but firmly hold the lobule and pull it *down* and *back*.

Ear wax impaction

Background

This is by far the most common external ear problem that pharmacists encounter and is the most common ear problem in the general population. It has been reported that GPs see between 5 and 50 patients per month requesting ear wax removal. However, many more patients self-diagnose and medicate without seeking GP assistance, therefore pharmacists have an important role in ensuring that treatment is appropriate. The high number of presentations might be due to patient misconception that ear wax needs to be removed. Ear wax performs a number of important functions, including, mechanical protection of the tympanic membrane and contributing to a slightly acidic medium that has been reported to exert protection against infection.

Prevalence and epidemiology

A number of patient groups appear to be more prone to ear wax impaction than the general population, for example, patients with congenital anomalies (narrowed ear canal) and mental retardation. Additionally, elderly people are probably more susceptible to impaction due to the decrease in cerumen-producing glands resulting in drier ear wax.

Table 3.2
Examination of the pinna and external auditory meatus: Possible causes of the presenting complaint

Patient presents with	Possible causes
Redness and swelling	Perichondritis, haematoma
Discharge	Otitis externa or otitis media. If discharge mucinous, discharge originates in the middle ear; the external auditory meatus does not have mucous glands
Pain in mastoid area	Otitis media, mastoiditis
Pain when pressing tragus or moving pinna	Otitis externa

Table 3.3
Specific questions to ask the patient: Ear wax

Question	Relevance
Course of symptoms	● The patient usually has a history of gradual hearing loss with ear wax impaction
Associated symptoms	● Dizziness and tinnitus indicates an inner ear problem and should be referred. Ear wax impaction rarely causes tinnitus, vertigo or true pain
History of trauma	● Check if the person has recently tried to clean the ears. This often leads to wax impaction
Use of medicines	● If a patient has used an appropriate OTC medication correctly this would necessitate referral for further investigation

Aetiology

The skin of the tympanic membrane is unusual. It is not simply shed as skin is from the rest of the body but is migratory. The skin moves outwards, away from the ear drum and out along the ear canal. This means that the ears are largely self-cleaning as the ear canal naturally sheds wax from the ear. However, this normal function can be interrupted, usually by misguided attempts to clean ears. Wax therefore becomes trapped, hampering its outward migration.

Arriving at a differential diagnosis

Careful questioning along with inspection of the EAM should mean that wax impaction is readily distinguished from other conditions (Table 3.3).

Clinical features of ear wax impaction

Patients present with varying degrees of ear discomfort, a feeling of fullness in the ear and slight hearing loss.

Conditions to eliminate

Trauma of EAM

It is common practice for people to use all manner of implements to try and clean the EAM of wax. Questioning should determine whether symptoms followed the insertion of a cleaning implement (e.g. cotton buds, hair-

grips and pens). Inspection of the EAM might reveal **laceration** of the ear canal and the patient could be experiencing greater **conductive deafness** because of the wax becoming further impacted. These cases are probably best referred so that the EAM can be viewed with an auroscope.

Foreign bodies

Usually, few symptoms are present, except ear canal blockage and potential conductive deafness. Children are the most likely age group to present with a foreign body in the EAM and suspected cases need to be referred for removal.

 TRIGGER POINTS indicative of referral: The ear

- Associated trauma-related conductive deafness
- Dizziness or tinnitus
- Foreign body in the EAM
- OTC medication failure
- Pain originating from the middle ear

Evidence base for over-the-counter medication

Cerumunolytics have been used for many years to help soften, dislodge and remove impacted ear wax. However, there is very little evidence to suggest that currently marketed products are more beneficial than warmed water. Olive and almond oils along with sodium bicarbonate ear drops are still advocated by the *British*

National Formulary as being safe and efficacious. This appears from the literature to be based on more anecdotal evidence than published trial data. One double-blind study that compared Cerumol, sodium bicarbonate and water showed all three treatments to be significantly better than no treatment at all but there were no differences in efficacy between the treatment groups. Cerumol has also been studied in vitro and shown to be significantly better than sodium bicarbonate, but these findings were not then taken into a clinical setting. Exterol (marketed as Otex to the general public) has also been investigated in a multicentre trial, the findings of which showed Exterol to be significantly better than its own vehicle and Cerumol. However, the study suffered from poor trial design, so the findings must be viewed with caution. A similar trial design comparing Earex with Cerumol has also been undertaken. The authors concluded that Earex was marginally better than Cerumol but the trial lacked a placebo control.

Docusate sodium (Waxsol) has also been claimed to be highly efficacious, although these claims are unsubstantiated.

Summary

The evidence from limited trial data suggests simple remedies such as water appear to be equally effective as

marketed ear wax products. Additionally, trial data does not clearly point to any product that has superior efficacy. In America, the FDA has approved a peroxide-based product as being an effective treatment for wax removal. In light of this information and the trial by Fahmy et al (1982) involving Exterol, peroxide-based products are probably first-line treatment.

Practical prescribing and product selection

Prescribing information relating to ear wax medicines reviewed in the section 'Evidence base for over-the-counter medication' is discussed and summarised in Table 3.4 and useful tips relating to patients presenting with ear wax are given in Hints and Tips Box 3.1.

Cerumunolytics

Although agents used to soften ear wax have limited evidence of efficacy, they are very safe. They can be given to all patient groups, do not interact with any medicines and can be used in children. They have very few side-effects, which appear to be limited to local irritation when first administered. They might, for a short while, increase deafness and the patient should be warned about this possibility.

Table 3.4
Practical prescribing: Summary of medicines for ear wax

Medicine	Use in children	Likely side-effects	Drug interactions of note	Patients in whom care should be exercised	Pregnancy
Cerumol	No lower	None	None	None	None
Exterol/Otex	age limit	Irritation			
Waxsol	stated				
Sodium bicarbonate		None			

HINTS AND TIPS BOX 3.1: EAR DROPS

Hypersensitivity reactions to ear drops	Local reactions to the active ingredient or constituents that might cause severe irritation and pain have been reported. If a person has had a previous reaction using ear drops then care must be exercised
Administration of ear drops	1. Hold the bottle in your hands for a few minutes prior to administration to warm the solution. This makes insertion more comfortable 2. Tilt your head to one side with the ear pointing toward the ceiling 3. With one hand, straighten the ear canal. Adults pull the pinna up and back and in children, pull down and back 4. With the dropper in the other hand, hold it as near as possible to the ear canal without touching it and place the correct number of drops into the ear canal 5. Keep the head in the tilted position for several minutes or insert a cotton wool plug 6. Return the head to the normal position and wipe away any excess solution with a clean tissue

Cerumol

The standard dose for adults and children is five drops in to the affected ear two or three times a day. In between administration a plug of cotton wool moistened with Cerumol or smeared with petroleum jelly should be applied to retain the liquid.

Peroxide-based products (Exterol and Otex)

For adults and children, five drops should be instilled once or twice daily for at least 3 to 4 days. Unlike Cerumol, the patient should be advised not to plug the ear but retain the drops in the ear for several minutes by keeping the head tilted and then wipe away any surplus. Patients might experience mild, temporary effervescence in the ear as the urea hydrogen peroxide complex liberates oxygen.

Docusate (Waxsol)

The manufacturers of Waxsol recommend that adults and children use enough ear drops to fill the affected ear on not more than two consecutive nights.

Sodium bicarbonate

This is only available as a non-proprietary product and should be instilled two to three times a day for up to 3 days.

Further reading

Corbridge R J 1998 Essential ENT practice. Edward Arnold, London

Fahmy S, Whitefield M 1982 Multicentre clinical trial of Exterol as a cerumenolytic. British Journal of Clinical Practice 36:197–204

Keane E M, Wilson H, McGrane D et al 1995 Use of solvents to disperse ear wax. British Journal of Clinical Practice 49:71–72

Sharpe J F, Nilson J A, Ross L et al 1990 Ear wax removal: a survey of current practice. British Medical Journal 301:1251–1253

Zivic R C, King S 1993 Cerumen-impaction management for clients of all ages. Nurse Practitioner 18:29, 33–36, 39

Otitis externa

Background

Otitis externa is a common, generalised inflammation of the EAM. It usually occurs as an acute episode but can become chronic in children.

Prevalence and epidemiology

The prevalence of otitis externa is largely unknown, although it has been reported that a GP will see one patient every fortnight. It is common in patients following prolonged exposure of the ear to water (e.g. swimmer's ear) and moist, humid environments predispose patients to ear canal infections.

Aetiology

Primary infection, contact sensitivity or a combination of both causes otitis externa. Certain local or general factors can precipitate otitis externa. Local causes include trauma or discharge from the middle ear and general causes include seborrhoeic dermatitis, psoriasis and skin infections.

Arriving at a differential diagnosis

In common with ear wax impaction, otitis externa is easily recognised providing a careful history and an examination has been conducted. However, other otological conditions can present with similar symptoms of pain and discharge. It is therefore important to differentiate between otitis externa and conditions that require referral. Table 3.5 highlights some of the questions that should be asked of the patient.

Clinical features of otitis externa

Otitis externa is characterised by irritation, which – depending on the severity – can become intense. This provokes the patient to scratch the skin of the EAM,

Table 3.5
Specific questions to ask the patient: The ear

Question	Relevance
Symptom presentation	● Generally patients first complain of irritation in otitis externa, which progresses to pain and discharge
Discharge	● Otitis media is the most common cause of ear discharge and is usually mucopurulent. If discharge is present with otitis externa, then discharge is not mucopurulent

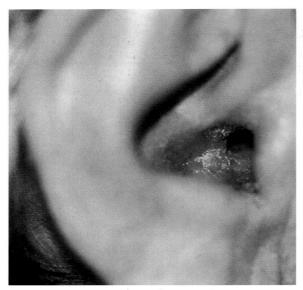

Fig. 3.3 Otitis externa. Reproduced from *Shared Care for ENT*, 1999, by C Milford and A Rowlands, Isis Medical Media Ltd, with permission from Martin Dunitz Publishers

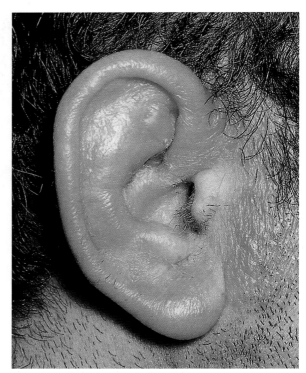

Fig. 3.4 Perichondritis. From *Essential ENT Practice*, 1998, by R Corbridge, reproduced by permission of Hodder Arnold

resulting in trauma and pain. Patients might not present until pain becomes a prominent feature. However, there should be a period when irritation is the only symptom apparent. Chewing and manipulation of the tragus and pinna can exacerbate pain. Otorrhoea (ear discharge) follows (Fig. 3.3) and the skin of the EAM can become **oedematous**, leading to conductive hearing loss.

Conditions to eliminate

Perichondritis

In severe cases of otitis externa the inflammation can spread from the outer ear canal to the pinna, resulting in perichondritis (Fig. 3.4). Referral is needed, as systemic antibiotics are required.

Trauma

Recent trauma (e.g. blow to the head) can cause an auricular haematoma. This is best known as a cauliflower ear and requires non-urgent referral.

Otalgia (earache)

Earache is normally due to a rapidly accumulating **effusion** in the middle ear (acute otitis media) and is most common in children aged 3 to 6 years old. Ear pain tends to be throbbing and signs of infection are often present (e.g. cough, cold or fever). In addition, the child might appear unwell. Pain resolves on rupture of the tympanic membrane, which releases a mucopurulent discharge. Inspection of the ear with a pen torch should reveal a red

and bulging tympanic membrane. Children can develop recurrent otitis media, which is known as 'glue ear'. The condition is symptomless apart from impaired hearing.

Malignant tumours

Skin, basal and squamous cell carcinomas can develop on the pinna of the ear. Typically they are slow growing and associated with increasing age. Any elderly patient presenting with an ulcerative or crusting lesion needs referral.

> ❗ **TRIGGER POINTS indicative of referral: Otitis externa**
>
> - Ear pain in children under 6 years of age (within 24 h)
> - Generalised inflammation of the pinna
> - If symptoms persist for 7 days or longer after initiation of treatment
> - Impaired hearing in children
> - Mucopurulent discharge
> - Pain on palpation of the mastoid area
> - Slow growing growths on the pinna in elderly people

Table 3.6
Practical prescribing: Summary of medicines for otitis externa

Medicine	Use in children	Likely side-effects	Drug interactions of note	Patients in whom care should be exercised	Pregnancy
Choline salicylate	> 1 year	None reported	None	None	OK
Acetic acid	> 12 years	Transient stinging or burning sensation			

Evidence base for over-the-counter medication

Unfortunately, OTC treatment of otitis externa is very limited. Inflammation of the EAM would respond to 1% hydrocortisone but current legislation dictates that this cannot be used on the face. This limits OTC options to either oral antihistamines – to try to combat itching and irritation – or analgesia to control pain. Choline salicylate is found in two proprietary products (Earex Plus, Audax). Two small trials comparing the analgesic effect of choline salicylate against aspirin and paracetamol have been conducted. Both trials concluded that choline salicylate reduced pain more quickly than oral analgesia.

In addition, a review article published in 2001 stated that acidification of the EAM using acetic acid combined with hydrocortisone is an effective treatment in most cases of otitis externa. However, it is unclear whether the efficacy of the regimen is attributable to acetic acid, hydrocortisone or a combination of both. One OTC product, Earcalm Spray, contains 2% acetic acid and is indicated for the treatment of superficial infections of the EAM. The *British National Formulary* states that it might be useful to treat mild otitis externa but there is a lack of trial data to support its use.

Practical prescribing and product selection

Prescribing information relating to otitis externa medicines reviewed in the section 'Evidence base for over-the-counter medication' is discussed below and summarised in Table 3.6.

Choline salicylate (Earex Plus and Audax)

Choline salicylate can be given to adults and children over the age of 1 year. The EAM should be filled completely with drops then plugged with cotton wool soaked with the ear drops. This should be repeated every 3 to 4 h.

Acetic acid (Earcalm Spray)

This can be given to adults and children aged 12 and over. The dose is one spray (60 mg) into each affected ear at least three times a day. The maximum dosage frequency is one spray every 2 to 3 h. Treatment should be continued until 2 days after symptoms have disappeared but if there is no clinical improvement after 7 days treatment should be discontinued.

Further reading
Bain J 1990 Childhood otalgia: acute otitis media. 2. Justification for antibiotic use in general practice. British Medical Journal 300:1006–1007
Hewitt H R 1970 Clinical evaluation of choline salicylate ear drops. The Practitioner 204:438–440
Milford C, Rowlands A 1999 Shared care for ENT. Isis Medical Media, Oxford
Lawrence N 1970 A comparison of analgesic therapies for the relief of acute otalgia. British Journal of Clinical Practice 24:478–479

Web sites
Prodigy:www.prodigy.nhs.uk/PILS

Self-assessment questions

The following questions are intended to supplement the text. Two levels of question are provided; multiple choice questions and case studies. The multiple-choice questions are designed to test factual recall and the case studies allow knowledge to be applied to a practice setting.

Multiple choice questions

3.1. Which of the following OTC treatments would you recommend for otitis media?

   a. Hydrocortisone
   b. An astringent
   c. Local analgesia
   d. Emollient
   e. None of the above

3.2. Otitis media is more prevalent in which age group?

   a. 0–3 years
   b. 3–6 years
   c. 6–9 years
   d. 9–12 years
   e. Over 12 years

3.3. If a patient complains of **tinnitus** and deafness, what is the most likely part of the ear to be affected?

   a. Outer ear
   b. Middle ear
   c. Inner ear
   d. Either middle or outer ear
   e. Either inner or middle

3.4. Which patient group is predisposed to otitis externa?

   a. Patients with seborrhoeic dermatitis
   b. Patients with acne vulgaris
   c. Patients with tinea corporis
   d. Patients with discoid eczema
   e. Patients with lichen planus

3.5. Symptoms suggestive of an inner ear problem are?

   a. Itch, pain and discharge
   b. Pain, discharge and deafness
   c. Deafness, dizziness and tinnitus
   d. Pain only
   e. Itch only

3.6. The best way to view the EAM of an adult is to?

   a. Pull the pinna up and back to straighten the EAM
   b. Pull the pinna down and back to straighten the EAM
   c. Pull the pinna up and forward to straighten the EAM
   d. Pull the pinna down and forward to straighten the EAM
   e. Pull the pinna back to straighten the EAM

3.7. Elderly people are more prone to ear wax because?

   a. Of an increase in cerumen production
   b. The skin migrates at a slower rate
   c. Decreased oestrogen concentrations cause less wax to be produced
   d. The number of cerumen glands decreases with age
   e. Greater immobility

3.8. Which of the following represents the best treatment for ear wax impaction?

   a. Nothing
   b. Peroxide-based products
   c. Removal with cotton buds
   d. Warm water
   e. Cerumolytics

Questions 3.9 to 3.11 concern the anatomy of the ear:

A. Mastoid area
B. The pinna
C. Tympanic membrane
D. External auditory meatus
E. Tragus

Select, from A to E, which of the above anatomical structures is most appropriate:

3.9. When painful on manipulation suggests external ear involvement

3.10. Serves to collect sound

3.11. Appears to bulge if an infection is present

Questions 3.12 to 3.14 concern the following OTC treatment options:

A. Hydrogen peroxide ear drops
B. Almond oil
C. Hydrocortisone 1% cream
D. Choline salicylate ear drops
E. Sodium bicarbonate ear drops

Select, from A to E, which of the above medicines:

3.12. Should not be used for children

3.13. Can reduce pain

3.14. Probably represents the most efficacious product to treat ear wax impaction

Questions 3.15 to 3.17: for each of the questions below, *one* or *more* of the responses is (are) correct. Decide which of the responses is (are) correct. Then choose:

A. If a, b and c are correct
B. If a and b only are correct
C. If b and c only are correct
D. If a only is correct
E. If c only is correct

Directions summarised

A	B	C	D	E
a, b and c	a and b only	b and c only	a only	c only

3.15. Which statements are associated with the EAM:

    a. The outer third consists mainly of cartilage
    b. To inspect the EAM of a child the pinna should be pulled down and back
    c. To inspect the EAM of an adult the pinna should be pulled down and back

3.16. Conductive deafness can be caused by:

    a. Insertion of a foreign body into the EAM
    b. Blockage of the eustachian tube
    c. Poor ear-cleaning technique

3.17. Otitis externa is characterised by:

    a. Intense ear pain
    b. Mucopurulent discharge
    c. Itch

Questions 3.18 to 3.20: these questions consist of a statement in the left-hand column followed by a statement in the right-hand column. You need to:

● decide whether the first statement is true or false
● decide whether the second statement is true or false

Then choose:

A. If both statements are true and the second statement is a correct explanation of the first statement
B. If both statements are true but the second statement is *not* a correct explanation of the first statement
C. If the first statement is true but the second statement is false
D. If the first statement is false but the second statement is true
E. If both statements are false

Directions summarised

	First statement	Second statement	
A	True	True	Second explanation is a correct explanation of the first
B	True	True	Second statement is *not* a correct explanation of the first
C	True	False	
D	False	True	
E	False	False	

	First statement	*Second statement*
3.18.	Swimmers often get otitis externa	Prolonged exposure to water predisposes people to EAM infections
3.19.	Perichondritis is a precursor to otitis externa	Topical antibiotics are ineffective
3.20.	All children with ear pain must be referred	Systemic antibiotics are needed

Case study

CASE STUDY 3.1

Mr SW has asked to speak to the pharmacist because his ear is bothering him.

a. Discuss the appropriately worded questions you will need to ask Mr SW to determine the diagnosis of his complaint.

Questions to ask include: duration; medication tried; whether the symptoms are getting better, worse or staying about the same; the degree of discomfort; whether there is any discharge. You should also check the order in which the symptoms presented, any precipitating factors, and if there is a previous history of symptoms.

b. How would a physical examination help to confirm or refute your diagnosis?

A physical examination will allow, along with questions, differentiation between middle and outer ear involvement.

You decide that Mr SW has impacted ear wax.

c. Compare and contrast the different products available to treat Mr SW's symptoms?

Cerumunolytics are the mainstay of treatment. However, the evidence base for efficacy is poor. The British National Formulary still advocates the use of simple agents such as olive and almond oil. Comparative trials have shown that these agents are no more effective than water. In the US, the FDA has approved peroxide-based products; these are probably first-line treatments.

CASE STUDY 3.2

Mrs PR asks to speak to the pharmacist about her 4-year-old son Luke. She wants some Calpol to treat his earache.

a. How do you respond?

The pharmacist needs to establish the severity of the earache and try to determine the cause of the pain.

b. What questions will you need to ask?

When was the onset of earache? Describe the pain. Is any discharge present? Are there any associated symptoms (e.g. cough and cold)? How is Luke's general condition compared to normal? Is this the first episode or is it a recurrent problem? Is there any loss of hearing? Is the earache associated with any trauma?

You find out that the earache has been present for a day or so and that Luke is more irritable than normal. Mrs PR says he has a temperature but that she hasn't actually taken it. Apart from this Luke has no other symptoms. However, he had this problem about a year ago and was given Calpol then and it seemed to help.

c. What course of action are you going to take?

It appears Luke has a middle ear infection. Examination of the tympanic membrane would confirm this and if possible should be carried out in the pharmacy. Instigation of Calpol seems reasonable and Mrs PR could buy some for Luke. If symptoms did not subside in the next 24 h then referral to the GP would be appropriate.

Answers to multiple choice questions

3.1 = e 3.2 = b 3.3 = c 3.4 = a 3.5 = b 3.6 = a 3.7 = d 3.8 = b 3.9 = e 3.10 = b,
3.11 = c 3.12 = c 3.13 = d 3.14 = a 3.15 = b 3.16 = d 3.17 = e 3.18 = a 3.19 = d 3.20 = e.

The central nervous system

Background

The number of patient requests for advice and or products to treat headache and insomnia make up a smaller proportion of pharmacist's workload than other conditions such as coughs and colds yet sales for analgesics and hypnotics are extremely high. The vast majority of patients will present with benign and non-serious conditions and in only very few cases will sinister pathology be responsible.

General overview of CNS anatomy

The central nervous system (CNS) comprises the brain and spinal cord. Its major function is to process and integrate information arriving from sensory pathways and communicate an appropriate response back via afferent pathways. CNS anatomy is complex and beyond the scope of this book. The reader is referred to any good anatomical text for a comprehensive description of CNS anatomy.

History taking

A differential diagnosis for all CNS conditions will be made solely from questions asked of the patient. It is especially important that a social and work-related history is sought alongside questions asking about the patient's presenting symptoms because pressure and stress are implicated in the cause of CNS conditions.

Headache

Background

Headache is not a disease state or a condition but rather a symptom, of which there are many causes. Headache can be the major presenting complaint, for example in migraine, tension and cluster headache, or one of many symptoms, for example in an upper respiratory tract infection.

Headache classification

If the pharmacist is to advise on appropriate treatment and referral then it is essential to make an accurate diagnosis. However, with so many disorders having headache as a symptom pharmacists should endeavour to follow an agreed classification system. The 1998 International Headache Society (IHS) classification (Table 4.1) is now almost universally accepted. The system first distinguishes between primary and secondary headache disorders. This is useful to the community pharmacist, as any secondary headache disorder is symptomatic of an underlying cause and would normally require referral. In the IHS system, primary headaches are classified on symptom profiles, relying on careful questioning coupled with epidemiological data on the distribution a particular headache disorder has within the population.

Prevalence and epidemiology

The exact prevalence of headache is not precisely known. However, virtually everyone will have suffered from a

Table 4.1
IHS Classification of headache

Primary headache disorders	Secondary headache disorders
Migraine	**Headache associated with head trauma**
Migraine without aura	Acute post-traumatic headache
Migraine with aura	Chronic post-traumatic headache
Ophthalmoplegic	**Headache associated with vascular disorders**
Tension-type headache	**Headache associated with non-vascular disorders**
Episodic tension-type headache	High cerebrospinal fluid pressure
Chronic tension-type headache	Low cerebrospinal fluid pressure
Cluster headache and chronic paroxysmal hemicrania	Intracranial infection
Cluster headache	Intracranial sarcoidosis and other non-infectious inflammatory disorders
episodic cluster headache	Headache related to intrathecal injections
chronic cluster headache	Intracranial neoplasm
Chronic paroxysmal hemicrania	**Headache associated with substances or their withdrawal**
Miscellaneous headaches unassociated with structural lesions	**Headache associated with non-cephalic infection**
Idiopathic stabbing headache	Viral infection
External compression headache	Bacterial infection
Cold stimulus headache	Headache related to other infection
Benign cough headache	**Headache associated with metabolic disorder**
Benign exertional headache	**Headache or facial pain associated with disorders of the cranium, neck, eyes, ears, nose, sinuses, teeth, mouth or other facial or cranial structures**
Headache associated with sexual activity	**Cranial neuralgias, nerve trunk pain and deafferentation pain**
	Headache not classifiable

Source: adapted from Silberstein et al 1999. Reproduced by permission of Martin Dunitz Ltd

headache at sometime; it is probably the most common pain syndrome experienced by humans. It has been estimated that up to 80 to 90% of the population will experience one or more headaches per year.

Tension headache has been reported to affect between 40 and 90% of people in Western countries. Migraine affects approximately 15% of women and is three times more common than in men. Conversely, cluster headache is five to six times more prevalent in men.

Aetiology

Considering headache affects almost everyone, the mechanisms that bring about headache are still poorly understood. Pain control systems modulate headaches of all types, independent of the cause. However, the exact aetiology of tension headache and migraine are still to be fully elucidated. Tension headache is commonly referred to as muscle contraction headache, as electromyography has shown **pericranial** muscle contraction, which is often exacerbated by stress. However, similar muscle contraction is noted in migraine sufferers and this theory has now fallen out of favour. Consequently, no current theory for tension headache is unanimously endorsed.

Traditionally, migraine was thought to be a result of abnormal blood flow but this vascular theory cannot explain all migraine symptoms. The use of 5-HT$_3$ antagonists to reduce and stop migraine attacks suggests some neurochemical pathophysiology. Migraine is therefore probably a combination of vascular and neurochemical changes that are rooted in a genetic abnormality; recent work has shown 55% of families have mutations located on chromosome 19.

Arriving at a differential diagnosis

Given that headache is extremely common, and most patients will self-medicate, any patient requesting advice should ideally be questioned by the pharmacist, as it is likely that the headache has either not responded to OTC medication or is troublesome enough for the patient to seek advice. Arrival at an accurate diagnosis will rely exclusively on questioning, therefore a number of headache-specific questions should be asked (Table 4.2). In addition to these symptom-specific questions, the pharmacist should also enquire about the person's social history because social factors – mainly stress – play a significant role in headache. Ask about the person's work and family status to determine if the person is suffering from greater levels of stress than normal.

Clinical features of headache

In a community pharmacy the overwhelming majority of patients (80–90%) will present with tension headache. A further 10% will have migraine. Very few will have other primary headache disorders and fewer still will have a secondary headache disorder. This text therefore concentrates on migraine, tension and cluster headache.

Tension headache

Tension headaches can be classed as either acute or chronic. Acute tension headache occurs when the patient experiences the headache for less than 15 days per month and has no persistent symptoms. Tension headache is classed as chronic when headaches occur for more than 15 days per month and last for more than 6 months. Patients generally present with a history of previous headaches over the last few days or weeks. They might have tried OTC medication without complete symptom resolution or say that the headaches are becoming more frequent. Pain is bifrontal or bioccipital, generalised and non-throbbing (Fig. 4.1). The patient might describe the pain as tightness or a weight pressing down on their head. The pain is gradual in onset and tends to worsen progressively through the day. Pain is normally mild to moderate and not aggravated by movement, although it is often worse under pressure or stress.

Migraine

There are an estimated 5 million migraine sufferers in the UK, half of whom have not been diagnosed by their GP. The peak onset for a person to have their first attack is

Table 4.2
Specific questions to ask the patient: Headache

Question	Relevance
Onset of headache	<ul><li>In early childhood or as young adult, primary headache is most likely. After 50 years of age the likelihood of a secondary cause is much greater</li><li>Headache and fever at the same time imply an infectious cause</li><li>Headache that follows head trauma might indicate post-concussive headache or intracranial pathology</li></ul>
Frequency and timing	<ul><li>Headache associated with the menstrual cycle or certain times, e.g. weekend or holidays, suggests migraine</li><li>Headaches that occur in clusters at same time of day/night suggest cluster headache</li><li>Headaches that occur on most days with same pattern suggest tension headache</li></ul>
Location of pain (see Fig. 4.1)	<ul><li>Cluster headache is nearly always unilateral in frontal, ocular or temporal areas</li><li>Migraine headache is unilateral in 70% of patients but can change from side to side from attack to attack</li><li>Tension headache is often bilateral, either in frontal or occipital areas, and described as a tight band</li><li>Very localised pain suggests an organic cause</li></ul>
Severity of pain	<ul><li>Mild to moderate dull and band-like suggests tension headache</li><li>Severe to intense ache or throbbing suggests haemorrhage or aneurysm</li><li>Piercing, boring, searing eye pain suggests cluster headache</li><li>Moderate to severe throbbing pain that often starts as dull ache suggests migraine</li></ul>
Triggers	<ul><li>Pain that worsens on exertion, coughing and bending suggests a tumour</li><li>Food (in 10% of sufferers), menstruation and relaxation after stress are indicative of migraine</li><li>Lying down makes cluster headache worse</li></ul>
Attack duration	<ul><li>Typically migraine attacks last between a few hours and 3 days</li><li>Tension headaches last between a few hours and several days, e.g. a week or more</li><li>Cluster headache will only normally last 2 to 3 h</li></ul>

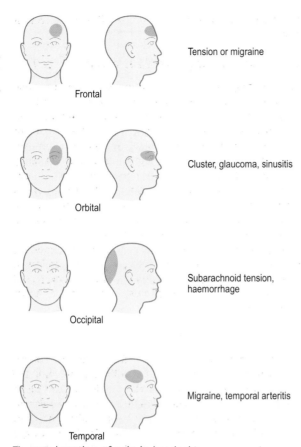

Tension or migraine

Frontal

Cluster, glaucoma, sinusitis

Orbital

Subarachnoid tension, haemorrhage

Occipital

Migraine, temporal arteritis

Temporal

Fig. 4.1 Location of pain in headache

often in adolescence or as a young adult. Migraines are rare over the age of 50 and anyone in this age group presenting for the first time with migraine-like symptoms should be referred to the GP to eliminate secondary causes of headache. If this is not their first attack they will normally have a history of recurrent and episodic attacks of headache. Attacks last anything between a few hours and up to 3 days. The average length of an attack is 24 h. The IHS classification recognises seven subtypes of migraine. However, for practical purposes migraines can be broadly divided into two types: migraine with aura (classical migraine) and migraine without aura (common migraine). A migraine attack can be divided into three phases:

● Phase one: premonitory phase (prodrome phase), which can occur hours or possibly days before the headache. The patient may complain of a change in mood or notice a change in behaviour. Feelings of well being, yawning, poor concentration and food cravings have been reported. These prodromal features are highly individual but are relatively consistent to each patient. Identification of 'triggers' is sometimes possible if a patient keeps a diary.

● Phase two: headache with or without aura
● Phase three: as the headache subsides the patient may feel lethargic, tired and drained before recovery, which may take several hours and is termed the resolution phase.

Headache with aura (classic migraine)

This accounts for less than 25% of migraine cases. The aura develops over 5 to 20 min and can last for up to 1 h. It can either be visual or neurological. Visual auras can take many guises, such as scotomas (blind spots), fortification spectra (zig-zag lines) or flashing and flickering lights. Neurological auras (pins and needles) typically start in the hand, migrating up the arm before jumping to the face and lips. Within 60 min of the aura ending the headache usually occurs. Pain is unilateral, throbbing and moderate to severe. Sometimes the pain becomes more generalised and diffuse. Physical activity and movement tends to intensify the pain. Nausea affects almost all patients but only a third will experience sickness. Photophobia (dislike of light) and phonophobia (dislike of noise) often make patients seek a dark quiet room to relieve their symptoms. The patient might also suffer from fatigue, find concentrating difficult and be irritable.

Headache without aura (common migraine)

The remaining 75% of sufferers do not experience an aura but do suffer from all other symptoms as described above.

Cluster headache

Cluster headache is predominantly a condition that affects men aged between the ages of 40 and 60. Typically the headache occurs at the same time each day and lasts between 10 min and 3 h, with 50% of patients experiencing night-time symptoms. Patients are woken 2 to 3 h after falling asleep with steady intense unilateral orbital boring pain, often described as being poked in the eye with a red-hot poker. Additionally, conjunctivitis and nasal congestion (which laterally becomes watery) is experienced on the same side of the head as the headache.

The condition is characterised by periods of acute attacks, typically lasting a number of weeks to a few months with sufferers experiencing between one to three attacks per day. This is then followed by periods of remission, which can last months or years. During acute phases, alcohol can trigger an attack. Nausea is usually absent and a family history uncommon.

Conditions to eliminate

All suspected secondary causes of headache except sinusitis need to be referred. In addition, patients suffering from cluster headache require referral, as OTC management is very unlikely to be effective.

Sinusitis

The pain tends to be relatively localised, usually orbital, unilateral and dull. A course of decongestants could be tried but if treatment failure occurs referral to the GP for possible antibiotic therapy would be needed. For further information on sinusitis, see page 11.

Eye strain

Patients who perform prolonged periods of close work, for example VDU operators, can suffer from frontal aching headache. In the first instance, patients should be referred to an optician for a routine eye check.

Glaucoma

Patients experience a frontal headache with pain in the eye. Sometimes, but not often, the eye appears red and is painful. Vision is blurred and the cornea can look cloudy. In addition, the patient might notice haloes around the vision. For further information on glaucoma see page 35.

Meningitis

Severe generalised headache associated with fever, an obviously ill patient, neck stiffness, a positive Kernig's sign (pain behind both knees when extended) and latterly a **purpuric rash** are classically associated with meningitis. However, meningitis is notoriously difficult to diagnose early and any child who has difficulty in placing the chin on the chest, has a headache and is running a temperature above 102°F (38.9°C) should be referred urgently.

Subarachnoid haemorrhage

The patient will experience very intense and severe pain, located in the occipital region. Nausea and vomiting are often present and a decreased lack of consciousness is prominent. Patients often describe the headache as the worse headache they have ever had. It is extremely unlikely that a patient would present in the pharmacy with such symptoms but if one did then immediate referral is needed.

Temporal arteritis

The temporal arteries that run vertically up the side of the head, just in front of the ear, can become inflamed. When this happens, they are tender to touch and might be visibly thickened. Unilateral pain is experienced and the person generally feels unwell with fever, **myalgia** and general malaise. It is most commonly seen in the elderly, especially women. Prompt treatment with oral corticosteroids is required because the retinal artery can become compromised, leading to blindness. Urgent referral is needed.

Conditions causing raised intracranial pressure

Space-occupying lesions (brain tumour, **haematoma** and abscess) can give rise to varied headache symptoms, ranging from severe chronic pain to intermittent moderate pain. Pain can be localised or diffuse and tends to be more severe in the morning, with a gradual improvement over the next few hours. Coughing, sneezing, bending and lying down can worsen the pain. Nausea and vomiting are common. After a prolonged period of time neurological symptoms start to become evident, such as drowsiness, confusion, lack of concentration, difficulty with speech and **paraesthesia**.

Any patient with a recent history (last 2 to 3 months) of head trauma, headache of long-standing duration or insidious worsening of symptoms, especially decreased consciousness and vomiting must be referred for fuller evaluation.

Trigeminal neuralgia

Pain follows the course of either the second (maxillary; supplying the cheeks) or third (mandibular; supplying the chin, lower lip and lower cheek) division of the nerve leading to pain experienced in the cheek, jaws, lips or gums. Pain is short lived, usually lasting only a couple of minutes but is severe and lancing and is almost always unilateral. It is three times more common in women than men.

Depression

Depression often presents with tension-like headaches. Check for loss of appetite, weight loss, decreased libido, sleep disturbances and constipation. If the patient exhibits these characteristics then referral to the GP

> **TRIGGER POINTS indicative of referral: Headache**
>
> - Headache unresponsive to analgesics
> - Headache in children under 12 with stiff neck or skin rash
> - Headache occurs after recent (1 to 3 months) trauma injury
> - Headache that has lasted for more than 2 weeks
> - Nausea and/or vomiting in the absence of migraine symptoms
> - Neurological symptoms, if migraine excluded, especially change in consciousness
> - New or severe headache in patients over 50
> - Progressive worsening of headache symptoms over time
> - Symptoms indicative of cluster headache
> - Very sudden and/or severe onset of headache

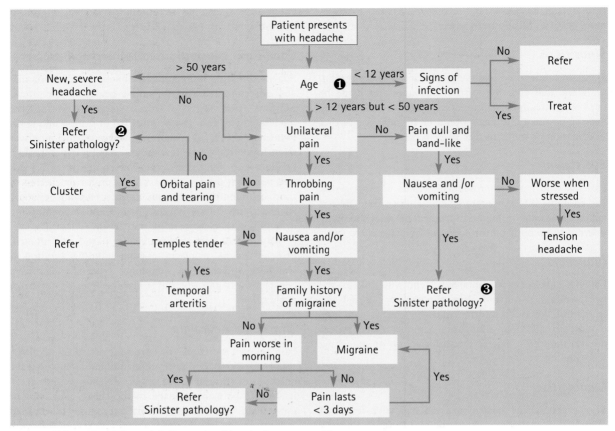

Fig. 4.2 Primer for differential diagnosis of headache

❶ Age
Caution should be exercised in children who present with headache. Although the majority of headaches will not have an organic cause, children under 12 are probably best referred if they show no signs of a systemic infection (e.g. fever, malaise).

❷ Referral for suspected sinister pathology
With increasing age it is more likely that a sinister cause of headache is responsible for the symptoms, especially if the patient has not experienced similar headache symptoms before. Mass lesions (tumours and haematoma) and temporal arteritis should be considered.

❸ Referral for suspected sinister pathology
Nausea and vomiting in the absence of migraine-like symptoms should be treated seriously. Mass lesions and subarachnoid haemorrhage need to be eliminated.

would be necessary to determine if the patient is suffering from depression. Recent changes to the patient's social circumstances, for example loss of job, might also support your differential diagnosis.

Figure 4.2 will help in the differentiation of serious and non-serious causes of headache.

Evidence base for over-the-counter medication

Three products are specifically formulated and marketed to aid relief from pain and nausea associated with migraine: Migraleve, Midrid and Buccastem. The evidence for these products is reviewed but products for tension headache, such as simple analgesia, are not covered.

Migraleve

Migraleve is available as either Migraleve Pink tablets, which contain a paracetamol codeine combination (500/8) plus buclizine 6.25 mg, or Migraleve Yellow tablets, which contain only the analgesic combination. A number of trials have investigated Migraleve Pink tablets against placebo, buclizine and ergotamine products in an attempt to establish clinical effectiveness.

A review of two trials involving Migraleve (one that compared Migraleve with buclizine and another that compared it with placebo) showed Migraleve was as effective as buclizine and superior to placebo in reducing severity of migraine attacks. Migraleve has also been compared to ergotamine-containing products; the standard drug at the time the trial was conducted. Results from a GP research group concluded that Migraleve was equally effective as Migril in treating migraine. However, results should be viewed with caution because the trial suffered from poor design, lacking randomisation, placebo or proper blinding. Trials by Carasso and Yehuda (1984) also reported beneficial effects of Migraleve.

The most recent trial (Adam 1987) was well designed, being double-blind, randomised and placebo controlled. The author concluded that, compared with placebo, Migraleve did reduce the severity of attacks significantly but not their total duration.

Midrid

Midrid capsules contain isometheptene mucate 65 mg and paracetamol 325 mg. A number of trials have investigated the effect of Midrid on reducing the severity of migraine attacks. Trials date back to 1948, although it was not until the 1970s that soundly designed trials were performed. Two studies – conducted in 1975 and 1976 – using similar methodology investigated isometheptene versus placebo and paracetamol. Both were double blind, placebo controlled and had identical inclusion criteria. The 1975 trial concluded that isometheptene was superior in relieving headache severity compared with placebo, although the dose of isometheptene used was double that found in Midrid. The 1976 trial also concluded that isometheptene was significantly superior to placebo and appeared to be better than paracetamol alone, but this did not reach statistical significance. A further trial in 1978 compared Midrid with placebo and ergotamine. Fifty patients who suffered four or more migraine attacks per month were recruited to the study.

Diary cards were completed for six attacks in which patients rated relief from headache on a four-point rating scale. The author concluded that Midrid was as effective as ergotamine and that both were more beneficial than placebo, although it is unclear whether this was statistically significant.

Summary

From the limited trial data reviewed it appears that Midrid and Migraleve are more effective than placebo. Therefore either could be recommended but it is not known which product is most efficacious. Further trials comparing the efficacy of Migraleve versus Midrid would be useful to establish if one was superior to another.

Prochlorperazine (Buccastem M)

The deregulation of prochlorperazine in 2001 represents a significant step forward in treatment options for pharmacists to manage migraine. It has been found to be a potent antiemetic in a number of conditions including migraine. It is administered via the buccal mucosa and therefore patients will need to be counselled on correct administration.

Practical prescribing and product selection

Prescribing information relating to specific products used to treat migraine in the section 'Evidence base for over-the-counter medication' is discussed and summarised in Table 4.3 and useful tips relating to patients presenting with migraine are given in Hints and Tips Box 4.1.

Table 4.3
Practical Prescribing: Summary of medicines for migraine

Medicine	Use in children	Likely side-effects	Drug interactions of note	Patients in whom care should be exercised	Pregnancy
Migraleve	> 10 years	Dry mouth, sedation and constipation	Increased sedation with alcohol, opioid analgesics, anxiolytics, hypnotics and antidepressants	Glaucoma, prostate enlargement	Avoid in the third trimester
Midrid	> 12 years	Dizziness, rash	Avoid concomitant use with MAOIs and moclobemide due to risk of hypertensive crisis Avoid in patients taking beta-blockers and TCAs	Control of hypertension and diabetes might be affected, although a short treatment course is unlikely to be clinically important	Avoid
Buccastem M	> 18 years	Drowsiness	Increased sedation with alcohol, opioid analgesics, anxiolytics, hypnotics and antidepressants	Patients with Parkinson's disease, epilepsy and glaucoma	OK

HINTS AND TIPS BOX 4.1: MIGRAINE

Administration of buccal tablets	1. Place the tablet either between the upper lip and gum above the front teeth or between the cheek and upper gum
	2. Allow the tablet to dissolve slowly
	3. The tablet should take between 3 to 5 h to dissolve. If food or drinks are to be consumed in this time, place the tablet between the upper lip and gum, above the front teeth
	4. The tablets should not be chewed, crushed, or swallowed
	5. Touching the tablet with the tongue, or drinking fluids, can cause the tablet to dissolve faster

Migraleve

Migraleve is recommended for children aged 10 and over. The dose for adults and children over 14 is two Migraleve Pink tablets taken when the attack is imminent or begun. If further treatment is required, one or two Migraleve Yellow tablets can be taken every 4 h. The dose for children aged between 10 and 14 is half that of the adult dose. The maximum adult dose is eight tablets (two Migraleve Pink and six Migraleve Yellow) in 24 h and for children aged between 10 and 14 years of age the maximum dose is four tablets (one Migraleve Pink and three Migraleve Yellow) in 24 h.

The buclizine component of Migraleve Pink tablets can cause drowsiness and antimuscarinic effects, whereas the codeine content might result in patients experiencing constipation. Buclizine and codeine can interact with POM and OTC medication, especially those that cause sedation. The combined effect is to potentiate sedation and it is important to warn the patient of this. It appears that Migraleve is safe in pregnancy but, because of the codeine component, it is best avoided in the third trimester.

Midrid

Midrid is licensed for use only in adults. The dose is two capsules at the start of an attack followed by one capsule every hour until relief is obtained. A maximum of five capsules can be taken in a 12-h period. It is a sympathomimetic agent, therefore, like decongestants, it interacts with MAOIs, which might lead to fatal hypertensive crisis, and it can affect diabetes and hypertension control (see page 65). Side-effects reported with Midrid include transient rashes and other allergic reactions.

Buccastem M

Buccastem M is indicated for previously diagnosed migraine sufferers aged 18 years and over who experience nausea and vomiting. The dose is one or two tablets twice daily. Side-effects include, drowsiness, dizziness, dry mouth, insomnia, agitation and mild skin reactions. Because it crosses the blood–brain barrier it will potentiate the effect of other CNS depressants and interact with alcohol. Prochlorperazine has been used safely in pregnancy, although the manufacturer advises avoidance unless absolutely necessary during the first trimester of pregnancy.

Further reading

Adam E I 1987 A treatment for the acute migraine attack. Journal of International Medical Research 15:71–75

[Anonymous] 1973 Reports from the general practitioner clinical research group. Migraine treated with an antihistamine-analgesic combination. Practitioner 211:357–361

Carasso R L, Yehuda S 1984 The prevention and treatment of migraine with an analgesic combination. British Journal of Clinical Practice 38:25–27

Coutin I B, Glass S F 1996 Recognizing uncommon headache syndromes. American Family Physician 54:2247–2252

Dowson A J 2002 Headache (1) Migraine. Pharmaceutical Journal 268:141–143

Dowson A J 2002 Headache (2) Non-migraine headache. Pharmaceutical Journal 268:176–178

Headache Classification Committee of the International Headache Society 1998 Classification and diagnostic criteria for headache disorders, cranial neuralgia and facial pain. Cephalagia 8:S1–S96

Mathew N T 1997 Cluster headache. Seminars in Neurology 17:313–323

Merrington D M 1975 Comments on Migraleve trial reports. Current Therapeutic Research, Clinical and Experimental 18:222–225

Silberstein S D, Lipton R B, Goadsby P J et al 1999 Headache in primary care. Isis Medical Media, Oxford

Web sites

International Headache Society: www.i-h-s.org/
Migraine Action Association: www.migraine.org.uk
The Migraine Trust: www.migrainetrust.org.uk

Insomnia

Background

Typically, an adult needs approximately 8 h sleep a day, although some people require as little as 3 h. In addition, sleep requirements also tend to decrease with increasing age. It is likely that everyone at some point will experience insomnia because this can arise from many different causes (Fig. 4.3) but for most people the problem will be of nuisance value only, affecting next-day alertness.

Insomnia is arbitrarily defined as transient (a few days), short term (less than 2 to 3 weeks) or chronic (greater than 3 weeks) in nature. Pharmacists can manage most patients with transient or short-term insomnia, however cases of chronic insomnia are best referred to the GP, as there is usually an underlying cause.

Prevalence and epidemiology

Approximately 20 to 40% of adults report occasional sleep difficulty and half of them consider it to be significant. However, it is reported that only 5% of patients go on to develop chronic insomnia. Insomnia is twice as common in women than men and is more prevalent, in both sexes, with increasing age.

Aetiology

Insomnia reflects disturbances of arousal and/or sleep systems in the brain. Their relative activities determine the degree of alertness during wakefulness and depth and quality of sleep. Therefore insomnia may be caused by any factor, which increases activity in arousal systems or decreases activity in sleep systems.

Arriving at a differential diagnosis

The key to arriving at a differential diagnosis is to take a detailed sleep history. Asking symptom-specific questions will help the pharmacist to determine if referral is necessary (Table 4.4). Two key features of insomnia need to be determined: the type of insomnia and how it affects the person. Transient insomnia is often caused by a change of routine, for example time zone changes or a

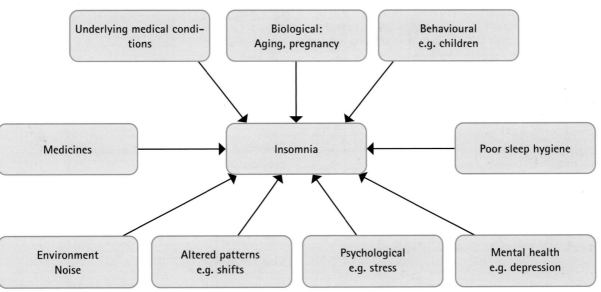

Fig. 4.3 Causes of insomnia

Table 4.4
Specific questions to ask the patient: Sleep

Question	Relevance
Pattern of sleep	• An emotional disturbance (predominantly anxiety) is commonly associated in patients who find it difficult to fall asleep; patients who fall asleep but wake early and cannot fall asleep again, or who are then restless, are sometimes suffering from depression
Daily routine	• Has there been any change to the work routine – changes to shift patterns, additional workload resulting in longer working hours and greater daytime fatigue
Underlying medical conditions	• Medical conditions likely to cause insomnia are GORD, pregnancy, pruritic skin conditions, asthma, Parkinson's disease, osteoarthritis and depression
Recent travel	• Time zone changes will affect the person's normal sleep pattern and it can take a number of days to re-establish normality

change to shift patterns, excessive noise, light or extremes of temperature. Short-term insomnia is usually related to acute stress such as sitting exams, bereavement, loss of job, forthcoming marriage or house move. Asking the patient to tell you what they are thinking about before they fall asleep and when they awake will give you a clue to the cause of the insomnia.

Clinical features of insomnia

Patients will complain of difficulty in falling asleep, staying asleep, poor quality of sleep or lack of refreshment by sleep.

Conditions to eliminate

Insomnia in children

Bedwetting is the most common sleep arousal disorder in children. If this is not the cause, then insomnia invariably stems from a problem such as fear of the dark, insecurity or nightmares. Children should not be given sleep aids but referred to their GP for further evaluation, as the underlying cause needs to be addressed.

Medicine-induced insomnia

Medication can cause all three types of insomnia (Table 4.5). The mild stimulant effects of caffeine, contained in chocolate, tea, coffee and cola drinks, are frequently implicated in causing transient insomnia. It is therefore advisable to instruct patients to avoid products containing caffeine after 6 or 7.00 p.m.

Underlying medical conditions

Many medical conditions can precipitate insomnia. It is therefore necessary to establish a medical history from the patient. A key role for the pharmacist in these

Table 4.5
Medication that can cause insomnia

Type of medication	Example
Stimulants	Caffeine, theophylline, sympathomimetics (e.g. pseudoephedrine), MAOIs
Antiepileptics	Carbamazepine, phenytoin
Alcohol	Low to moderate amounts can promote sleep but when taken in excess or over long periods of time it can disturb sleep
Propranolol	Can cause nightmares
Fluoxetine	
Griseofulvin	

situations is to ensure that the condition is being treated optimally and check that the medication regime is appropriate. If improvements to prescribing could be made then the prescriber should be contacted to discuss possible changes to the patient's medication.

Depression

It is well known that between one-third and two-thirds of patients suffering from chronic insomnia will have a recognisable psychiatric illness; most commonly depression. The patient will complain of having difficulty in staying asleep and suffer from early morning waking. The pharmacist should look for other symptoms of depression, such as fatigue, loss of interest and appetite, feelings of guilt, low self-esteem, difficulty in concentrating and constipation.

Figure 4.4 will help in the differential diagnosis of the different types of insomnia.

TRIGGER POINTS indicative of referral: Insomnia

- Children under 12
- Duration of more than 3 weeks
- Insomnia for which no cause can be ascertained
- Previously undiagnosed medical conditions
- Symptoms suggestive of anxiety or depression

Evidence base for over-the-counter medication

Many cases of transient and short-term insomnia should be managed initially by non-pharmacological measures. If these fail to rectify the problem then short-term use of sedating antihistamines can be tried.

Sleep hygiene

The term 'sleep hygiene' is used to refer to patient behaviour and practice that affects sleep. Patients should be encouraged to maintain a routine, with a regular bedtime and wakening time. Food snacks, alcoholic and caffeine-containing drinks should be avoided. Patients should also be told to avoid sleeping in very warm rooms and not to exercise near bedtime. Elderly patients should also try to stop taking daytime naps because these further reduce their sleep need at night.

Medication

The sedating antihistamines diphenhydramine and promethazine are the mainstay of pharmacological treatment.

Diphenhydramine

A substantial body of evidence exists to support the clinical effectiveness of diphenhydramine (DPH) as a

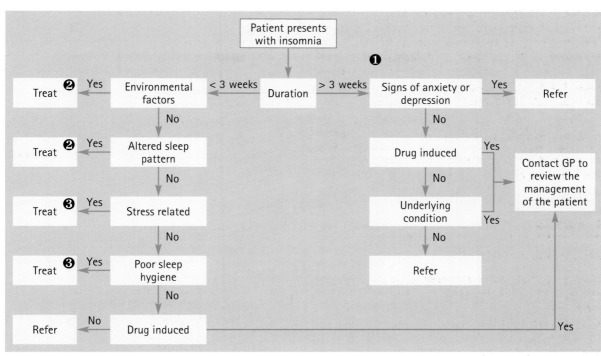

Fig. 4.4 Primer for differential diagnosis of insomnia

❶ No cases of insomnia lasting longer than 3 weeks should be treated with OTC medication. If a previously undiagnosed medical condition is suspected, most often anxiety or depression or if insomnia has been possibly caused by the patients pre-existing condition/medicines, then the GP should be consulted and treatment options discussed/suggested.

❷ Patients should not take antihistamines for more than 7 to 10 continuous days as tolerance to their effect can develop.

❸ In the first instance, strategies to manage the patient's insomnia should be suggested rather than issuing medication.

sleep aid. At doses of 50 mg DPH has been shown to be consistently superior to placebo in inducing sleep, and as effective as 60 mg of sodium pentobarbital. Doses higher than 50 mg DPH do not produce statistically superior clinical effect and night-time doses should therefore not exceed this amount.

Promethazine

Promethazine is widely accepted to cause sedation when used for its licensed indications, however, only one trial that investigated its use as a hypnotic could be found. This study by Adam & Oswald (1986) recruited 12 healthy volunteers who took placebo or promethazine 20 or 40 mg in a blinded fashion. The authors concluded that both doses of promethazine increased the length of sleep and that sleep disturbances were reduced compared with placebo. However, it was not clear if this reached statistical significance.

Summary

Of the two sedating antihistamines, DPH has by far the stronger evidence base to substantiate its use as a hypnotic. It therefore seems prudent to use this as the treatment of choice.

Herbal remedies

Herbal remedies containing hops, German chamomile, skullcap, wild lettuce, passiflora and valerian are available and widely used. In one study of elderly patients, over 11% of respondents had used herbal remedies within the last year. However, there is little evidence to support their use. The majority of information available in the literature relates to hypothesised action of chemical constituents or studies in animals. Valerian appears to be the only product for which more than one trial has been conducted on humans; a number of whom reported a sedative effect.

Practical prescribing and product selection

Prescribing information relating to medicines for insomnia in the section 'Evidence base for OTC medication' is discussed and summarised in Table 4.6 and useful tips relating to patients presenting with insomnia are given in Hints and Tips Box 4.2.

Both the antihistamines that are used for insomnia are first-generation antihistamines and interact with other sedating medication, resulting in potentiation of sedation. Additionally, they possess antimuscarinic side-

Table 4.6
Practical Prescribing: Summary of medicines for insomnia

Medicine	Use in children	Likely side-effects	Drug interactions of note	Patients in whom care should be exercised	Pregnancy
Diphenhydramine Promethazine	> 16 years	Dry mouth, sedation, and grogginess next day	Increased sedation with alcohol, opioid analgesics, anxiolytics, hypnotics and antidepressants	Glaucoma, prostate enlargement	BNF states OK, although some manufacturers advise avoidance.

HINTS AND TIPS BOX 4.2: INSOMNIA

Antihistamines	Tolerance can develop with continuous use
Patients who self treat for depression	St John's wort (hypericum) is used by many patients to treat depression. There is a growing body of evidence that it is more effective than placebo for mild depression and is comparable in effect to TCAs. However, pharmacists should not recommend it routinely. If depression is suspected then the patient should be referred for further assessment. St John's Wort also interacts with other medicines, including warfarin, SSRIs, antiepileptics, digoxin, ciclosporin, theophylline and contraceptives.

---

effects, which commonly lead to dry mouth and possibly to constipation. It is these antimuscarinic properties that mean patients with glaucoma and prostate enlargement should ideally avoid their use as it could lead to increased intraocular pressure and precipitation of urinary retention.

Diphenhydramine (e.g. Nytol, Nightcalm)

Diphenhydramine is made by a number of manufacturers to aid the relief of temporary sleep disturbance. It is licensed only for adults and children over 16 years of age, and should be taken 20 min before going to bed.

Promethazine

Proprietary brands of promethazine on sale to the public include, Sominex (20 mg) and Phenergan Nightime (25 mg). Adults and children over 16 years of age should take one tablet an hour before bedtime.

Further reading
Adam K, Oswald I 1986 The hypnotic effects of an antihistamine: promethazine. British Journal of Clinical Pharmacology 22:715–717
Anderson E G 1992 Night people: avoiding the quick fix for insomnia. Geriatrics 47:65–66
Gillin J C, Byerley W F 1990 The diagnosis and management of insomnia. New England Journal of Medicine 322:239–248
Mellinger G D, Balter M B, Uhlenhuth E H 1985 Insomnia and its treatment. Prevalence and correlates. Archives of General Psychiatry 42:225–232

Newall C A, Anderson L A, Phillipson J D 1996 Herbal medicines: a guide for health-care professionals. Pharmaceutical Press, London
Rickels K, Morris R J, Newman H et al 1983 Diphenhydramine in insomniac family practice patients: a double-blind study. Journal of Clinical Pharmacology 23:234–242
Sproule B A, Busto U E, Buckle C et al 1999 The use of non-prescription sleep products in the elderly. International Journal of Geriatric Psychiatry 10:851–857

Web sites
National Sleep Foundation: www.sleepfoundation.org/

Nausea and vomiting

Background

Nausea and vomiting are common symptoms of many disorders, especially gastrointestinal conditions. However, infection, acute alcohol ingestion, anxiety, severe pain, labyrinth and cardiovascular causes can also produce nausea and vomiting.

Recent deregulation of a number of POMs means that community pharmacists can now more effectively manage nausea and vomiting. Until deregulation of domperidone and prochlorperazine, treatment choices were limited to anticholinergics and first-generation antihistamines, used as prophylactic agents for the prevention of motion sickness (see page 226).

Prevalence and epidemiology

Nausea and vomiting are symptoms of other conditions and therefore their prevalence and epidemiology within the population are determined by that condition. Needless to say, nausea and vomiting is common and most people at some point in time will experience these symptoms.

Aetiology

Nausea occurs because activity in the vomiting centre (located in the medulla oblongata) increases. Information received from the receptor cells in the walls of the gastrointestinal tract and parts of the nervous system reach a 'threshold value' that induces the vomiting reflex. Additionally, further input is received at the vomiting centre from an area known as the chemoreceptor trigger zone. This is highly sensitive to certain circulating chemicals, for example substances released by damaged tissues as a result of bacterial infection.

Arriving at a differential diagnosis

Nausea and/or vomiting rarely occur in isolation. Other symptoms are usually present and should therefore allow a differential diagnosis to be made. Most cases will have a gastrointestinal origin, with gastroenteritis being the most common acute cause in all age groups. However, questioning the patient about associated symptoms should be made as other causes of nausea and vomiting need to be eliminated. (Table 4.7)

Clinical features of nausea and vomiting

Nausea is an unpleasant sensation, which might be a precursor to the forceful expulsion of gastric contents (vomiting). Currently, nausea associated with gastritis and migraine can be treated with OTC medicines.

Gastritis

Gastritis is often alcohol or medicine induced and can present as acute or chronic nausea and vomiting. Epigastric pain is usually present. For further information on gastritis, see page 107.

Nausea and vomiting associated with headaches

Vomiting, and especially nausea, are common symptoms in patients who suffer from migraines. However, other causes of headache, such as raised intracranial pressure, can also cause vomiting and nausea. For further information on nausea and vomiting associated with headaches, see page 63.

Conditions to eliminate

Nausea and vomiting in neonates (up to 1 month old)

Vomiting in neonates should always be referred because it suggests some form of congenital disorder, for example Hirschsprung's disease.

Nausea and vomiting in infants (1 month to 1 year old)

In the first year of life the most common causes of nausea and vomiting are feeding problems, gastrointestinal and urinary tract infection. Vomiting in infants needs to be differentiated from regurgitation. Regurgitation is an effortless back flow of small amounts of liquid and food between meals or at feed times; vomiting is the forceful expulsion of gastric contents. The infant will usually have a fever and be generally unwell if vomiting is associated with infection. If projectile vomiting occurs in an infant under 3 months of age then pyloric stenosis should be considered.

Table 4.7
Specific questions to ask the patient: Nausea and vomiting

Question	Relevance
Presence of abdominal pain	● Certain abdominal conditions, e.g. appendicitis, cholecystitis and cholelithiasis, can also cause nausea and vomiting. However, for all three conditions abdominal pain would be the presenting symptom and not nausea and vomiting. The severity of the pain alone would trigger referral
Timing of nausea and vomiting	● Early morning vomiting is often associated with pregnancy. If vomiting occurs immediately after food this suggests gastritis and if vomiting begins 1 or more hours after eating food then peptic ulcers are possible
Signs of infection	● Acute cases of gastroenteritis will normally have other associated symptoms, e.g diarrhoea, fever and abdominal discomfort. If infection is due to food contamination then other people are often affected at the same time

Nausea and vomiting in children (1 year to 12 years old)

Children under 12 who experience nausea and vomiting will usually have gastroenteritis, fever or otitis media. In most instances the conditions are self-limiting and medication designed to reduce pain and temperature (analgesia), and replace fluid (oral rehydration therapy; ORT) will help resolve symptoms.

Pregnancy

Pregnancy should always be considered in women of childbearing age if nausea and vomiting occur in the absence of other symptoms. Sickness tends to be worse in the first trimester and in the early morning.

Excess alcohol consumption

The patient should always be asked about recent alcohol intake, as excess quantities are associated with nausea and early morning vomiting.

Medicine-induced nausea and vomiting

Many medications can cause nausea and vomiting. Frequently implicated medicines are cytotoxics, opiates, iron, antibiotics, NSAIDs, potassium supplements, selective serotonin reuptake inhibitors (SSRIs), nicotine gum (ingestion of nicotine rather than buccal absorption), theophylline and digoxin toxicity. If medication is suspected then the pharmacist should contact the prescriber to discuss alternative treatment options.

Middle ear diseases

Any middle ear disturbance or imbalance can produce nausea and vomiting. Tinnitus, dizziness and vertigo are suggestive of Menière's disease.

 TRIGGER POINTS indicative of referral: Nausea and vomiting

- Children who fail to respond to OTC treatment
- Severe abdominal pain
- Suspected pregnancy
- Unexplained nausea and vomiting in any age group
- Vomiting in children under 1 year old

Evidence base for over-the-counter medication

Currently, only two medicines available OTC have licensed indications for the treatment of nausea and vomiting.

Domperidone

Domperidone is licensed for pharmacy sale for the relief of postprandial symptoms that include nausea. A number of small studies have suggested that domperidone is more effective than placebo. However, the studies were of variable design, with differing inclusion criteria and methodology, making judgement on the effectiveness of domperidone difficult to determine. However, it remains the only medication available to pharmacists to treat nausea associated with over eating and, as such, is a useful treatment option.

Prochlorperazine

Prochlorperazine is licensed for the relief of nausea and vomiting associated with migraine. This represents a significant step forward in treatment options for pharmacists to manage migraine. It has potent antiemetic properties in a number of conditions including migraine.

Practical prescribing and product selection

Prescribing information relating to medicines for nausea and vomiting in the section 'Evidence base for over-the counter medication' is discussed and summarised in Table 4.8.

Domperidone (Motilium 10)

Motilium 10 is licensed for use in adults and children aged over 16 years. The dose is one tablet four times a day, preferably after meals. Its safety in pregnant women has not been established, although there appear to be no reports of domperidone being teratogenic. Side-effects are rare but galactorrhoea and, less frequently gynaecomastia, breast enlargement or soreness, reduced libido, dystonia and rash have been reported.

Domperidone does not appear to have any important clinical interactions, however, as it is a dopamine antagonist it could theoretically alter the peripheral actions of dopamine agonists such as bromocriptine.

Prochlorperazine (Buccatem M)

For dosing and counselling on Buccatem M, see page 65.

Further reading

Bekhti A, Rutgeerts L 1979 Domperidone in the treatment of functional dyspepsia in patients with delayed gastric emptying. Postgraduate Medicine 55:S30–S32

Dollery C 1999 Therapeutic drugs, 2nd edn. Churchill Livingstone, Edinburgh

Haarmann K, Lebkuchner F, Widmann A et al 1979 A double-blind study of domperidone in the symptomatic treatment of chronic post prandial upper gastrointestinal distress. Postgraduate Medicine 55:S24–S27

Sarin S K, Sharma P, Chawla Y K et al 1986 Clinical trial on the effect of domperidone on non-ulcer dyspepsia. Indian Journal of Medical Research 83:623–628

Table 4.8
Practical Prescribing

Medicine	Use in children	Likely side-effects	Drug interactions of note	Patients in whom care should be exercised	Pregnancy
Domperidone	>16 years	None	None	None	Manufacturer states to avoid
Prochlorperazine	>18 years	Drowsiness	Increased sedation with alcohol, opioid analgesics, anxiolytics, hypnotics and antidepressants	Patients with Parkinson's disease, epilepsy and glaucoma	OK

Self-assessment questions

The following questions are intended to supplement the text. Two levels of question are provided; multiple choice questions and case studies. The multiple-choice questions are designed to test factual recall and the case studies allow knowledge to be applied to a practice setting.

Multiple choice questions

4.1. The most common cause of nausea and vomiting is?

  a. Migraine
  b. Gastroenteritis
  c. Gastritis
  d. Medicine induced
  e. Excess alcohol consumption

4.2. Which product does not contain an ingredient that can be useful for nausea?

  a. Mintec
  b. Midrid
  c. Motilium 10
  d. Migraleve
  e. Buccastem M

4.3. Cluster headache could be best described as?

  a. Piercing pain behind both eyes that lasts for a matter of only minutes
  b. Piercing pain behind one eye that lasts for a matter of only minutes
  c. Unilateral orbital piercing pain with associated unilateral nasal congestion
  d. Bilateral orbital piercing pain with associated nasal congestion
  e. Bilateral orbital piercing pain only

4.4. Nausea and vomiting is associated with?

  a. Tension headache
  b. Trigeminal neuralgia
  c. Cluster headache
  d. Subarachnoid haemorrhage
  e. Sinusitis

4.5. What herbal remedy is used to help treat insomnia?

  a. Golden rod
  b. Tolu balsam
  c. Burdock
  d. Mugwort
  e. Passion flower

4.6. Which trigger sign or symptom warrants referral?

  a. Headache lasting 7 to 10 days
  b. Headache described as 'vice like'
  c. Headache associated with the workplace environment
  d. Headache in a child under 12 with no sign of infection
  e. Headache associated with fever

4.7. The amount of sleep needed with increasing age?

  a. Increases
  b. Decreases
  c. Stays the same

4.8. Which of these statements is true when giving advice on sleep hygiene?

  a. Drinking coffee and tea is OK before bedtime
  b. Try to vary the time when you go to bed
  c. Sleep in a warm room
  d. Try not to nap through the day
  e. Take light exercise before going to bed

Questions 4.9 to 4.11 concern the following anatomical locations of the brain:

A. Orbital
B. Temporal
C. Occipital
D. Generalised
E. Unilateral and frontal

Select, from A to E, which of the above locations:

4.9. Is associated with cluster headache

4.10. Is associated with subarachnoid haemorrhage

4.11. Is associated with tension headache

Questions 4.12 to 4.14 concern the following medicines:

A. Motilium 10
B. Midrid
C. Maxolon
D. Marvelon
E. Migraleve

Select, from A to E, which of the above medicines:

4.12. Should be avoided by patients taking paracetamol

4.13. Is only licensed for nausea associated with migraine

4.14. Has been linked to causing migraine

Questions 4.15 to 4.17: for each of the questions below, *one* or *more* of the responses is (are) correct. Decide which of the responses is (are) correct. Then choose:

A. If a, b and c are correct
B. If a and b only are correct
C. If b and c only are correct
D. If a only is correct
E. If c only is correct

Directions summarised

A	B	C	D	E
a, b and c	a and b only	b and c only	a only	c only

4.15. Tension headache can be described as:

   a. Dull ache, not normally throbbing
   b. Worsening as the day progresses
   c. Unilateral

4.16. Symptoms of the aura associated with migraine include:

   a. Scotomas
   b. Flashing lights
   c. Pins and needles

4.17. Which statements relating to headache are true:

   a. Common migraine is more common in women than men
   b. Cluster headache is more common in women than men
   c. Temporal arteritis affects mainly middle-aged men.

Questions 4.18 to 4.20: these questions consist of a statement in the left-hand column followed by a statement in the right-hand column. You need to:

● decide whether the first statement is true or false
● decide whether the second statement is true or false

Then choose:

A. If both statements are true and the second statement is a correct explanation of the first statement
B. If both statements are true but the second statement is not a correct explanation of the first statement
C. If the first statement is true but the second statement is false
D. If the first statement is false but the second statement is true
E. If both statements are false

Directions summarised

	First statement	Second statement	
A	True	True	Second explanation is a correct explanation of the first
B	True	True	Second statement is *not* a correct explanation of the first
C	True	False	
D	False	True	
E	False	False	

	First statement	**Second statement**
4.18.	Common migraine is more common in women than men	Trigger factors can precipitate attacks
4.19.	Insomnia can be caused by depression	Early morning wakening contributes to sleeplessness
4.20.	Headache in VDU operators is common	Throbbing headache is caused by the flickering of VDU screens

Case study

CASE STUDY 4.1

Mrs PC, a 36-year-old woman, asks you for something to treat her headache. On questioning you find out the following:

- She has had the headache for about 5 days.
- The pain is located mainly behind left eye and front of head but is also at back of head.
- Mrs PC is experiencing aching, but no sickness or visual disturbances.
- She has tried paracetamol, which helps for a while but the pain comes back after a few hours.
- She has not had this type of headache before.
- Work at the moment is busy because of a conference she is organising.
- She takes nothing from her GP except the mini-pill.
- There is no recent history of head trauma.
- The pain gets worse as day goes on.

a. What is the likely differential diagnosis, and why?

Tension headache, probably as a result of additional stress at work while organising the conference.

b. From the above responses, which symptoms allowed you to rule out other conditions?

The following symptoms allowed you to rule out other causes of headache:

- *Age (36): most likely causes are tension and migraine headaches based solely on age.*
- *Sex (female): women experience more migraines than men, and fewer cluster headaches. Therefore migraine is a possibility.*
- *Duration (5 days): most migraines do not last beyond 72 h; cluster headache duration even less. More sinister causes of headache tend to last longer than 5 days. Therefore tension headache is likely.*
- *Location (behind eye and back of head): the pain seems fairly generalised, which is indicative of tension headache.*

- *Nature of pain (ache): again, tension headaches are often described as non-throbbing. The pain does not appear to be severe, which means sinister pathology less likely.*
- *Associated symptoms (none): no nausea or vomiting. This tends to exclude migraine and conditions causing raised intracranial pressure.*
- *Medication (paracetamol): this appears to work but doesn't really help in establishing the cause of the headache.*
- *New headache (yes): the patient has not suffered from this type of headache before, a fact that might be suggestive of a more serious cause of headache. Further questioning is needed to make a judgement on whether referral would be appropriate.*
- *Lifestyle (work is busy): stress is a contributing factor to tension headache. It appears the patient is suffering from more stress than normal and this could be a cause of the headache.*
- *Medication from GP (mini pill): unlikely to cause the headache but further questions should be asked of the patient about how long they have been taking the medication. Most ADRs normally coincide with new medication or an alteration to the dosage regimen.*
- *Recent trauma (none): this tends to exclude headache caused by space-occupying lesions. It is worth remembering that symptoms manifest themselves only once pressure is exerted on adjacent structures by a haematoma, tumour or abscess. It might therefore take several weeks for the patient to notice symptoms. Therefore always ask about trauma over the last 6 to 12 weeks.*
- *Periodicity (worse as the day goes on): this is suggestive of tension headache. It therefore appears that the majority of questions point to tension headache as the most likely cause of headache.*

CASE STUDY 4.2

Mr FD, a 55-year-old man, asks you for a strong painkiller for his headache. He has had the headache for a few days but it doesn't seem to be going away.

a. Based solely on epidemiological data what are the most likely causes of his headache?

Tension headache followed by migraine and cluster headache. His age also means that other more sinister causes of headache such as temporal arteritis, cancer and haematoma are more likely.

After talking to Mr FD, you find out the following:

● The headache is located in the frontal area and is bilateral.
● He describes the pain as throbbing.
● He has never had a headache like this before.
● He has not suffered from migraines in the past.
● There are no associated symptoms of upper respiratory tract infection.
● He is retired and has a non-stressful lifestyle.
● He has tried paracetamol but without much success.
● He takes atenolol for hypertension.

b. What do you think is causing his headaches?

It appears that tension headache and migraine can be ruled out. Cluster headache is a possibility but the type of pain and location is not right. This suggests that the headache might be a secondary type of headache requiring referral. Sinusitis is a secondary cause of headache but the patient shows no recent symptoms of upper respiratory tract infection.

Because you believe the headache could be caused by a sinister pathology, you recommend that Mr FD sees his GP straight away. The next day he presents with a prescription for prednisolone.

c. What differential diagnosis did the GP arrive at?

Temporal arteritis.

d. What extra information could you have got from the patient to help you arrive at the same diagnosis?

Enquire about tenderness in the temple region or if the scalp was tender to touch.

Answers to multiple choice questions
4.1 = b   4.2 = a   4.3 = c   4.4 = d   4.5 = e   4.6 = d   4.7 = b   4.8 = d   4.9 = a   4.10 = c,
4.11 = d 4.12 = e   4.13 = a   4.14 = d   4.15 = b   4.16 = a   4.17 = d   4.18 = b   4.19 = a   4.20 = c.

Women's health

Background

Women have unique healthcare needs, ranging from pregnancy to menstrual disorders. Most of these conditions are outside the remit of the community pharmacist and specialist care is needed. However, a small number of conditions can be adequately treated OTC, providing an accurate diagnosis is made. This chapter explores such conditions and attempts to outline when referral should be made.

History taking

As with all conditions that present in the community pharmacy, it is essential to take an accurate history from the patient. However, for conditions affecting women's health this is especially important. The pharmacist will rely entirely on information gained by thorough questioning. There are no opportunities for any form of physical examination or access to diagnostic tests, unlike the GP. Additionally, the patient might feel uncomfortable or embarrassed about discussing symptoms especially in a busy pharmacy. Male pharmacists could find that this level of embarrassment is heightened.

Cystitis

Background

Cystitis literally means inflammation of the bladder. The majority of patients who present in the community pharmacy will have accurately self-diagnosed cystitis but

confirmation of the patient diagnosis is essential to eliminate other potential causes. Before moving on to discuss cystitis in women further it is prudent to mention that men can also suffer from cystitis. However, in men cystitis is uncommon because of the longer urethra, which provides a greater barrier to bacteria entering the bladder; fluid from the **prostate gland** also confers some antibacterial property. This is especially so in men under the age of 50. After 50 years of age urinary tract infections in men become more common due to prostate enlargement.

Prevalence and epidemiology

Patients aged between 15 and 34 account for the majority of cases seen within a primary care setting and it is estimated that 20 to 50% of all women will experience at least one episode of cystitis in their lifetime; half of whom will have further attacks. A number of these patients who suffer recurrent cystitis will have identifiable risk factors that predispose them to reoccurrence such as pregnancy, prior infections of the upper urinary tract (kidneys and ureters), undiagnosed diabetes, the use of contraceptive devices and increased or more vigorous sexual activity.

Aetiology

Infection is caused, in the majority of cases, by the patient's own bowel flora that ascend the urethra from the **perineal** and **perianal** areas. Bacteria are thus transferred to the bladder where they proliferate. The most common bacterial organisms implicated in cystitis are *Escherichia coli, Staphylococcus* and *Enterococci*.

However, several studies have shown that up to 50% of women do not have positive urine cultures according to traditional criteria (> 10^5 bacteria per mL of urine), although they do have 'low count **bacteriuria**' and therefore do have a urinary tract infection.

Arriving at a differential diagnosis

The majority of patients presenting to the community pharmacist will have acute uncomplicated cystitis. The pharmacist's aims are therefore to confirm a patient self-diagnosis, rule out **pyelonephritis** and identify patients who are at risk of complications as a result of cystitis. Asking symptom-specific questions will help the pharmacist determine whether referral is needed (Table 5.1).

Clinical features of acute uncomplicated cystitis

Cystitis is characterised by **dysuria**, urinary frequency, urgency, **nocturia** and **haematuria**. However, only a small minority of patients will present with all symptoms. In addition, the patient might report passing only small amounts of urine, with pain worsening at the end of voiding urine. Symptoms usually start suddenly. Low back pain and **suprapubic** discomfort can also be present but are not common. Haematuria, although common, should be viewed with caution because it might indicate stones or a tumour. Such cases are best referred.

Conditions to eliminate

Pyelonephritis

Involvement of the ureter or kidney by the invading pathogen is the most frequent complication and results from the bacteria ascending from the bladder to these higher anatomical structures. The patient will show signs of systemic infection such as fever, chills, flank pain and possibly nausea and vomiting. Referral is needed to confirm the diagnosis, exclude pelvic inflammatory disease (PID) and issue appropriate treatment.

Vaginitis

Vaginitis exhibits similar symptoms to cystitis, in that dysuria, nocturia, and frequency are common. However, all patients should be questioned about an associated vaginal discharge. The presence of vaginal discharge is highly suggestive of vaginitis and referral is needed.

Chemical vaginitis
This is a common cause of dysuria in younger women. The patient should be asked about the use of vaginal sprays and toiletries (e.g. bubble baths).

Sexually transmitted diseases

Sexually transmitted diseases (STDs) can be caused by a number of pathogens, for example *Chlamydia trachomatis* and *Neisseria gonorrhoea*. Symptoms are similar to acute uncomplicated cystitis but they tend to be more gradual in onset and last for a longer period of time. In addition pyuria (pus in the urine) is usually present.

Medicine-induced cystitis

Non-steroidal anti-inflammatory agents (especially tiaprofenic acid) and cyclophosphamide have been shown to cause cystitis.

Oestrogen deficiency

Postmenopausal **women** experience thinning of the endometrial lining as a result of a reduction in the levels of circulating oestrogen in the blood. This increases the

Table 5.1 Specific questions to ask the patient: Cystitis	
Question	**Relevance**
Duration	● Symptoms that have lasted longer than 5 to 7 days should be referred because of the risk that the person might have developed pyelonephritis
Age of the patient	● Cystitis is unusual in children and should be viewed with caution. It might be a sign of a structural urinary tract abnormality. Referral is needed ● Elderly female patients have a higher rate of complications associated with cystitis and are therefore best referred
Presence of fever	● Referral is needed if the person presents with fever associated with dysuria, frequency and urgency as fever is a sensitive indicator of an upper urinary tract infection
Vaginal discharge	● If a patient reports vaginal discharge then the likely diagnosis is not cystitis but a vaginal infection
Location of pain	● Pain experienced in the loin area suggests an upper urinary tract infection

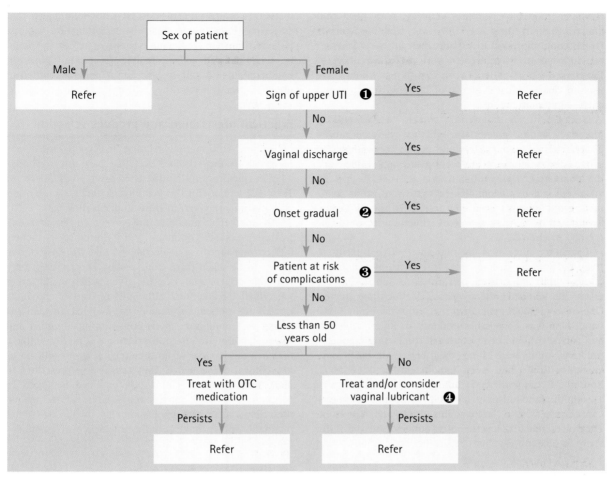

Fig. 5.1 Primer for differential diagnosis of cystitis

❶ **Involvement of the higher urinary tract structures**
Symptoms such as fever, flank pain, nausea and vomiting suggest conditions such as pyelonephritis.

❷ **Gradual onset**
STDs should be considered in patients whose symptoms are not sudden.

❸ **At-risk patients**
Patients at risk of developing upper UTI include diabetics, pregnant women, the immunocompromised, the elderly and those patients in whom symptoms have been present for more than 5 to 7 days.

❹ **Patients over 50 years old**
Oestrogen deficiency might account for the patient's symptoms resulting in local atrophy of the vagina.

likelihood of irritation or trauma leading to cystitis symptoms. If the symptoms are caused by intercourse, symptomatic relief can be gained with a lubricating product. Referral for possible hormone replacement therapy or a topical oestrogen would be appropriate if the symptoms recur.

Figure 5.1 will aid the differentiation of cystitis from other conditions.

Evidence base for over-the-counter medication

OTC treatment is limited to products that contain alkalinising agents, namely sodium citrate, sodium bicarbonate and potassium citrate. They are used to return the urine pH to normal, thus relieving symptoms of dysuria.

> **❗ TRIGGER POINTS** indicative of referral: Cystitis
>
> - Children under 12
> - Diabetics
> - Duration longer than 7 days
> - Elderly women
> - Immunocompromised patients
> - Men
> - Patients with associated fever, nausea, vomiting and flank pain
> - Pregnancy
> - Vaginal discharge

However, they have dubious efficacy, with little trial data to support their use. Only one trial by Spooner (1984) could be found to support their efficacy. Spooner concluded that, when treated with a 2-day course of Cymalon, 80% of patients with cystitis for whom there was no clear clinical evidence of bacterial infection did gain symptomatic relief.

Because it is impossible within a community pharmacy setting to determine whether cystitis is caused by a bacterial pathogen, it would not be unreasonable to offer a 2-day course of an alkalinising agent, provided the pharmacist was confident that the patient had an acute episode of uncomplicated cystitis. If, after treatment, symptoms persisted then referral to the GP should be advised as a 3-day course of trimethoprim would be therapy of choice.

Cranberry juice is a popular alternative remedy to treat and prevent urinary tract infections, although few clinical trials have been performed to substantiate or refute its clinical effectiveness. A Cochrane review (Jepson et al 2000) concluded that, from the limited trial data, there was no reliable evidence of its effectiveness and patients should be discouraged from using cranberry products until such time that better designed and evaluated trials had been conducted. In June 2001, Kontiokari et al published findings from a well-designed 12-month randomised trial that compared cranberry concentrate with a lactobacillus drink and a control. They concluded that cranberry concentrate did offer some protection against recurrence of urinary tract infections. Based on this latest trial it would appear that cranberry juice might offer some protection against UTIs but further trial data is needed before it should be recommended as a credible treatment. However, cranberry juice is safe to take and if patients wanted to use such products then they will not come to any harm.

Practical prescribing and product selection

Prescribing information relating to cystitis medicines reviewed in the section 'Evidence base for over-the-counter medication' is discussed and summarised in Table 5.2 and useful tips relating to patients presenting with cystitis are given in Hints and Tips Box 5.1.

All marketed products are presented as a 2-day treatment course. The majority are presented as sachets (Effercitrate are dissolvable tablets) and the dose is one sachet to be taken three times a day. They possess very few side-effects and can be given safely with other prescribed medication, although in theory products containing potassium should be avoided in patients taking ACE inhibitors, potassium-sparing diuretics and spironolactone. However, in practice it is highly unlikely that a 2-day course of an alkalinising agent will be of any clinical consequence. They can also be prescribed to most patient groups (Table 5.2) and can be given in pregnancy, although most manufacturers advise against prescribing in pregnancy, presumably on the basis that pregnant women have a higher incidence of complications resulting from cystitis.

Table 5.2
Practical Prescribing: Summary of Medicines for Cystitis

Medicine	Use in children	Likely side-effects	Drug interactions of note	Patients in whom care should be exercised	Pregnancy
Potassium citrate					
Effercitrate	> 1 year	Gastric irritation	None	Patients taking ACE inhibitors, potassium-sparing diuretics and spironolactone	OK, but best avoided
Cystopurin	> 6 years	None			
Sodium citrate					
Cymalon	Not recommended	None reported	None	Patients with heart disease, hypertension or renal impairment	OK, but best avoided
Cystemme					
Canesten Oasis					

HINTS AND TIPS BOX 5.1: CYSTITIS

Fluid intake	Patients should be advised to drink about 5 L fluid during every 24-h period. This will help promote bladder voiding, which is thought to help 'flush' bacteria out of the bladder
Product taste	The taste of potassium citrate mixture is unpleasant. Patients should be advised to dilute the mixture with water to make the taste more acceptable

Further reading

Forland M 1993 Urinary tract infection. How has its
management changed? Postgraduate Medicine 93:71–74,
77–78, 84–86

Jepson R G, Mihaljevic L, Craig J 2000 Cranberries for
preventing urinary tract infections. Cochrane Database
Systems Review 2:CD001321

Kontiokari T, Sundqvist K, Nuutinen M et al 2001 Randomised
trial of cranberry–lingonberry juice and Lactobacillus GG
drink for the prevention of urinary tract infections in
women. British Medical Journal 322:1571

Reisman A B, Stevens D L 2002 Telephone medicine. A guide
for the practicing physician. Philadelphia: ACP-ASIM

Spooner J B 1984 Alkalinisation in the management of cystitis.
Journal of International Medical Research 12:30–34

Web sites

General site on women's health: www.womenshealthlondon.
org.uk

Vaginal discharge

Background

Patients of any age can experience vaginal discharge.
The three most common causes of vaginal discharge are
bacterial vaginosis, vulvovaginal candidiasis (thrush) and
trichomoniasis. Because thrush is the only condition that
can be treated OTC, the text concentrates on differentiating this from other conditions.

Prevalence and epidemiology

It has been reported that 75% of females will experience
at least one episode of thrush during their childbearing
years. The condition is uncommon in prepubertal girls
unless they have been receiving antibiotics. In adolescents it is the second most common cause of vaginal
discharge after bacterial vaginosis.

Aetiology

The vagina naturally produces a watery discharge, the
amount and character of which varies depending on
many factors, such as pregnancy, hormonal status and
concurrent medication. At the time of ovulation the
discharge is greater in quantity and of higher viscosity.
Normal secretions have no odour. The epithelium of the
vagina contains glycogen, which is broken down by
enzymes and bacteria (most notably lactobacilli) into
acids. This maintains the low vaginal pH, creating an
environment inhospitable to pathogens. The glycogen
concentration is controlled by oestrogen production;
therefore any changes in oestrogen levels will result in
either increased or decreased glycogen concentrations. If
oestrogen levels decrease glycogen concentration also
decrease giving rise to an increased vaginal pH and
making the vagina more susceptible to opportunistic
infection such as *Candida albicans*.

Arriving at a differential diagnosis

Many patients will self-diagnose their condition. The
availability of efficacious OTC products and direct
consumer mass marketing by pharmaceutical companies
will mean that the pharmacists' role will often be to
confirm a self-diagnosis of thrush. This is very important
as misdiagnosis can have important consequences
because other conditions can result in greater health
concerns. For example, bacterial vaginosis has been
linked with PID and an increased risk of preterm birth
and *C. trachomatis* can cause infertility. Symptoms of
pruritus, burning and discharge are common to all three
common causes of vaginal discharge. Therefore no one
symptom can be relied upon with 100% certainty to
differentiate between thrush, bacterial vaginosis and
trichomoniasis. However, certain symptom clusters are
strongly suggestive of diagnosis. Asking symptom-
specific questions will help the pharmacist to determine
if referral is needed (Table 5.3).

Table 5.3
Specific questions to ask the patient: Vaginal discharge

Question	Relevance
Discharge	● Any discharge with a strong odour should be referred. Bacterial vaginosis is associated with a white discharge that has a strong fishy odour and trichomoniasis is malodorous with a green–yellow discharge. By contrast, discharge associated with thrush is often described as 'curd-like' or 'cottage-cheese-like' with little or no odour
Age	● Thrush can occur in any age group, unlike bacterial vaginosis and trichomoniasis, which are rare in premenarchal girls. In addition, trichomoniasis is also rare in women aged over 60
Pruritus	● Vaginal itching tends to be most prominent in thrush compared with bacterial vaginosis and trichomoniasis
Onset	● In thrush, the onset of symptoms is sudden, whereas the onset of bacterial vaginosis and trichomoniasis tends to be less sudden

Clinical features of thrush

The dominant feature of thrush is vaginal itching. This is often accompanied with soreness of the vulval lips and discharge in up to 20% of patients. The discharge has little or no odour and is curd-like. Symptoms are generally acute in onset.

Conditions to eliminate

Bacterial vaginosis

The exact cause of bacterial vaginosis is unknown although *Gardnerella vaginalis* is often implicated. Roughly 50% of patients will have a thin white discharge with a strong fishy odour, which may be worse during menses.

Trichomoniasis

Trichomoniasis, a protozoan infection, is primarily transmitted through sexual intercourse. Women usually present with profuse, frothy, greenish-yellow and malodorous discharge accompanied by vulvar itching. Other symptoms may include vaginal spotting, dysuria and urgency.

Cystitis

Dysuria can affect up to one in three women with vaginal infection. However, the patient will often be able to sense that it is an external discomfort, rather than an internal discomfort located in the urethra or bladder that occurs with urinary tract infections.

Recurrent thrush

After treatment a minority of patients will present with recurrent symptoms. This may be due to poor compliance, misdiagnosis, resistant strains of *Candida*, undiagnosed diabetes or the patient having a mixed infection (it has been reported that 14% of women have mixed infections of thrush, bacterial vaginosis or trichomonas). Such cases require referral.

Atrophic vaginitis

Symptoms consistent with thrush in elderly women, especially vaginal itching and burning, may be due to atrophic vaginitis. However, clinically significant atrophic vaginitis is uncommon in postmenopausal women, but should be referred to rule out this problem.

There are also several factors that predispose women to thrush, which require consideration prior to instigating treatment.

Medicine-induced thrush

Broad-spectrum antibiotics, corticosteroids and medication affecting the oestrogen status of the patient (oral contraceptives, HRT, tamoxifen and raloxifene) can predispose women to thrush.

Diabetes

Patients with poorly controlled diabetes (type 1 or 2) are more likely to suffer from thrush because hyperglycaemia can enhance production of protein surface receptors on *C. albicans* organisms. This hinders phagocytosis by neutrophils, making thrush more difficult to eliminate.

Pregnancy

Hormonal changes during pregnancy will alter the vaginal environment and have been reported to make eradication of *Candida* more difficult. Topical agents are safe and effective in pregnancy but OTC licensed indications do not allow sale to pregnant women and therefore these patients must be referred to the GP.

Chemical and mechanical irritants

Ingredients in feminine hygiene products, for example bubble baths, vaginal sprays and douches can precipitate attacks of thrush by altering vaginal pH. Condoms have also been found to irritate and alter the vaginal pH.

Figure 5.2 will help in the differentiation of vaginal thrush from other conditions in which vaginal discharge is a major presenting complaint.

 TRIGGER POINTS indicative of referral: Vaginal thrush

- Diabetics
- Discharge that has a strong smell
- OTC medication failure
- Pregnant women
- Recurrent attacks
- Women under 16 and over 60

Evidence base for over-the-counter medication

Topical imidazoles and one systemic triazole (fluconazole) are available OTC to treat vaginal thrush. They are potent and selective inhibitors of fungal enzymes necessary for the synthesis of ergosterol, which is needed to maintain the integrity of cell membranes.

All antifungals used to treat vaginal thrush have proven and comparable efficacy with clinical cure rates between 85 and 90%. Additionally, cure rates between single or multiple dose therapy and multiple day therapy show no differences. Treatment choice will therefore be driven by patient acceptability. However, oral antifungals (fluconazole) should not be used as first-line therapy, but reserved for severe cases, as indiscriminate use of

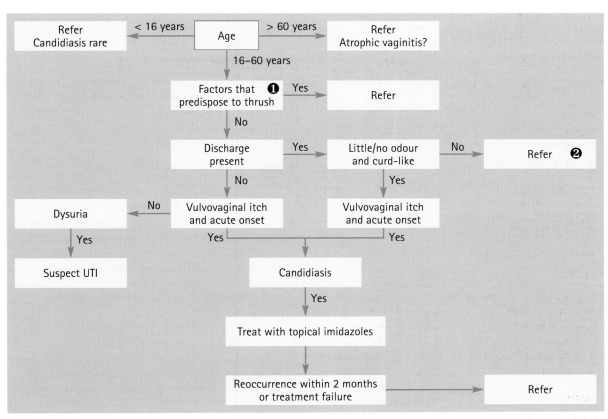

Fig. 5.2 Primer for differential diagnosis of vaginal thrush

❶ If the person is pregnant or has diabetes then referral is the most appropriate option. If the person is suffering from medicine-induced candidiasis the prescriber should be contacted to discuss suitable treatment options and, if appropriate, alternative therapy.

❷ Discharge that has a strong odour and is not white and curd-like should be referred, as trichomoniasis or bacterial vaginosis are more likely causes.

fluconazole can lead to fluconazole resistance. In addition, fluconazole also exhibits a greater side-effect profile than topical imidazoles and interacts with other medicines.

Practical prescribing and product selection

Prescribing information relating to medicines for thrush reviewed in the section 'Evidence base for over-the-counter medication' is discussed below and summarised in Table 5.4; useful tips relating to patients presenting with thrush are given in Hints and Tips Box 5.2.

Topical imidazoles (clotrimazole, econazole, miconazole)

A number of formulations are available for local application, including creams, vaginal tablets and pessaries. Pharmacists and the public are probably most familiar with the Canesten range of products. All internal preparations should be administered at night. This gives the medicine time to be absorbed and eliminates the possibility of accidental loss, which is more likely

to occur if the person is mobile. Slight irritation on application is infrequently reported (about 5% of users) and has been linked to the vehicle and not the active ingredient. There are no interactions of note due to being locally applied, although they may damage latex condoms and diaphragms. Consequently the effectiveness of such contraceptives may be reduced.

Fluconazole (Diflucan One, Canesten Oral)

Fluconazole is a single oral dose that can be taken at any time of the day. It is generally well tolerated but fluconazole can cause gastrointestinal disturbances, such as nausea, abdominal discomfort, diarrhoea and flatulence in up to 10% of patients. There are a number of established clinically important drug interactions with fluconazole. These include anticoagulants, ciclosporin, rifampicin, phenytoin and tacrolimus. However, these drug interactions relate to the use of multiple-dose fluconazole and the relevance to single-dose fluconazole has not yet been established. However, it would be prudent to avoid these combinations until further evidence is available with single-dose fluconazole.

Table 5.4
Practical prescribing: Summary of medicines for thrush

Medicine	Use in children	Likely side-effects	Drug interactions of note	Patients in whom care should be exercised	Pregnancy
Canesten	Not applicable	Irritation	None	None	OK but pregnant women should be referred
Fluconazole/ Diflucan One, Canesten Oral		GI disturbances	Anticoagulants, ciclosporin, rifampicin, phenytoin, tacrolimus		Avoid

HINTS AND TIPS BOX 5.2: THRUSH

Administration of pessaries	As the dosage is taken at night, patients should be advised to use the pessary when in bed
	1. Remove the pessary from the packaging and place firmly into applicator (the end of the applicator needs to be squeezed gently to allow the pessary to fit)
	2. Lying on your back, with knees drawn towards the chest, insert the applicator as deeply as is comfortable into the vagina
	3. Slowly press the plunger of the applicator until it stops. Remove and dispose of the applicator
	4. Remain in the supine position
Use of yoghurt	Some people recommended live yoghurt as a 'natural' treatment. This is based on sound rationale because lactobacilli contained in the yoghurt produce lactic acid, which inhibits the growth of Candida
General advice to help prevent infection	Avoid tight clothing, e.g. underwear, jeans, etc. Use simple non-perfumed soaps when washing
Symptom resolution	The symptoms of thrush (burning, soreness or itching of the vagina) should disappear within 3 days of treatment. If no improvement is seen after 7 days the patient should be referred to the GP
Vaginal douching	This should not be encouraged and avoided wherever possible

Further reading
Brown D, Binder G L, Gardner H L et al 1980 Comparison of econazole and clotrimazole in the treatment of vulvovaginal candidiasis. Obstetrics and Gynecology 56:121–123
Eschenbach D A, Hillier S, Critchlow C et al 1988 Diagnosis and clinical manifestations of bacterial vaginosis. American Journal of Obstetrics and Gynecology 158:819–828
Ferris D G, Dekle C, Litaker M S 1996 Women's use of over-the-counter antifungal medications for gynecologic symptoms. Journal of Family Practitioners 42:595–600
Fidel P L, Sobel J D 1996 Immunopathogenesis of recurrent vulvovaginal candidiasis. Clinical Microbiological Reviews 9:335–348
Floyd R, Hodgson C 1986 One-day treatment of vulvovaginal candidiasis with a 500-mg clotrimazole vaginal tablet compared with a three-day regimen of two 100-mg vaginal tablets daily. Clinical Therapeutics 8:181–186
Lebherz T B, Ford L C, Kleinkopf V 1981 A comparison of a three-day and seven-day clotrimazole regimen for vulvovaginal candidiasis. Clinical Therapeutics 3:344–348
Lebherz T B, Goldman L, Wiesmeier E et al 1983 A comparison of the efficacy of two vaginal creams for vulvovaginal candidiasis, and correlations with the presence of Candida species in the perianal area and oral contraceptive use. Clinical Therapeutics 5:409–416
Smith M A, Shimp L A 2000 20 common problems in women's health care. McGraw-Hill, New York
Sobel J D, Faro S, Force R W et al 1998 Vulvovaginal candidiasis: epidemiologic, diagnostic, and therapeutic considerations. American Journal of Obstetrics and Gynecology 178:203–211
Tobin M J 1995 Vulvovaginal candidiasis: topical vs. oral therapy. The American Family Physician 51:1715–1720, 1723–1724.

Web sites
Embarrassing problems.com: www.embarrassingproblems.com/pages2/vaginalprobs1.htm

Primary dysmenorrhoea (period pain)

Background

Menstruation spans the years between **menarche** to menopause. Typically this will last 30 to 40 years, starting around the age of 12 and ceasing around the age of 50. The menstrual cycle usually lasts 28 days but this varies and it can last anything between 21 and 45 days. Menstruation itself lasts between 3 and 7 days. Individuals can also exhibit differences in menstrual cycle length and blood flow.

Prevalence and epidemiology

Primary dysmenorrhoea (PD) affects between 30 to 60% of menstruating women, with 7 to 15% reporting severe and debilitating pain, which is associated with school and work absence.

Aetiology

PD is characterised by the overproduction of prostaglandin E_2, which increases uterine activity causing muscle contraction experienced by the patient as pain.

Arriving at a differential diagnosis

The main consideration of the community pharmacist is to exclude causes other than PD. PD can be defined as pain in the absence of pelvic pathology, and can be treated OTC. PD is a diagnosis based on exclusion. It is essential to take a detailed history of the patient's menstrual history. This should be done in a quiet area of the pharmacy away from other patients because of the potential for embarrassment. The frequency, severity and relationship of symptoms to the menstrual cycle need to be established. Asking symptom-specific questions will help the pharmacist to determine if referral is needed (Table 5.5).

Clinical features of PD

A typical presentation of PD is of lower abdominal cramping pains shortly before (6 h) and for 2 or possibly 3 days after the onset of bleeding. Associated back pain, nausea and/or vomiting can also occur in up to 50% of patients. It is classically associated with young women who have recently started having regular periods. However, there may be a gap of months or years between menarche and onset of symptoms. This is due to as many as 50% of women being **anovulatory** in the first year (and still 10% of women 8 years after the menarche). This is important to know, as anovulatory cycles are usually pain free.

Conditions to eliminate

Endometriosis (presence of endometrial tissue outside of the uterus)

The exact incidence of endometriosis is unclear, however it is the most common cause of secondary dysmenorrhoea. Reports suggest it may occur in up to 50% of menstruating women but many are asymptomatic. Any person over the age of 30 presenting for the first time with dysmenorrhoea should be viewed with caution. Patients' experience lower abdominal pain (aching rather than cramping), that usually starts 5 to 7 days before menstruation begins and can be constant and severe. The pain often worsens at the onset of menstruation. Referred pain into the back and down the thighs is also possible.

Dysfunctional uterine bleeding

Dysfunctional uterine bleeding is a non-specific medical term defined as abnormal uterine bleeding that is not due to structural or systemic disease and includes conditions such as **amenorrhoea** (lack of menstruation) and menorrhagia (heavy periods); with the majority of cases attributable to menorrhagia. The pharmacist should ask the patient if their periods are different than usual.

Table 5.5
Specific questions to ask the patient: Primary dysmenorrhoea

Question	Relevance
Age	● PD is most common in adolescents and women in their early twenties. Secondary dysmenorrhoea usually affects women many years after the menarche, typically after the age of 30
Nature of pain	● A great deal of overlap exists between PD and secondary dysmenorrhoea but generally PD results in cramping whereas secondary causes are usually described as dull, continuous diffuse pain
Severity of pain	● Pain is rarely severe in PD; the severity decreases with the onset of menses. Any patient presenting with severe lower abdominal pain should be referred
Onset of pain	● PD starts very shortly before the onset of menses and rarely lasts for more than 3 days. Pain associated with secondary causes of dysmenorrhoea typically starts a few days before the onset of menses

Table 5.6
Medication that can alter menstrual bleeding
Anticoagulants
Cimetidine
Monoamine oxidase inhibitors
Phenothiazines
Steroids
Thyroid hormones

Pelvic inflammatory disease

PID is associated with dysmenorrhoea, however other symptoms such as fever, malaise, vaginal discharge, and **dyspareunia** are present.

Medicine-induced menstrual bleeding

Occasionally, medicines can change menstrual bleeding patterns (Table 5.6). If an adverse drug reaction (ADR) is suspected then the pharmacist should contact the prescriber and discuss other treatment options. Additionally, the incidence of menstrual pain is higher in patients who have had an intrauterine device fitted.

Endometrial carcinoma

This is characterised by inappropriate uterine bleeding and usually occurs in postmenopausal women. All unexplained bleeding in postmenopausal women should be referred because up to one third of cases are due to endometrial carcinoma.

TRIGGER POINTS indicative of referral: Primary dysmenorrhoea

- Heavy or unexplained bleeding
- Pain experienced before menses
- Pain that increases at the onset of menses
- Signs of systemic infection (e.g. fever, malaise)
- Vaginal bleeding in postmenopausal women
- Women over the age of 30

Evidence base for over-the-counter medication

Non-steroidal anti-inflammatories

The use of non-steroidal anti-inflammatories (NSAIDs) would be a logical choice because raised prostaglandin levels cause PD. In multiple clinical trials these agents, when given orally, have been shown to be effective in 80 to 85% of women with PD. Currently the only systemic NSAID available OTC is ibuprofen.

Hyoscine butylbromide (Buscopan) and Hyoscine hydrobromide (Feminax)

Although both products are marketed for PD there appears to be little or no evidence to support the manufacturers' claims of efficacy.

In one study, Buscopan was given to 17 patients in a double-blind, placebo-crossover trial. The study failed to demonstrate a significant effect compared to placebo or the comparator drug – aspirin, although in the author's opinion Buscopan was a good alternative to NSAIDs.

No trials could be found in the public domain to support the efficacy of Feminax. Feminax is a combination product of hyoscine (0.1 mg per tablet) and paracetamol and codeine. However, the dose of hyoscine is so low that it is unlikely to have a pharmacological action and therefore any effect Feminax may have will be exerted by the analgesic content and not hyoscine.

Low-dose combined oral contraceptives

Although not available OTC, oral contraceptives have been found to be effective in treating PD. Therefore if standard OTC treatment is not controlling symptoms adequately the patient is best referred as contraceptives provide an alternative treatment option.

Practical prescribing and product selection

Prescribing information relating to the medicines reviewed in the section 'Evidence base for over-the-counter medication' is discussed and summarised in Table 5.7; useful tips relating to patients presenting with PD are given in Hints and Tips Box 5.3.

Ibuprofen

Ibuprofen should be used as first-line therapy unless the patient is contraindicated from using an NSAID. A trial of two to three cycles should be long enough to determine if NSAID therapy is successful.

There are a plethora of marketed ibuprofen products (e.g. Nurofen, Cuprofen, Advil) all of which have a standard dose for the relief of PD. Adults should take 200 to 400 mg (one or two tablets) three times a day, although most patients will need the higher dose of 400 mg three times a day. Because ibuprofen is only used for a few days each cycle it is generally well tolerated. However, gastric irritation is possible and ibuprofen can cause peptic ulcers and bronchospasm in asthmatics with a history of hypersensitivity to aspirin or any other NSAID. It is therefore contraindicated in these patient groups. Ibuprofen can interact with many medicines although the vast majority are not clinically significant (see Table 5.7).

Buscopan

The dosage frequency for Buscopan in adults is two tablets four times a day, commencing 2 days before the

Table 5.7
Practical Prescribing: Summary of medicines for primary dysmenorrhoea

Medicine	Use in children	Likely side-effects	Drug interactions of note	Patients in whom care should be exercised	Pregnancy
Ibuprofen	Not recommended	GI discomfort, nausea and diarrhoea	Lithium, anticoagulants, methotrexate	Elderly (increased risk of side-effects)	Not applicable because patients do not menstruate when pregnant and therefore would not suffer from PD
Buscopan		Dry mouth, sedation and constipation	Increase in side-effects with anticholinergic medicines, e.g. TCAs	Glaucoma	
Feminax		Constipation	None	None	

HINTS AND TIPS BOX 5.3: PRIMARY DYSMENORRHOEA

Hot water bottles	The application of warmth to the lower abdomen can confer some relief of the pain

---

expected onset of the period and continuing for 3 days after menstruation has begun. It is contraindicated in patients with narrow-angle glaucoma and myasthenia gravis and care should be exercised in patients whose conditions are characterised by tachycardia, for example hyperthyroidism and cardiac problems. Anticholinergic side-effects such as dry mouth, visual disturbances and constipation may be experienced but are generally mild and self-limiting. Side-effects are potentiated if Buscopan is given with tricyclic antidepressants, anti-histamines, butyrophenones, phenothiazines and disopyramide.

Feminax

Adults should be advised to take two tablets every 4 h, to a maximum of eight in 24 h. Feminax has very few side-effects but the codeine component can cause constipation. Theoretically, because of its hyoscine component the same interactions, cautions, contraindications and side-effects would be equally applicable to Feminax as is the case with Buscopan but as the dose is so low then they are not applicable.

Further reading

Avant R F 1988 Dysmenorrhea. Primary Care 15:549–559

Brenner P F 1996 Differential diagnosis of abnormal uterine bleeding. American Journal of Obstetrics and Gynecology 175:766–769

Bromham D R Endometriosis in primary medical care. British Journal of Clinical Practice, Suppl. 72:54–58

Harlow S D, Ephross S A 1995 Epidemiology of menstruation and its relevance to women's health. Epidemiological Review 17:265–286

Kemp J H 1972 'Buscopan' in spasmodic dysmenorrhoea. Current Medical Research Opinions1:19–25

Nabrink M, Birgersson L, Colling-Saltin A S et al 1990 Modern oral contraceptives and dysmenorrhoea. Contraception 42:275–283

Web sites

Cancerbacup: cancer information service: www.cancerbacup. org.uk/questions/specific/womens/endometrial.htm

National Endometriosis Society: www.endo.org.uk/

Premenstrual syndrome

Background

Premenstrual syndrome (PMS) is a broad term that encompasses a wide range of symptoms – both physical and psychological. Symptoms start around the time of ovulation and are apparent to the patient a week or more before menstruation begins. Symptoms can range from mild to very severe, and in the unfortunate few can cause extreme morbidity.

Prevalence and epidemiology

Because of varying definitions of what constitutes PMS, the prevalence and epidemiology is unclear. Surveys have shown that over 90% of women have experienced PMS symptoms at some time, with 30 to 40% of patients suffering moderately, although fewer than 10% exhibit severe symptoms.

Aetiology

Controversy surrounds the aetiology of PMS. It is probably multifactorial, although some authors state it has a physiological cause whereas others support a psychological cause. Current thinking favours a psychological cause, as serotonin levels are abnormal in the luteal phase of the menstrual cycle and treatment with serotonin reuptake inhibitors has had some success.

Arriving at a differential diagnosis

Due to the varying and wide-ranging symptoms associated with PMS the pharmacist must endeavour to differentiate PMS from other gynaecological and mental health disorders. Careful questioning of when the symptoms occur and what symptoms are experienced will hopefully give rise to a differential diagnosis of PMS, although this might not be easy. It is important not to focus on one cycle's symptoms but ask the patient to describe their symptoms over previous cycles. A diary over three cycles should be maintained to allow a fuller picture of symptoms to be elucidated. Asking symptom-specific questions will help the pharmacist to determine if referral is needed (Table 5.8).

Clinical features of PMS

The most common presenting symptoms of PMS are irritability, moodiness, agitation, nervousness and anxiety. Breast tenderness, bloating, water retention, abdominal pain and headache usually accompany these symptoms.

Conditions to eliminate

Primary dysmenorrhoea

Some of the physiological symptoms of PMS, for example abdominal pain, also occur in patients with PD. However, other symptoms of PMS should be present and the onset of symptoms is days before menses and not hours as is the case with PD.

Mental health disorders

Depression and anxiety are common mental health disorders, which are often undiagnosed and may be

encountered by community pharmacists. Patients with PMS may experience symptoms similar to such conditions, namely low or sad mood, loss of interest or pleasure and prominent anxiety or worry. Other symptoms include disturbed sleep and appetite, dry mouth and poor concentration. However, the symptoms are not cyclical and are not associated with other symptoms of PMS such as breast tenderness and bloatedness.

TRIGGER POINTS indicative of referral:
Premenstrual syndrome

- Psychological symptoms alone
- Severe or disabling symptoms
- Symptoms that either worsen or stay the same after the onset of menses
- Women under the age of 30

Evidence base for over-the-counter medication

A number of dietary supplements are marketed for PMS-like symptoms. Most notably, vitamin B_6 has been widely touted as an effective therapy for PMS. A recent meta-analysis concluded that symptoms of irritability, fatigue and bloating were favourably reduced with vitamin B_6 supplementation. Vitamin B_6 might therefore be worth trying for those patients who experience relatively minor symptoms. For patients who exhibit moderate to severe symptoms, referral should be made as treatment with selective serotonin reuptake inhibitors (SSRIs) has proven to be effective in many cases.

Other dietary supplements that have been suggested to offer relief of PMS symptoms include vitamin E, magnesium, evening primrose oil and calcium. However, only calcium supplementation, at doses of 1200 to 1600 mg per day, appears to have any evidence of efficacy. Evening primrose oil is widely advocated as a treatment for PMS but trial data is conflicting. A recent review of clinical trial data by Budeiri et al (1996) concluded that evening primrose oil had little or no clinical benefit.

Table 5.8
Specific questions to ask the patient: Premenstrual syndrome

Question	Relevance
Onset of symptoms	● Symptoms that are experienced 7 to 14 days before, and that disappear a few hours after the onset of menses, are suggestive of PMS
Age of patient	● PMS is most common in women aged in their thirties and forties
Presenting symptoms	● Patients with PMS will normally have symptoms suggestive of mental health disorders, such as low mood, insomnia and irritability. This can make excluding mental health disorders such as depression difficult. However, other symptoms such as breast tenderness, bloatedness and fluid retention are also often present

Table 5.9
Practical Prescribing: Summary of medicines used in premenstrual syndrome

Medicine	Use in children	Likely side-effects	Drug interactions of note	Patients in whom care should be exercised	Pregnancy
Pyridoxine	Not applicable	Very high doses can cause toxicity (> 500 mg daily)	Levodopa when administered alone	None	Not applicable because patients do not menstruate when pregnant and therefore would not suffer from PMS
Calcium		Nausea and flatulence	None	Renally impaired patients	

Practical prescribing and product selection

Prescribing information relating to medicines for PMS reviewed in the section 'Evidence base for over-the-counter medication' is discussed and summarised in Table 5.9.

Vitamin B_6 (pyridoxine)

There is no definitive dose of vitamin B_6 required to alleviate symptoms of PMS. However, doses of up to 100 mg daily have been shown to help reduce symptoms. Side-effects are extremely rare with doses at this level, although neurological symptoms for example, numbness has been linked with vitamin B_6. A number of drug interactions have been observed in patients taking vitamin B_6, most notably with phenytoin, phenobarbitone and levodopa. However, only the vitamin B_6/levodopa interaction is significant and should be avoided. Although doses as low as 5 mg vitamin B_6 will reduce the effects of levodopa, the problem of this interaction in clinical practice is almost always negated because combinations of levodopa/carbidopa (Sinemet) or levodopa/benserazide (Madopar) are unaffected by vitamin B_6.

Calcium

Calcium supplementation should provide at least 1200 mg of elemental calcium per day. It is important to ensure that a product taken by the patient provides the required amount of elemental calcium. For example, a calcium lactate 300-mg tablet provides only 39 mg of elemental calcium; calcium carbonate 1.25 mg tablets (e.g. Calcichew) provide 500 mg of elemental calcium per tablet. Calcium supplements can cause mild gastrointestinal disturbances such as nausea and flatulence. If the patient is taking tetracycline antibiotics or iron then a 2-h gap should elapse between doses to avoid decreased absorption of the antibiotic or iron.

Further reading

Budeiri D, Po A L, Dornan J C 1996 Is evening primrose oil of value in the treatment of premenstrual syndrome? Control Clinical Trials 17:60

Korzekwa M I, Steiner M 1997 Premenstrual syndromes. Clinics in Obstetrics and Gynecology 40:564–576

Smith M A, Youngkin E Q 1986 Managing the premenstrual syndrome. Clinical Pharmacology 5:788–797

Ward M W, Holimon T D 1999 Calcium treatment for premenstrual syndrome. Annals of Pharmacotherapy 33:1356–1358

Wyatt K M, Dimmock P W, Jones P W et al 1999 Efficacy of vitamin B-6 in the treatment of premenstrual syndrome: systematic review. British Medical Journal 318:1375–1381

Web sites

National Association for Premenstrual Syndrome: www.pms.org.uk/

Self-assessment questions

The following questions are intended to supplement the text. Two levels of question are provided; multiple choice questions and case studies. The multiple choice questions are designed to test factual recall and the case studies allow knowledge to be applied to a practice setting.

Multiple choice questions

5.1. Primary dysmenorrhoea affects?

   a. 10 to 20% of women
   b. 20 to 30% of women
   c. 30 to 60% of women
   d. 40 to 60% of women
   e. 50 to 70% of women

5.2. When do PMS symptoms usually begin?

   a. Before ovulation
   b. At the start of ovulation
   c. Before menstruation
   d. At the start of menstruation
   e. None of the above

5.3. What percentage of women of childbearing age will experience an episode of thrush?

   a. 50%
   b. 55%
   c. 60%
   d. 70%
   e. 75%

5.4. What medication can precipitate thrush?

   a. Aspirin
   b. Propranolol
   c. Ampicillin
   d. Ramipril
   e. Levothyroxine (thyroxine)

5.5. What conditions predispose patients to pyelonephritis?

   a. Hypertension
   b. Rheumatoid arthritis
   c. Diabetes mellitus
   d. Hyperlipidaemia
   e. Asthma

5.6. Dysuria accompanied with fever and flank pain is indicative of?

   a. Cystitis
   b. Trichomoniasis
   c. Pyelonephritis
   d. Vaginitis
   e. Endometriosis

5.7. What symptoms are commonly associated with primary dysmenorrhoea?

   a. Lower abdominal cramping pain that starts 7 to 10 days before onset of the period
   b. Lower abdominal cramping pain that starts 2 to 3 days before onset of period
   c. Lower abdominal cramping pain that starts 6 to 12 hours before onset of period
   d. Lower abdominal gripping pain that starts 2 to 3 days before onset of period
   e. Lower abdominal gripping pain that starts 6 to 12 hours before onset of period

5.8. Which of the following medicines can interact with phenytoin?

   a. Fluconazole
   b. Hyoscine
   c. Potassium citrate
   d. Paracetamol
   e. Codeine

Questions 5.9 to 5.11 concern the following patient groups:

A. Children under 12 years old
B. Women over 30 years old
C. Women between the ages of 12 and 50
D. Women aged over 60 years old
E. Women between the ages of 40 and 60

Select, from A to E, which of the patient groups:

5.9. Are most likely to suffer from endometriosis

5.10. Are unlikely to suffer from cystitis

5.11. Should be referred automatically if they have vaginal discharge

Questions 5.12 to 5.14 concern the following conditions:

A. Vaginal thrush
B. Bacterial vaginosis
C. Trichomoniasis
D. Atrophic vaginitis
E. Cystitis

Select, from A to E, which of the conditions:

5.12. Has a fishy-smelling discharge

5.13. Is rare in patients aged over 60 years old

5.14. Has a cottage-cheese-like discharge

Questions 5.15 to 5.17: for each of the questions below, *one* or *more* of the responses is (are) correct. Decide which of the responses is (are) correct. Then choose:

A. If a, b and c are correct
B. If a and b only are correct
C. If b and c only are correct
D. If a only is correct
E. If c only is correct

Directions summarised

A	B	C	D	E
a, b and c	a and b only	b and c only	a only	c only

5.15. Pharmacists should refer a patient with vaginal candidiasis when:

a. She has had more than two attacks in the last 6 months
b. She is aged under 16 years old
c. She is taking antibiotics

5.16. Which of the following symptoms are associated with premenstrual syndrome?

a. Fatigue
b. Irritability
c. Breast tenderness

5.17. Which of the following medicines can cause menstrual bleeding?

a. Levothyroxine
b. Sertraline
c. Amoxicillin

Questions 5.18 to 5.20: these questions consist of a statement in the left-hand column followed by a statement in the right-hand column. You need to:

- decide whether the first statement is true or false
- decide whether the second statement is true or false

Then choose:

A. If both statements are true and the second statement is a correct explanation of the first statement
B. If both statements are true but the second statement is not a correct explanation of the first statement
C. If the first statement is true but the second statement is false
D. If the first statement is false but the second statement is true
E. If both statements are false

Directions summarised

	First statement	Second statement	
A	True	True	Second explanation is a correct explanation of the first
B	True	True	Second statement is *not* a correct explanation of the first
C	True	False	
D	False	True	
E	False	False	

	First statement	Second statement
5.18.	Cystitis is uncommon in men	They have a shorter urethra than women
5.19.	Vaginal discharge is uncommon in children under 12	Antibiotic therapy can precipitate attacks in this age group
5.20.	PMS symptoms tend to be less severe in older women	The incidence increases with increasing age

Case study

CASE STUDY 5.1

Ms PR, a 26-year-old woman, presents to the pharmacy one Saturday afternoon asking for something for cystitis. The counter assistant finds out that she has had the symptoms about 3 days and has tried no medication to relieve the symptoms. At this point Ms PR is referred to the pharmacist.

a. What other questions do you need to ask?

The questions to ask are:

- *Location, nature and severity of the pain.*
- *Nature of the pain.*
- *Severity of the pain.*
- *Associated symptoms.*
- *Previous history.*
- *Any factors that might have precipitated the attack.*
- *Medical history, including any regular medication currently taking.*
- *Presence of any vaginal discharge.*

You find out that Ms PR is suffering from pain on urination, discomfort and that she is going to the toilet frequently but has no other symptoms. She has had these symptoms previously about 2 years ago but they went on their own after a day or two. She takes no medicine from her GP.

b. What course of action are you going to take and why?

Symptoms suggest an uncomplicated acute urinary tract infection and empirical treatment could be instigated. However, the patient needs to be told that if treatment fails then she should visit the GP. Advice about adequate fluid intake should also be given.

Ms PR returns to the pharmacy on Monday evening with a prescription for erythromycin 250 mg qds × 20.

c. Is this an appropriate antibiotic for a urinary tract infection?

Trimethoprim is normally the medicine of choice. This is because Escherichia coli, Staphylococcus and Enterococci are the usual causative agents of cystitis and trimethoprim has activity against all of these. Alternatives to trimethoprim include broad-spectrum antibiotics such as amoxicillin. Erythromycin has a similar spectrum of activity to amoxicillin broad-spectrum antibiotics and could therefore be used.

CASE STUDY 5.2

A 29-year-old woman – Ms SY – explains that she has an intense itching around the vagina and would like some treatment for it. She had a similar problem about a year ago. On questioning, Ms SY says that she has a clear odourless discharge coming from her vagina, slight pain on urination and is suffering from intense itching in the vagina.

a. What is the likely condition that Ms SY is suffering from?

Vaginal candidiasis (thrush).

b. How can this condition be differentiated from other conditions affecting the vagina?

Bacterial infection has a fishy odour and trichomoniasis produces copious green–yellow discharge.

c. What factors predispose patients to this condition?

Pregnancy, certain medication, tight undergarments, diabetes mellitus, irritant local applications.

d. Under what circumstances would you decide to refer Ms SY rather than sell her an OTC treatment?

The following factors would require referral rather than OTC treatment:

- *First time sufferer.*
- *Previous history of sexually transmitted disease or exposure to partner with STD.*
- *More than two attacks in the last 6 months.*
- *Pregnancy or suspected pregnancy.*
- *Patient aged under 16 or over 60.*

- *Abnormal or irregular vaginal bleeding.*
- *Pain in the lower abdomen.*
- *Previous reaction to anti-candidial products.*
- *Dysuria.*
- *Vulval or vaginal sores, ulcers or blisters.*

Note: the above are the licence restrictions imposed on manufacturers by the Medicines Control Agency.

e. Giving examples, discuss the OTC treatment of this condition.

OTC treatment will involve topical imidazoles: intravaginal and/or external use. These include clotrimazole (Canesten), econazole (Ecostatin, Pevaryl), miconazole (Daktarin). A variety of formulations is available, all of which have similar efficacy.
Single-dose products are more convenient and might promote compliance.
    Fluconazole is a single-dose oral product. Use it as second-line therapy because of resistance and drug interactions.

f. What counselling tips would you give Ms SY about her treatment and methods to prevent the reoccurrence of the condition?

The following are helpful for women with thrush:

- *Products used in the vagina (PV products) should be used at night.*
- *Finish the course.*
- *Use the cream tds for 2 weeks.*
- *Eating natural yoghurt is thought to help prevent recolonisation from the rectum.*

Answers to multiple choice questions

5.1 = c 5.2 = b 5.3 = e 5.4 = c 5.5 = c 5.6 = c 5.7 = c 5.8 = a 5.9 = b 5.10 = a,
5.11= a 5.12 = b 5.13 = c 5.14 = a 5.15 = b 5.16 = a 5.17 = d 5.18 = c 5.19 = a 5.20 = e.

Gastroenterology

Background

The main function of the gastrointestinal (GI) tract is to break food down into a suitable energy source to allow normal physiological function of cells. Needless to say, the process is complex and involves many different organs. Consequently, there are many conditions that affect the GI tract, some of which are acute and self-limiting and respond well to OTC medication, and others that are serious and require referral.

General overview of the anatomy of the GI tract

It is vital that pharmacists have a sound understanding of the anatomy of the GI tract. Many conditions will present with similar symptoms from similar locations, for example abdominal pain, and the pharmacist will need a basic knowledge GI tract anatomy – and in particular of where each organ of the GI tract is located – to facilitate a correct differential diagnosis.

Oral cavity

The oral cavity comprises of the cheeks, hard and soft palates and tongue.

Stomach

The stomach is roughly J-shaped and receives food and fluid from the oesophagus. It empties into the duodenum. It is located slightly left of midline and anterior (below) to the rib cage. The lesser curvature of the stomach sits adjacent to the liver.

Liver

The liver is located below the diaphragm and located mostly right of midline in the upper right quadrant of the abdomen. The liver performs many functions, including carbohydrate, lipid and protein metabolism and the processing of many medicines.

Gall bladder

The gall bladder is a pear-shaped sac that lies deep to the liver and hangs from the lower front margin of the liver. Its function is to store and concentrate bile made by the liver.

Pancreas

The pancreas lies behind the stomach. It is essential for producing digestive enzymes transported to the duodenum via the pancreatic duct and secretion of hormones such as insulin.

History taking and the physical exam

A thorough patient history is essential as physical examination of the GI tract in a community pharmacy is limited to inspection of the mouth. This should allow confirmation of the diagnoses for conditions such as mouth ulcers and oral thrush. A detailed description of how to examine the oral cavity appears in the following section.

Conditions affecting the oral cavity

Background

The process of digestion starts in the oral cavity. The tongue and cheeks position large pieces of food so that the teeth can tear and crush food into smaller particles. Saliva moistens, lubricates and begins the process of digesting carbohydrates (by secreting amylase enzymes) prior to swallowing.

The physical exam

The oral cavity can easily be examined in the pharmacy provided the mouth can be viewed with a good light source, preferably a pen torch (Fig. 6.1). The patient will usually present with some form of oral lesion and/or pain in a particular part of the mouth. The pharmacist should examine this area carefully, but the rest of the oral cavity should also be inspected. Checks for periodontal disease (bleeding gums) and other sites of mouth soreness should be performed. The floor of the mouth and underside of

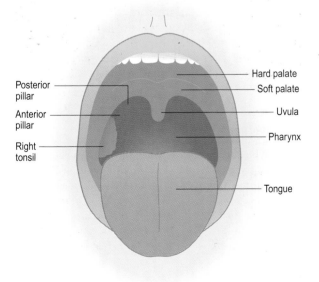

Fig. 6.1 The oral cavity

the tongue can be viewed by asking the patient to curl the tongue toward the roof of the mouth; the buccal mucosa is best observed when the patient half opens the mouth.

Mouth ulcers

Background

The majority of patients (80%) presenting with ulceration will have minor aphthous ulcers (MAU). It is the community pharmacist's role to exclude more serious pathology, for example systemic causes and carcinoma.

Prevalence and epidemiology

The prevalence and epidemiology of MAU is poorly understood. They occur in all ages but it has been reported that they are more common in patients aged between 20 and 40. It is estimated that one in five of the general population is affected. Smokers have been shown to have a lower incidence of mouth ulcers, but smoking is not advocated!

Aetiology

The aetiology of MAU is unknown. A number of theories have been put forward to explain why people get MAU, including stress, trauma, food hypersensitivities, nutritional deficiencies (iron, zinc and vitamin B_{12}) and infection, but none have so far been proven.

Arriving at a differential diagnosis

There are three main clinical presentations of ulcers: minor, major and herpetiform. Although, it is likely the patient will be suffering from MAU it is essential that other causes are recognised and referred to the GP for further evaluation. A number of ulcer-specific questions should always be asked of the patient to aid in diagnosis (Table 6.1). After questioning the patient, the oral cavity should be inspected to confirm the diagnosis.

Clinical features of minor aphthous ulcers

The ulcers of MAU are roundish, grey–white in colour and painful. They are small – usually less than 1 cm in diameter – and shallow. They rarely occur on the gingival mucosa and occur singly or in small crops of up to five ulcers. It normally takes 7 to 14 days for the ulcers to heal (Fig. 6.2).

Conditions to eliminate

Major aphthous ulcers

Characterised by large (greater than 1 cm in diameter) numerous ulcers, in crops of 10 or more. The ulcers often

Table 6.1
Specific questions to ask the patient: Ulcers

Question	Relevance
Number of ulcers	• MAU occur singly or in small crops. A single large ulcerated area is indicative of more serious pathology • Patients with numerous ulcers are more likely to be suffering from other forms of ulceration such as major or herpetiform ulcers rather than MAU
Location of ulcers	• Ulcers on the side of the cheeks, tongue and inside of the lips are likely to be MAU • Ulcers located toward the back of the mouth are more consistent with major or herpetiform ulcers
Size and shape	• Irregular-shaped ulcers tend to be caused by trauma. If trauma is not the cause then referral is necessary to exclude sinister pathology • If ulcers are large or very small then they are unlikely to be caused by MAU
Associated pain	• Any patient presenting with a painless ulcer in the oral cavity must be referred. This can indicate sinister pathology
Age	• MAU commonly occur between the ages of 10 and 40. MAU in young children is uncommon and other causes such as primary infection with herpes simplex should be excluded. If MAU is suspected in children under 10 and it is the first time the patient has had the ulcers then referral should be considered to confirm the diagnosis

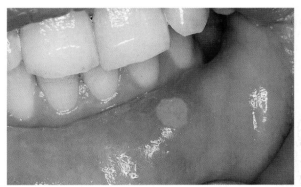

Fig. 6.2 Minor aphthous ulcer. Reproduced from *Cawson's Essentials of Oral Pathology and Oral Medicine* by R Cawson et al, 2002, Churchill Livingstone, with permission

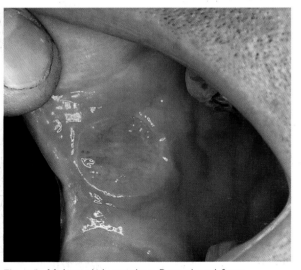

Fig. 6.3 Major aphthous ulcer. Reproduced from *Cawson's Essentials of Oral Pathology and Oral Medicine* by R Cawson et al, 2002, Churchill Livingstone, with permission

coalesce to form one large ulcer. The ulcers heal slowly and can persist for many weeks (Fig. 6.3).

Herpetiform ulcers

Herpetiform ulcers are pinpoint and occur in large crops of up to 100 at a time. They usually heal within a month and often occur in the posterior part of the mouth, an unusual location for MAU (Fig. 6.4).

Trauma

Trauma to the oral mucosa will result in damage and ulceration. Trauma can be mechanical or thermal, resulting in ulcers with an irregular border. Patients should have no history of ulceration or signs of systemic infection (Fig. 6.5).

Oral thrush

Oral thrush usually presents as creamy-white soft elevated patches. It is covered in more detail in the next section and the reader is referred to page 103 for differential diagnosis of thrush from other oral lesions.

Herpes simplex

Herpes simplex virus is a common cause of oral ulceration in children. Primary infection results in ulceration of

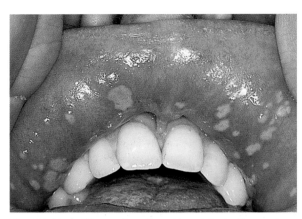

Fig. 6.4 Herpetiform ulcer. Reproduced from *Cawson's Essentials of Oral Pathology and Oral Medicine* by R Cawson et al, 2002, Churchill Livingstone, with permission

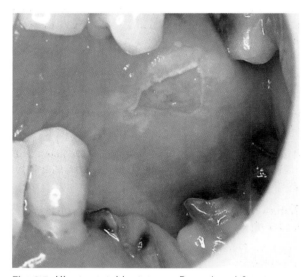

Fig. 6.5 Ulcer caused by trauma. Reproduced from *Textbook of General and Oral Medicine,* by D Wray et al, 1999, Churchill Livingstone, with permission

any part of the oral mucosa, especially the gums, tongue and cheeks. The ulcers tend to be small and discrete and many in number. Prior to the eruption of ulcers the person might show signs of systemic infection such as fever and pharyngitis.

Squamous cell carcinoma

Squamous cell carcinoma is the most common oral malignant lesion, with approximately 2000 people diagnosed each year in the UK. Smokers are at increased risk and account for 75% of cases, therefore patients should always be asked about their smoking history. It is most common in people over the age of 50 and initially presents as a painless ulcer that, over time, becomes

painful. The majority are noted on the side of the tongue, mouth and lower lip. The ulcer is likely to have been present for a number of weeks before the patient presents to a healthcare practitioner.

Erythema multiforme (Stevens Johnson syndrome)

Infection or drug therapy can cause erythema multiforme, although in about 50% of cases no cause can be found. Symptoms are sudden in onset causing widespread ulceration of the oral cavity. In addition, the patient might have **annular** and symmetric erythematous skin lesions located toward the extremities. Conjunctivitis and eye pain are also common.

Behçet's syndrome

Most patients will suffer from recurrent, painful major aphthous ulcers that are slow to heal. Lesions are also observed in the genital region and eye involvement (iridocyclitis) is common.

Figure 6.6 will aid the differentiation between serious and non-serious conditions that cause mouth ulcers.

> **❗ TRIGGER POINTS indicative of referral: Mouth ulcers**
>
> ● Children under 10
> ● Duration longer than 14 days
> ● Painless ulcer
> ● Signs of systemic illness, e.g. fever
> ● Ulcers greater than 1 cm in diameter
> ● Ulcers in crops of five to ten, or more

Evidence base for over-the-counter medication

A wide range of products are marketed for the temporary relief and treatment of mouth ulcers. These contain corticosteroids, local anaesthetics, astringents and antiseptics.

Products containing corticosteroids

Triamcinolone acetonide 0.1% in Orabase

Triamcinolone acetonide was deregulated from POM to P status in 1994. It has been suggested as a useful preparation to treat MAU by a number of authors, although there is a lack of clinical evidence from trial data. A study by Browne et al (1968) failed to demonstrate statistically significant improvement in the time it took to heal ulcers, although subjective improvements were noted by patients using triamcinolone in Orabase and not by those using Orabase alone. The improvements were minor and the authors suggest that triamcinolone in Orabase should not be used for routine use but be reserved for severe

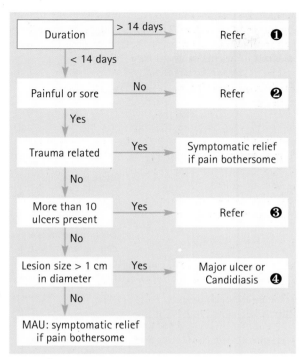

Fig. 6.6 Primer for differential diagnosis of mouth ulcers

❶ Duration
MAU normally resolve in 7 to 14 days. Ulcers that fail to heal within this time need referral to exclude other causes.

❷ Painless ulcers
These can indicate sinister pathology, especially if the patient is over 50 years old. In addition, it is likely that the ulcer will have been present for some time before the patient presented to the pharmacy.

❸ Numerous ulcers
Crops of 5 to 10 or more ulcers are rare in MAU. Referral is necessary to determine the cause.

❹ Major ulcer or Candidiasis
See Fig. 6.7 for primer for differential diagnosis of oral thrush.

episodes. A further trial, which evaluated triamcinolone, Orabase, betametasone 0.1 mg tablets and carbenoxolone gel failed to demonstrate statistical improvement for any of the treatments.

Hydrocortisone sodium succinate (Corlan) pellets
Only one trial could be found that investigated the efficacy of hydrocortisone sodium succinate pellets (Truelove & Morris-Owen 1958). At the request of the authors, a specific tablet formulation of hydrocortisone was made, which could be placed on the surface of the ulcer. The request was made because attempts using hydrocortisone ointment were largely unsuccessful as oral fluids washed the ointment away. The authors recruited 52 patients suffering from various forms of oral ulceration; 23 of the patients were suffering from minor aphthous ulceration. The authors stated that 22 of the 23

patients obtained rapid relief of pain and the healing rate of the ulcers was accelerated. However, the study lacked randomisation, a placebo or blinding. Due to the limited data and poor trial design it is difficult to say whether hydrocortisone sodium succinate pellets are effective, better than placebo or indeed have any effect at all.

Products containing anaesthetic or analgesics

There is very little trial data to support the pain-relieving effect of anaesthetics or analgesics in MAU, apart from choline salicylate. However, these preparations are clinically effective in other painful oral conditions. It is therefore not unreasonable to expect some relief of symptoms to be shown when using these products to treat MAU.

Choline salicylate
Choline salicylate has been shown to exert an analgesic effect in a number of small-scale studies. However, only one study by Reedy (1970) involving 27 patients evaluated choline salicylate in the treatment of oral aphthous ulceration. No significant differences were found between choline salicylate and placebo in ulcer resolution but choline salicylate was found to be significantly superior to placebo in relieving pain.

Practical prescribing and product selection

Prescribing information relating to the medicines used for ulcers reviewed in the section 'Evidence base for over-the-counter medication' is discussed and summarised in Table 6.2; useful tips relating to patients presenting with ulcers are given in Hints and Tips Box 6.1.

Triamcinolone acetonide 0.1% in Orabase (Adcortyl in Orabase 0.1%)

Adcortyl should be applied between two and four times a day for up to 5 days. All patient groups can use the product and it is well tolerated, with no side-effects reported. Because it is applied locally there are no drug interactions. The manufacturers state there is inadequate evidence of safety in pregnancy, although there have been no reports of teratogenic effects.

Hydrocortisone sodium succinate (Corlan) pellets

Each pellet contains 2.5 mg hydrocortisone. The dose for adults and children over 12 is one pellet to be sucked four times a day in close proximity to the ulcers. It does not interact with any medicines, can be taken by all patient groups, has no side-effects and appears to be safe in pregnancy.

Choline salicylate (e.g. Bonjela, Dinnefords Teejel Gel)

Choline salicylate is licensed from 4 months upwards for the treatment of soreness in the mouth (e.g. teething

Table 6.2
Practical prescribing: Summary of medicines for ulcers

Medicine	Use in children	Likely side-effects	Drug interactions of note	Patients in whom care should be exercised	Pregnancy
Adcortyl in Orabase	Yes but manufacturers do not state a lower age limit	None	None	None	OK
Corlan	> 12 years	None			OK, although manufacturer states there is inadequate evidence
Choline salicylate	> 10 year.*				OK
Lidocaine		Can cause sensitisation reactions			Neonatal respiratory depression in large doses. Avoid in the third trimester
Benzocaine					

* Age limit is arbitrarily set by author. Marketed products do have licences for use in younger people

HINTS AND TIPS BOX 6.1: ULCERS

Application of Adcortyl	Apply after food, as food is likely to rub off the paste

pain), however, it would be good practice to refer children under 10 years old presenting with MAU for the first time. Adults and children over 10 years old should apply the gel, using a clean finger, over the ulcer every 3 to 4 h or when needed. It is a very safe medicine and can be given to all patient groups, including pregnant women. It is not known to interact with any medicines or to cause any side-effects.

Local anaesthetics (e.g. lidocaine: Anbesol Adult Strength Gel (2.0%)/Liquid (0.9%) and Benzocaine: Rinstead Adult Gel)

All local anaesthetics have a short duration of action, frequent dosing is therefore required to maintain the anaesthetic effect. They are thus best used on a when-needed basis although, depending on the concentration of anaesthetic included in products, the upper limit on the number of applications allowed does vary. In most instances the products should not be used more than eight times in a day. They appear to be free from any drug interactions, have minimal side-effects and can be given to most patients. A small percentage of patients might experience a hypersensitivity reaction with lidocaine or benzocaine; this appears to be more common with benzocaine. These products should be avoided in the third trimester of pregnancy.

Further reading

Browne R M, Fox E C, Anderson R J 1969 Topical triamcinolone acetonide in recurrent aphthous stomatitis. A clinical trial. Lancet 1:565–567

Davis G 1996 CPPE distance learning. Oral health, vol 2. Recognition and treatment of orofacial problems. Outset Publishing, London

MacPhee I T, Sircus W, Farmer E D et al 1968 Use of steroids in treatment of aphthous ulceration. British Medical Journal 2(598):147–149

Reedy B L 1970 A topical salicylate gel in the treatment of oral aphthous ulceration. Practitioner 204:846–850

Scully C, Porter S 2000 ABC of oral health. Oral cancer. British Medical Journal 321:97–100

Truelove S C, Morris-Owen R M 1958 Treatment of aphthous ulceration of the mouth. British Medical Journal 1:603–607

Zakrzewska J M 1999 Fortnightly review: oral cancer. British Medical Journal 318:1051–1054

Web sites

General site on oral health: www.nlm.nih.gov/medlineplus/mouthandteeth.html

The Behçet's Syndrome Society: www.behcets-society.fsnet.co.uk/looklike.html

Oral thrush

Background

Oral thrush is an unusual infection in healthy adults. If thrush is suspected in this population the pharmacist should be suspicious of underlying pathology or identifiable risk factors that might have caused the oral thrush.

Prevalence and epidemiology

The very young and the very old are most likely to suffer from oral thrush. It has been reported that 5% of newborn infants and 10% of debilitated elderly patients suffer from oral thrush. Most other cases will be associated with underlying pathology such as immuno-compromisation, diabetes, xerostomia (dry mouth) or be attributable to identifiable risk factors such as recent antibiotic therapy, inhaled corticosteroids, and ill-fitting dentures.

Aetiology

Up to 40% of people carry *Candida albicans* in the oral cavity. Changes to the normal environment in the oral cavity will allow *C. albicans*, an opportunistic infection, to proliferate.

Arriving at a differential diagnosis

Oral thrush is not too difficult to diagnose with the aid of a careful history and an oral examination. It is the role of the pharmacist to eliminate underlying pathology and exclude risk factors. A number of oral thrush specific questions should always be asked of the patient to aid in diagnosis (Table 6.3). After questioning the pharmacist should inspect the oral cavity to confirm the diagnosis.

Clinical features of oral thrush

The classical presentation of oral thrush is of creamy-white soft elevated patches that can be wiped off revealing underlying erythematous mucosa. Pain and soreness is often present and the lesions can occur anywhere in the oral cavity.

Conditions to eliminate

Leukoplakia

Leukoplakia is a precancerous state that presents as a symptomless white patch and typically occurs over the age of 50. The patch cannot be wiped off, unlike oral

thrush. All elderly patients should be evaluated carefully for risk factors and if none is present referral is needed.

Mouth ulcers and squamous cell carcinoma

Mouth ulcers and squamous cell carcinoma are covered in more detail on pages 000 and the reader is referred to this section for differential diagnosis of these from oral thrush.

Figure 6.7 will aid the differentiation of thrush from other oral lesions.

TRIGGER POINTS indicative of referral: Oral thrush

- Diabetics
- Duration greater than 3 weeks
- Immunocompromised patients
- Painless lesions

Evidence base for over-the-counter medication

Only Daktarin oral gel (miconazole) is available OTC to treat oral thrush. It has proven efficacy and appears to have clinical cure rates between 80 and 90%. In comparative trials, Daktarin appears to have superior cure rates than the POM Nystatin.

Practical prescribing and product selection

Prescribing information relating to Daktarin Oral gel reviewed in the section 'Evidence base for over-the-counter medication' is discussed and summarised in Table 6.4; useful tips relating to the application of Daktarin are given in Hints and Tips Box 6.2.

The dose of gel varies depending on the age of patient and the distribution of the lesions. If lesions are localised then a small amount of gel can be applied directly to the area with a clean finger. For more generalised infections the dose should be given by way of a 5 mL spoon. For adults and children over 6 years, 5 mL of the gel should be applied four times a day and 5 mL used twice a day in children under six. For infants and children under 2 the

	Table 6.3 **Specific questions to ask the patient: Oral thrush**	

Question	Relevance
Size and shape of lesion	• Typically, patients with oral thrush present with 'patches'. They tend to be irregularly shaped and vary in size from small to large
Associated pain	• White, painless patches, especially in the elderly, should be referred to exclude sinister pathology
Location of lesions	• Oral thrush often affects the tongue and cheeks, although if precipitated by inhaled steroids the lesions appear on the pharynx

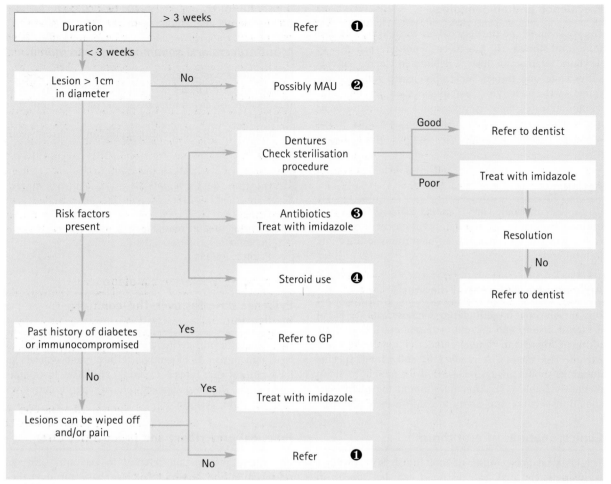

Fig. 6.7 Primer for differential diagnosis of oral thrush

❶ Duration
Any lesion lasting greater than 3 weeks must be referred to exclude sinister pathology.

❷ MAU
See Fig. 6.6 for primer for differential diagnosis of mouth ulcers.

❸ Antibiotics
Broad-spectrum antibiotics, e.g. amoxicillin and macrolides, can precipitate oral thrush by altering normal flora of the oral cavity.

❹ Inhaled corticosteroids
High-dose inhaled corticosteroids can cause oral thrush. Patients should be encouraged to use a spacer and wash their mouth out after inhaler use to minimise this problem.

Table 6.4
Practical Prescribing: Summary of medicines for oral thrush

Medicine	Use in children	Likely side-effects	Drug interactions of note	Patients in whom care should be exercised	Pregnancy
Daktarin	Infants upwards	Nausea and vomiting	Warfarin	None	OK

HINTS AND TIPS BOX 6.2: DAKTARIN

Application of Daktarin	Patients should be advised to hold the gel in the mouth for as long as possible to increase contact time between the medicine and the infection
Duration of treatment	Treatment should be continued for up to 2 days after the symptoms have cleared to prevent relapse and reinfection

dose is 2.5 mL twice a day. It can occasionally cause nausea and vomiting but these side-effects are rare. The manufacturers state that it can interact with a number of medicines, namely terfenadine, astemizole, mizolastine, cisapride, triazolam, midazolam, quinidine, pimozide, HMG-CoA (beta-hydroxy beta-methyl glutaryl coenzyme A) reductase inhibitors and anticoagulants. However, there is a lack of published data to determine how clinically significant these interactions are except with warfarin. Coadministration of warfarin with miconazole increases warfarin levels markedly and the patient's international normalised ratio (INR) should therefore be monitored closely. The manufacturers also state that Daktarin should be avoided in pregnancy, although published data do not support an association between miconazole and congenital defects.

Further reading

Hoppe J E 1997 Treatment of oropharyngeal candidiasis in immunocompetent infants: a randomized multicenter study of miconazole gel vs. nystatin suspension. The Antifungals Study Group. Pediatric Infectious Diseases Journal 16:288–293

Hoppe J E, Hahn H 1996 Randomized comparison of two nystatin oral gels with miconazole oral gel for treatment of oral thrush in infants. Antimycotics Study Group. Infection 24:136–139

Parvinen T, Kokko J, Yli-Urpo A 1994 Miconazole lacquer compared with gel in treatment of denture stomatitis. Scandinavian Journal of Dental Research 102:361–366

Web sites

General information: www.netdoctor.co.uk/diseases/facts/oralthrush.htm

Gingivitis

Background

Gingivitis simply means inflammation of the gums and is caused by an excess build-up of plaque on the teeth. The condition is entirely preventable if regular tooth brushing is undertaken. Despite this, dental caries and gum disease still affect almost everyone.

Prevalence and epidemiology

It is estimated 50% of the UK population are affected by gum disease and that more than 85% of people over 40 will experience gingival disease. Men more than women tend to suffer from severe gingivitis, which might be due to women practising better oral hygiene.

Aetiology

Following tooth brushing, the teeth soon become coated in a mixture of saliva and gingival fluid. Oral bacteria adhere to this coating and begin to proliferate, forming plaque; subsequent brushing of the teeth removes this plaque build up. However, if plaque is allowed to build up for 3 or 4 days, bacteria begin to undergo internal calcification producing calcium phosphate, better known as tartar (or calculus). This adheres tightly to the surface of the tooth and retains bacteria in situ. The bacteria release enzymes and toxins that invade the gingival mucosa, causing inflammation of the gingiva (gingivitis). If the plaque is not removed the inflammation travels downwards, involving the periodontal ligament and associated tooth structures (periodontitis). A pocket forms between the tooth and the gum and, over a period of years, the root of the tooth and bone are eroded until such time that the tooth becomes loose and lost. This is the main cause of tooth loss in people over 40 years of age.

Arriving at a differential diagnosis

Gingivitis often goes unnoticed because symptoms can be very mild and painless. This often explains why a routine check-up at the dentist reveals more severe gum disease than patients thought they had. A dental history needs to be taken from the patient, in particular details of tooth brushing routine and technique, as well as the frequency of visits to their dentist. The mouth should be inspected for tell-tale signs of gingival inflammation. A number of gingivitis-specific questions should always be asked of the patient to aid in diagnosis (Table 6.5).

Clinical features of gingivitis

Gingivitis is characterised by swelling and reddening of the gums, which bleed easily with slight trauma, for example when brushing teeth. Plaque might be visible; especially on teeth that are difficult to reach when tooth brushing. **Halitosis** might also be present.

Conditions to eliminate

Periodontitis

If gingivitis is left untreated it will progress in to periodontitis. Symptoms are similar to gingivitis but the patient will experience spontaneous bleeding and taste disturbances, and periodontal pockets might be visible. Referral to a dentist is needed for removal of tartar and plaque.

Spontaneous bleeding

A number of conditions can produce spontaneous gum bleeding, for example agranulocytosis and leukaemia. Other symptoms should be present, for example progressive fatigue, weakness and signs of systemic illness such as fever. Immediate referral to the GP is needed.

Table 6.5
Specific questions to ask the patient: Gingivitis

Question	Relevance
Tooth-brushing technique	● Overzealous tooth brushing can lead to bleeding gums and gum recession. Make sure the patient is not overcleaning the teeth
Bleeding gums	● Gums that bleed without exposure to trauma and is unexplained or unprovoked need referral to exclude underlying pathology

Medicine-induced gum bleeding

Medicines such as warfarin, heparin and NSAIDs can produce gum bleeding. Consultation with the prescriber to suggest alternative medication would be needed.

TRIGGER POINTS indicative of referral: Gingivitis

- Foul taste associated with gum bleeding
- Signs of systemic illness
- Spontaneous gum bleeding

Evidence base for over-the-counter medication

Put simply, there is no substitute for good oral hygiene. Prevention of plaque build-up is the key to healthy gums and teeth. Once daily brushing, with or without toothpaste, is adequate to maintain oral hygiene at adequate levels. If the patient brushes more regularly than this then this should not be discouraged. Brushing teeth should preferably take place after eating, and flossing is recommended to reach areas that a toothbrush might miss.

However, there is a plethora of oral hygiene products marketed for general sale to the public, whether through a pharmacy outlet or a general store. These products should be reserved for established gingivitis.

Mouthwashes contain chlorhexidine, hexetidine, hydrogen peroxide, sodium perborate and povidone–iodine. Of these, chlorhexidine in concentrations of either 0.1 or 0.2% has been proven the most effective antibacterial in reducing plaque formation and gingivitis. In clinical trials it has been shown to be consistently more effective than placebo and comparator medicines, and there appears to be no difference in effect between concentrations. It has even been used as a positive control.

Povidone–iodine has antiseptic properties and is beneficial in oral infection but has failed to show a significant effect in decreasing gingivitis and plaque formation except when combined with hydrogen peroxide. Hydrogen peroxide and povidone–iodine might therefore work synergistically because both products alone have failed to demonstrate effectiveness in inhibition of plaque formation.

Practical prescribing and product selection

Prescribing information relating to the medicines used for gingivitis reviewed in the section 'Evidence base for over-the-counter medication' is discussed and summarised in Table 6.6.

All mouthwashes, except those containing iodine, appear to be free from any drug interactions, have minimal side-effects and can be used by all patient groups. They are rinsed around the mouth for between 30 s and 1 min and then spat out. Information relating to iodine mouthwashes are given in Hints and Tips Box 6.3.

Table 6.6
Practical prescribing: Summary of medicines for gingivitis

Medicine	Use in children	Likely side-effects	Drug interactions of note	Patients in whom care should be exercised	Pregnancy
Chlorhexidine	No age limit stated	None	None	None	OK
Povidone-iodine	> 6 years			Patients with thyroid disease	Avoid if possible
Hexetidine	> 6 years	Mild irritation or numbness of tongue		None	OK

HINTS AND TIPS BOX 6.3: IODINE MOUTHWASH

Regular use of iodine-containing mouthwashes	Regular use in pregnant women should be avoided because prolonged use can lead to iodine crossing the placental barrier and absorption by the fetus of a significant amount of iodine. This can result in hypothyroidism and goitre in the fetus and newborn

Chlorhexidine gluconate (e.g. Corsodyl 0.2%, Eludril 0.1%)

The standard dose for adults and children is 10 mL twice a day. Although it is free from side-effects, patients should be warned that prolonged use might stain the tongue and teeth brown. Corsodyl is also available as a gel and spray.

Povidone–iodine (Betadine)

Adults and children over 6 years of age should use a 10 mL dose four times a day, either undiluted or diluted with an equal volume of water. Because of its iodine content it should not be used for periods longer than 14 days because a significant amount of iodine is absorbed. Pregnant women and patients with thyroid disorders should avoid its use.

Hexetidine (Oraldene)

Adults and children over 6 years of age should use a 15 mL dose two or three times a day.

Further reading
Addy M, Dummer P M, Hunter M L et al 1990 The effect of tooth brushing frequency, tooth brushing hand, sex and social class on the incidence of plaque, gingivitis and pocketing in adolescents: a longitudinal cohort study. Community Dental Health 7:237–247
Brecx M, Brownstone E, MacDonald L et al 1992 Efficacy of Listerine, Meridol and chlorhexidine mouthrinses as supplements to regular tooth cleaning measures. Journal of Clinical Periodontology 19:202–207
Ernst C P, Prockl K, Willershausen B 1998 The effectiveness and side effects of 0.1% and 0.2% chlorhexidine mouthrinses: a clinical study. Quintessence International 29:443–448
Greenstein G 1999 Povidone–iodine's effects and role in the management of periodontal diseases: a review. Journal of Periodontology 70:1397–1405
Hase J C, Ainamo J, Etemadzadeh H et al 1995 Plaque formation and gingivitis after mouthrinsing with 0.2% delmopinol hydrochloride, 0.2% chlorhexidine digluconate and placebo for 4 weeks, following an initial professional tooth cleaning. Journal of Clinical Periodontology 22:533–539
Jones C M, Blinkhorn A S, White E 1990 Hydrogen peroxide, the effect on plaque and gingivitis when used in an oral irrigator. Clinical Preventive Dentistry 1990; 12:15–18.

Kelly M 2000 Adult dental health survey: oral health in the United Kingdom 1998. The Stationery Office, London
Lang N P, Hase J C, Grassi M et al 1998 Plaque formation and gingivitis after supervised mouthrinsing with 0.2% delmopinol hydrochloride, 0.2% chlorhexidine digluconate and placebo for 6 months. Oral Diseases 4:105–113
Maruniak J, Clark W B, Walker C B et al 1992 The effect of 3 mouthrinses on plaque and gingivitis development. Journal of Clinical Periodontology 19:19–23

Web sites
The American Academy of Periodontology: www.perio.org/

Dyspepsia

Background

'Dyspepsia' is an umbrella term generally used by health-care professionals to refer to a group of upper abdominal symptoms that arise from five main conditions:

- non-ulcer dyspepsia (indigestion)
- reflux (heartburn)
- gastritis
- duodenal ulcers
- gastric ulcers.

These five conditions represent 90% of dyspepsia cases that present to the GP.

Prevalence and epidemiology

The exact prevalence of dyspepsia is unknown. This is largely because of the number of people who self medicate or do not report mild symptoms to their GP. However, it is clear that dyspepsia is extremely common. A quarter of the general population in Western society have been reported to suffer from dyspepsia and virtually everyone at some point in their lives will experience an episode of dyspepsia. Estimates suggest that 10% of people suffer on a weekly basis and that 5% of all GP consultations are for dyspepsia. The prevalence of dyspepsia is modestly higher in women than men.

Aetiology

The aetiology of dyspepsia differs depending on which condition the patient is suffering from. Lower oesophageal sphincter incompetence is the principal cause of reflux oesophagitis. Increased acid production results in inflammation of the stomach (gastritis) and is usually attributable to *Helicobacter pylori* infection, NSAID or acute alcohol ingestion. The presence of *H. pylori* is central to duodenal and gastric ulceration as *H. pylori* is present in nearly all individuals. The mechanism by which it affects the aetiology of peptic ulcers is still unclear but the bacteria is thought to secrete certain chemical factors that result in gastric mucosal damage. Finally, when no specific cause can be found for a patient's symptoms the complaint is said to be non-ulcer dyspepsia. (Some authorities do not advocate the use of this term, preferring instead the term 'functional dyspepsia'.)

Arriving at a differential diagnosis

Overwhelmingly, patients who present with dyspepsia are likely to be suffering from reflux, gastritis or non-ulcer dyspepsia. Despite this, a thorough medical and drug history should be taken to enable the community pharmacist to rule out serious pathology and diagnose dyspepsia. A number of dyspepsia specific questions should always be asked of the patient to aid in diagnosis (Table 6.7).

Clinical features of dyspepsia

Patients with dyspepsia present with a range of symptoms commonly involving:

- vague abdominal discomfort (aching) above the umbilicus associated with belching
- bloating
- flatulence
- a feeling of fullness
- heartburn.

Reflux oesophagitis is likely if heartburn is the dominant upper abdominal symptom.

Conditions to eliminate

Peptic ulceration

Ruling out peptic ulceration is probably the main consideration for community pharmacists when assessing patients with symptoms of dyspepsia. Ulcers are classed as either gastric or duodenal. They occur most commonly in patients aged between 30 and 50, although patients over the age of 60 account for 80% of deaths even though they only account for 15% of cases. Typically the patient will have well localised mid-epigastric pain described as 'constant', 'annoying' or 'gnawing'.

Table 6.7
Specific questions to ask the patient: Dyspepsia

Question	Relevance
Age	• The incidence of dyspepsia decreases with advancing age and therefore young adults are likely to suffer from dyspepsia with no specific pathological condition, unlike patients over 50 years of age, in whom a specific pathological condition becomes more common
Location	• Dyspepsia is experienced as pain above the umbilicus and centrally located (epigastric area). Pain below the umbilicus will not be due to dyspepsia • Pain experienced behind the sternum (breastbone) is likely to be heartburn • If the patient can point to a specific area of the abdomen then it is unlikely to be dyspepsia and could be caused by another GI condition, or could be musculoskeletal in origin
Nature of pain	• Pain associated with dyspepsia is described as aching or discomfort. Pain described as gnawing, sharp or stabbing is unlikely to be dyspepsia
Radiation	• Pain that radiates to other areas of the body is indicative of more serious pathology and the patient must be referred. The pain might be cardiovascular in origin, especially if it is felt down the inside aspect of the left arm
Severity	• Pain described as debilitating or severe must be referred to exclude more serious conditions
Associated symptoms	• Persistent vomiting with or without blood is suggestive of ulceration or even cancer and must be referred • Black and tarry stools indicate a bleed in the GI tract and must be referred
Aggravating or relieving factors	• Pain aggravated by food can indicate a gastric ulcer, whereas pain relieved by food can indicate a duodenal ulcer
Social history	• Bouts of excessive drinking are commonly implicated in dyspepsia. Likewise, eating food on the move or too quickly is often the cause of the symptoms. A person's job is often a good clue to whether these are contributing to their symptoms

In gastric ulcers the pain comes on whenever the stomach is empty, usually an hour or so after eating; it is generally not relieved by antacids or food and is aggravated by alcohol and caffeine. Gastric ulcers are also more commonly associated with weight loss and GI bleeds than duodenal ulcers. Patients can experience weight loss of 5 to 10 kg and although this could indicate carcinoma, especially in people aged over 40, on investigation a benign gastric ulcer is found most of the time.

The pain associated with duodenal ulcers often wakes the patient a few hours after falling asleep but subsides by morning and is relieved after eating. This is not commonly noticed in gastric ulceration.

Medicine-induced dyspepsia

A number of medicines can cause gastric irritation leading to or provoking GI discomfort. Patients should be questioned about medication, especially the use of aspirin and NSAIDs, which provoke dyspepsia in 25% of patients. Table 6.8 lists other medicines commonly implicated in causing dyspepsia.

Irritable bowel syndrome

Patients younger than 45, who have uncomplicated dyspepsia and also lower abdominal pain and altered bowel habits are likely to have irritable bowel syndrome (IBS). For further details on IBS see page 124.

Gastric carcinoma

Gastric carcinoma is the third most common GI malignancy after colorectal and pancreatic cancer. However, only 2% of patients who are referred by their GP for an endoscopy have malignancy. It is therefore a rare condition and community pharmacists are extremely unlikely to encounter a patient with carcinoma. Usually, the patient will experience upper abdominal discomfort with nausea and vomiting. Other symptoms associated with carcinoma are GI bleeding, fatigue, unexplained weight loss and dysphagia.

| Table 6.8 |
Medicines that commonly cause dyspepsia
ACE inhibitors
Alcohol (in excess)
Iron
Macrolide antibiotics
Metronidazole
Oestrogens
Theophylline

Oesophageal carcinoma

In its early stages, oesophageal carcinoma might go unnoticed. Over time, however, as the oesophagus becomes constricted, patients will complain of difficulty in swallowing and experience a sensation of food sticking in the oesophagus. As the disease progresses weight loss becomes prominent despite the patient maintaining a good appetite.

Atypical angina

Not all cases of angina have the classic textbook presentation of pain in the retrosternal area with radiation to the neck, back or left shoulder that is precipitated by temperature changes or exercise; patients can complain of dyspepsia-like symptoms and feel generally unwell. These symptoms might be brought on by a heavy meal. In such cases antacids will fail to relieve symptoms and referral is needed.

Figure 6.8 will aid differentiation of the causes of dyspepsia.

TRIGGER POINTS indicative of referral: Dyspepsia

- Dark or tarry stools
- Long-standing change in bowel habit
- Pain described as severe, debilitating or that wakes the patient in the night
- Persistent vomiting (with or without blood)
- Referred pain
- Sensation that food is 'sticking' in the throat
- Treatment failure
- Unexplained weight loss

Evidence base for over-the-counter medication

Each year an estimated £450 million is spent on proton pump inhibitors, H_2 antagonists and antacid drugs in the UK. OTC antacids and H_2 antagonists are the principal compounds in the drug management of dyspepsia.

Antacids

Antacids have been used for many decades to treat dyspepsia and have proven efficacy in neutralising stomach acid. However, the neutralising capacity of each antacid varies according to the metal salt used. In addition, the solubility of each metal salt differs, which affects their onset and duration of action. Sodium and potassium salts are the most highly soluble, which makes them quick but short acting. Magnesium and aluminium salts are less soluble and so have a slower onset but greater duration of action. Calcium salts have the advantage of being quick acting yet have a prolonged action.

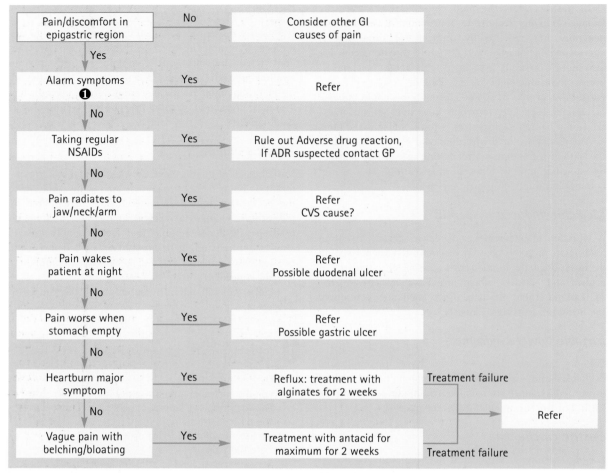

Fig. 6.8 Primer for differential diagnosis of dyspepsia

❶ **Alarm symptoms**
These include, dark stools, persistent vomiting, loss of weight and altered bowel habit.

It is therefore commonplace for manufacturers to combine two or more antacid ingredients to ensure a quick onset (generally sodium salts, e.g. sodium bicarbonate) and prolonged action (aluminium, magnesium or calcium salts).

Alginates

For patients suffering from heartburn and reflux an alginate product should be first-line treatment. When in contact with gastric acid the alginate precipitates out, forming a sponge-like matrix that floats on top of the stomach contents. In clinical trials alginate containing products have demonstrated superior symptom control compared to placebo and antacids.

H₂ antagonists

Two H_2 antagonists are currently available OTC in the UK: ranitidine and famotidine. Cimetidine was also available OTC until recently but it has been withdrawn

from sale, presumably because of poor sales. There is no doubt that, at POM doses, these agents work. However, lower doses are used for the licensed OTC indications and the question is whether at these lower doses the agents are still effective. There is a paucity of publicly available trial data supporting their use at non-prescription doses. Famotidine appears to have the greatest body of accessible trial data. A number of trials have been conducted in patients suffering from heartburn who regularly self-medicate with antacids. Famotidine was shown to be more effective than placebo and equally effective to antacids. No trials involving ranitidine could be found on public databases that involved patients taking OTC doses.

However, the inhibitory effects of OTC doses of ranitidine on gastric acid have been investigated in healthy volunteers. Trials showed conclusively that ranitidine, and its comparator drug famotidine, did significantly raise intragastric pH compared to placebo, although antacids (calcium carbonates) had a significantly quicker onset of action but with shorter duration. Despite ranitidine appearing to have no trial data relating to patients, it is assumed that the product license holders had enough evidence for their product to be granted a licence.

Summary

Antacids will work for the majority of people presenting at the pharmacy with dyspeptic symptoms. They should be used as first-line therapy unless heartburn predominates, when an alginate or alginate/antacid combination should be used. H_2 antagonists appear to be equally effective as antacids but are considerably more expensive. They should be reserved for patients who know they will suffer from dyspepsia after meals because their long-acting effect could be used as prophylactic cover.

Practical prescribing and product selection

Prescribing information relating to the medicines used for dyspepsia reviewed in the section 'Evidence base for over-the-counter medication' is discussed and summarised in Table 6.9.

Antacids

The majority of marketed antacids are combination products containing two, three or even four constituents. The rationale for combining different salts appears to be two-fold. First, to ensure the product has quick onset (containing sodium or calcium) and a long duration of action (containing magnesium, aluminium or calcium). Second, to minimise any side-effects that might be experienced from the product. For example, magnesium salts tend to cause diarrhoea and aluminium salts constipation, however, if both are combined in the same product then neither side-effect is noticed. Useful tips relating to antacids are given in Hints and Tips Box 6.4.

Antacids can affect the absorption of a number of medications via chelation and adsorption. Commonly affected medicines include tetracyclines, quinolones, imidazoles, phenytoin, penicillamine and bisphosphonates. In addition, the absorption of enteric-coated preparations can be affected due to antacids increasing the stomach pH. The majority of these interactions are easily overcome by leaving a minimum gap of 1 h between the respective doses of each medicine.

Most patient groups can take antacids, although patients on salt-restricted diets (patients with coronary heart disease) should ideally avoid sodium-containing antacids. In addition, antacids should not be recommended for children because dyspepsia is unusual in children under 12. Indeed, most products are licensed for use only for children aged 12 and over. However, there are a few exceptions (e.g. Aludrox, Asilone, Gaviscon), which can be prescribed for children as young as six.

Table 6.9
Practical prescribing: Summary of medicines for dyspepsia

Medicine	Use in children	Likely side-effects	Drug interactions of note	Patients in whom care should be exercised	Pregnancy
Antacids					
Sodium only	> 12 years	None	None	Patients with heart disease	OK
Calcium only		Constipation	Tetracyclines, quinolones, imidazoles, phenytoin, penicillamine and bisphosphonates	None	OK
Magnesium only		Diarrhoea			
Aluminium only		Constipation			
Alginates					
Gaviscon	> 6 years (Advance Liquid > 12 years)	None	None	Patients with heart disease	OK
Asilone Heartburn	> 6 years				
H_2 antagonists					
Pepcid AC	> 16 years	Diarrhoea, constipation, headache or rash	None	None	Not recommended
Zantac 75					

HINTS AND TIPS BOX 6.4: ANTACIDS

Type of formulation	Ideally, antacids should be given in the liquid form because the acid-neutralising capacity and speed of onset is greater than that of tablet formulations
Overuse of antacids	Misuse and chronic use of antacids will result in significant systemic absorption leading to various unwanted medical conditions. Milk-alkali syndrome has been reported with chronic abuse of calcium containing antacids, as has osteomalacia with aluminium-containing products. It is therefore important to determine patient use of antacids prior to recommending a specific product. Antacid therapy should ideally not be longer than 2 weeks. If symptoms have not resolved in this time then other treatments and/or evaluation from the GP should be recommended
When is the best time to take antacids?	Antacids should be taken after food because gastric emptying is delayed in the presence of food. This allows antacids to exert their effect for up to 3 h
The elderly	Avoid constipating products, the elderly are prone to constipation

Alginates (e.g. the Gaviscon range, Algicon)

Products containing alginates are combination preparations that contain an alginate with antacids. They are best given after each main meal and before bedtime, although they can be taken on a when-needed basis. They can be given in pregnancy and to most patient groups but, as with antacids, patients on salt-restricted diets should ideally avoid sodium-containing alginate preparations (e.g. Gaviscon and Asilone Heartburn). They are reported not to have any side-effects or interactions with other medicines.

H₂ antagonists

Sales of H_2 antagonists are restricted to adults and children over the age of 16. They cannot be given to pregnant women and are restricted to short-term use. They possess no clinically important drug interactions and side-effects are rare. Safety concerns were raised on deregulation of H_2 antagonists about the potential to mask serious underlying conditions and the possibility of increased adverse reactions. These fears appear to have been unfounded as follow-up studies and postmarketing surveillance has not shown any increase in risk associated with greater availability. Indeed, H_2 antagonists are now available as general sales list medicines.

Famotidine (Pepcid AC)

The dose for famotidine is one tablet to be taken straight away and, if symptoms persist, an additional dose can be repeated after 1 h. The maximum dose is 20 mg (two tablets) in 24 h.

Famotidine is also available as PepcidTwo. This is a combination of famotidine, calcium carbonate and magnesium hydroxide. The dose for PepcidTwo is the same for Pepcid AC. It has the additional advantage of quicker onset of action conferred by the antacid component of the product when compared to Pepcid AC.

Ranitidine (Zantac 75)

Dosing for Zantac 75 is similar to Pepcid AC in that one tablet should be taken straight away but if symptoms persist then a further tablet should be taken 1 h later. The maximum dose is 300 mg (four tablets) in 24 h. The General Sales List version of ranitidine, Zantac 75 Relief, has a slightly different licence in that it cannot be used for prevention of heartburn and the maximum dose is only two tablets in 24 h.

Further reading

Castell D O, Dalton C B, Becker D et al 1992 Alginic acid decreases postprandial upright gastroesophageal reflux. Comparison with equal-strength antacid. Digestive Diseases and Sciences 37:589–593

Drake D, Hollander D 1981 Neutralizing capacity and cost effectiveness of antacids. Annals of Internal Medicine 94:215–217

Feldman M 1996 Comparison of the effects of over-the-counter famotidine and calcium carbonate antacid on postprandial gastric acid. A randomized controlled trial. Journal of the American Medical Association 275:1428–1431

Halter F 1983 Determination of neutralization capacity of antacids in gastric juice. Zeitschrift fur Gastroenterologie 21:S33–S40

Heatley R 1995 Dyspepsia: GP guide to drug management. Prescriber; 6:39–50

Kinnear M, Ghosh S 1998 Peptic ulcer disease. Pharmaceutical Journal 260:825–829

Kinnear M, Ghosh S, Hudson S 1999 Gastro-oesophageal reflux disease. Pharmaceutical Journal 263:241–250

Li Wan Po A 1994 H_2 antagonists for the relief of dyspepsia. Pharmaceutical Journal 252:84–87

Muris J W, Starmans R, Pop P et al 1994 Discriminant value

of symptoms in patients with dyspepsia. Journal of Family Practice 38:139–143

Netzer P, Brabetz-Hofliger A, Brundler R et al 1998 Comparison of the effect of the antacid Rennie versus low dose H_2 receptor antagonists (ranitidine, famotidine) on intragastric acidity. Alimentary Pharmacology and Therapeutics 12:337–342.

Rao S S C 1997 Belching, bloating and flatulence. Postgraduate Medicine 101:263–278

Reilly T G, Singh S, Cottrell J et al 1996 Low dose famotidine and ranitidine as single post-prandial doses: a three-period placebo-controlled comparative trial. Alimentary Pharmacology and Therapeutics 10:749–755

Rigas B, Spiro H M 1995 Clinical gastroenterology, 4th edn. McGraw-Hill, New York

Smart H L, Atkinson M 1990 Comparison of a dimethicone/antacid (Asilone gel) with an alginate/antacid (Gaviscon liquid) in the management of reflux oesophagitis. Journal of the Royal Society of Medicine 83:554–556

Soo S, Moayyedi P, Deeks J et al 2000 Pharmacological interventions for non-ulcer dyspepsia (Cochrane Review). In: The Cochrane Library, Issue 3. Update Software, Oxford

Web sites

The British Society of Gastroenterology: www.bsg.org.uk

Diarrhoea

Background

Diarrhoea can be defined as an increase in frequency of the passage of soft or watery stools relative to the usual bowel habit for that individual. It can be classed as acute (less than 7 days), persistent (more than 14 days) or chronic (lasting longer than a month). Most patients will present to the pharmacy with a self-diagnosis of acute diarrhoea. It is necessary to confirm this self-diagnosis because patients' interpretations of their symptoms might not match up with the medical definition of diarrhoea.

Prevalence and epidemiology

The exact prevalence and epidemiology of diarrhoea is not well known. This is probably due to the number of patients who do not seek care or who self medicate. However, acute diarrhoea is extremely common and has been reported as being the second most common medical problem in households in the US, with all age groups experiencing between one to two episodes per year.

Aetiology

The aetiology of diarrhoea depends on its cause. Acute gastroenteritis, the most common cause of diarrhoea in all age groups, is usually viral in origin. Commonly implicated viruses are the rotavirus, the Norwalk virus

and the Norwalk-like virus. Rotaviruses are the most common cause of diarrhoea in children under the age of 2. The faecal–oral route transmits all three types of virus. Viral replication results in blunting of the villi of the upper small intestine decreasing the absorptive surface.

Bacterial causes, for example *Shigella* and *Salmonella* species are invasive, penetrating the mucosa of the small intestine, whereas *Escherichia coli* (the cause of traveller's diarrhoea) and *Bacillus* produce toxins stimulating the active secretion of electrolytes into the intestinal lumen. Bacterial causes of diarrhoea are normally a result of eating contaminated food or drink.

Arriving at a differential diagnosis

Acute diarrhoea is rarely life threatening. The most common causes of diarrhoea are viral or bacterial infection and the community pharmacist can appropriately manage the vast majority of cases. The main priority is identifying those patients who need referral and how quickly they need to be referred. Dehydration is the main complicating factor, especially in the very young and very old. Questions aimed at establishing the frequency, fluidity and nature of the stools should enable a patient self-diagnosis to be rejected or confirmed. A number of diarrhoea specific questions should always be asked of the patient to aid in diagnosis (Table 6.10).

Clinical features of acute diarrhoea

Symptoms are normally rapid in onset, with the patient having a history of prior good health. Nausea and vomiting might be present prior to or during the bout of acute diarrhoea. Abdominal cramping and tenderness is also often present. If rotavirus is the cause then the patient might also experience viral prodromal symptoms such as cough and cold. Acute infective diarrhoea is usually watery in nature with no blood present. Complete resolution of symptoms should be observed in 2 to 4 days. However, diarrhoea caused by the rotavirus can persist for longer.

Conditions to eliminate

Giardiasis

Giardiasis, a protozoal infection of the small intestine, is contracted through drinking contaminated drinking water. It is an uncommon cause of diarrhoea in Western society. However, with more people taking exotic foreign holidays, enquiry about recent travel should be made. The patient will present with watery and foul-smelling diarrhoea accompanied by symptoms of bloating, flatulence and epigastric pain. If giardiasis is suspected the patient must be referred to the GP quickly for confirmation and appropriate antibiotic treatment.

Table 6.10
Specific questions to ask the patient: Diarrhoea

Question	Relevance
Frequency and nature of the stools	<ul><li>Patients with acute, self-limiting diarrhoea will be passing watery stools more frequently than normal</li><li>Diarrhoea associated with blood and mucus requires referral to eliminate invasive infection, such as *Shigella,* and conditions such as inflammatory bowel disease</li></ul>
Periodicity	<ul><li>A history of recurrent diarrhoea of no known cause should be referred for further investigation</li></ul>
Duration	<ul><li>A person who presents with a history of chronic diarrhoea should be referred. The most frequent causes of chronic diarrhoea are IBS, inflammatory disease and colon cancer</li></ul>
Onset of symptoms	<ul><li>Ingestion of bacterial pathogens can give rise to symptoms in a matter of a few hours after eating contaminated food (toxin-producing bacteria) or up to 3 days later. It is therefore important to ask about food consumption over the last few days, establish if anyone else ate the same food and to check the status of his or her health</li></ul>
Timing of diarrhoea	<ul><li>Patients who experience diarrhoea first thing in the morning might have underlying pathology such as IBS</li><li>Nocturnal diarrhoea is often associated with inflammatory bowel disease</li></ul>
Recent change of diet	<ul><li>Changes in diet can cause changes to bowel function, for example when away on holiday. If the person has recently been to a non-Western country then giardiasis is a possibility</li></ul>
Signs of dehydration	<ul><li>Mild (< 5%) dehydration is characterised by slightly dry mucous membranes, loss of skin turgor and sunken eyes</li><li>Moderate (5 to 10%) dehydration is characterised by sunken fontanelle and eyes, dry mouth, decreased urine output and the patient will be moderately thirsty</li></ul>

Irritable bowel syndrome

Patients younger than 45 with lower abdominal pain and a history of alternating diarrhoea and constipation are likely to have IBS. For further details on IBS see page 124.

Medicine-induced diarrhoea

A variety of medicines – both POM and OTC – can induce diarrhoea (Table 6.11). If medication is suspected as the cause of the diarrhoea the GP should be consulted and an alternative suggested.

Ulcerative colitis and Crohn's disease

Both conditions are characterised by chronic inflammation at various sites in the GI tract and follow periods of remission and relapse. They can affect any age group, although peak incidence is between 20 and 30 years of age. In mild cases of both conditions, diarrhoea is one of the major presenting symptoms, although blood in the stool is usually present. Patients might also find that they have urgency, nocturnal diarrhoea and early morning rushes. In the acute phase patients will appear unwell and have malaise.

Malabsorption syndromes

Lactose intolerance is often diagnosed in infants under 1 year old. In addition to more frequent loose bowel

Table 6.11
Medicines that commonly cause diarrhoea

Magnesium containing antacids
Broad-spectrum antibiotics
NSAIDs
Digoxin at high doses
Excessive alcohol or caffeine ingestion
Proton-pump inhibitors
Thiazide diuretics

movements symptoms such as fever, vomiting, perianal excoriation and a failure to gain weight might occur.

Coeliac disease has a bimodal incidence: first, in early infancy when cereals become a major constituent of the diet, and second, during the fourth and fifth decades. Steatorrhoea (fatty stools) is common and might be observed by the patient as frothy or floating stools in the toilet pan. Bloating and weight loss in the presence of a normal appetite might also be observed.

Faecal impaction

Faecal impaction is most commonly seen in the elderly and those with poor mobility. Patients might present with continuous soiling as a result of liquid passing around hard stools and mistakenly believe they have diarrhoea. On questioning, the patient might describe the passage of regular poorly formed hard stools that are difficult to pass. Referral is needed because manual removal of the faeces is often required.

Colorectal cancer

Any middle-aged patient presenting with a longstanding change of bowel habit must be viewed with suspicion. Persistent diarrhoea accompanied by a feeling that the bowel has not really been emptied is suggestive of neoplasm. This is especially true if weight loss is also present.

Figure 6.9 will aid differentiation of diarrhoeal cases that require referral.

Evidence base for over-the-counter medication

Acute infectious diarrhoea still remains one of the leading causes of death in developing countries, despite

> **! TRIGGER POINTS indicative of referral: Diarrhoea**
>
> - Change in bowel habit in patients over 50
> - Diarrhoea following recent travel to tropical or subtropical climate
> - Duration longer than 2 to 3 days in children and elderly
> - Patients unable to drink fluids
> - Presence of blood or mucus in the stool
> - Rectal bleeding
> - Signs of dehydration
> - Severe abdominal pain
> - Steatorrhoea
> - Suspected faecal impaction in the elderly

advances in its treatment. In developed and Western countries diarrhoeal disease is primarily of economic and socially disruptive significance. Goals of OTC treatment in the UK are therefore concentrated on relief of symptoms.

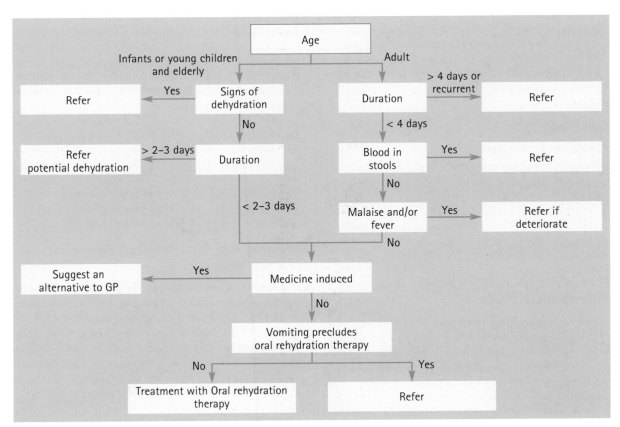

Fig. 6.9 Primer for differential diagnosis of diarrhoea

Oral rehydration therapy

Oral rehydration therapy (ORT) represents one of the major advances in medicine. It has proved to be a simple, highly effective treatment that has decreased mortality and morbidity associated with acute diarrhoea in developing countries. Solutions of glucose and electrolytes were first used in the 1940s but it wasn't until the 1970s and 1980s that a standardised solution was adopted and actively promoted by the World Health Organization (WHO). The standard WHO ORT provides 90 mEq/L sodium, 20 mEq/L potassium, 80 mEq/L chloride, 30 mEq/L bicarbonate and 111 mmol/L glucose. Constituents in proprietary products available in the UK have a lower sodium content (50 to 60 mEq/L) than the WHO ORT formula as people in Western society tend not to suffer sodium loss. ORT with 50 mEq/L sodium or less do, however, satisfactorily rehydrate otherwise healthy children who are mildly or moderately dehydrated. Products with lower sodium concentrations are also less likely to cause hypernatraemia, which has been observed when the WHO formula has been given as maintenance therapy after initial rehydration.

Rice-based ORT

In many developing countries a glucose substitute was added to electrolytes because of glucose unavailability. These products were found to be quite successful. Clinical trials have subsequently shown rice-based ORT to be highly efficacious, well tolerated and potentially more effective than conventional ORT.

Loperamide

Loperamide is thought to exert its action via opiate receptors slowing intestinal tract time and increasing the capacity of the gut. It has been extensively researched, with many published trials investigating its effectiveness in acute infectious diarrhoea. The majority of well-designed double-blind placebo-controlled trials have consistently shown it to be significantly better than placebo and comparable to diphenoxylate.

Bismuth subsalicylate

Bismuth-containing products have been used for many decades. Its use has declined over time as other products have become more popular. However, bismuth subsalicylate has been shown to be effective in treating traveller's diarrhoea. A review paper by Steffen (1990) concluded that bismuth subsalicylate was clinically superior to placebo, decreasing the number of unformed stools and increasing the number of patients who were symptom free. However, two of the trials reviewed showed bismuth subsalicylate to be significantly slower in symptom resolution than its comparator drug loperamide.

Kaolin and morphine

This product has no evidence to support its use and should not be recommended. However, it remains a popular home remedy, especially with the elderly.

Rotavirus vaccine

The US FDA approved a licence in August 1998 for the first rotavirus vaccine (RotaShield). In controlled trials this was found to prevent at least 50% of all rotavirus cases and nearly 100% of associated dehydration. A rare side-effect of intussusception (intestinal obstruction) occurred in just five of approximately 10 000 vaccine recipients but this number was not significantly higher than among those who had received placebo. Post-marketing surveillance revealed 15 cases of intussusception in an estimated 1.5 million doses and led to the vaccine being withdrawn from the market in the autumn of 1999. However, a *Lancet* article in 2001 questioned this finding, stating that the benefit:risk ratio favours its use in developing countries and recommending that the worldwide withdrawal of the vaccine should be reviewed.

Summary

ORT is effective in re-establishing normal fluid balance and should be first-line treatment for all age groups, especially children. Loperamide is a useful adjunct in reducing the number of bowel movements but should be reserved for those patients who will find it very inconvenient to have to go to the toilet. It is probably the medicine of choice for adults who want to be rid of symptoms as soon as possible.

Practical prescribing and product selection

Prescribing information relating to the medicines used for diarrhoea reviewed in the section 'Evidence base for over-the-counter medication' is discussed and summarised in Table 6.12; useful tips relating to patients presenting with diarrhoea are given in Hints and Tips Box 6.5.

ORT (e.g. Dioralyte, Rehydrat, Electrolade, Diocalm Replenish)

ORT can be given to all patient groups, has no side-effects or drug interactions. The volume of solution given depends on how much fluid has been lost. As infants and the elderly are more at risk of developing dehydration they should be encouraged to drink as much ORT as possible. Children and adults should usually take between 200 and 400 mL after each loose motion and parents should give 1 to $1^1/_2$ times the usual feed volume to infants.

Loperamide (e.g. Arret, Diocalm Ultra, Imodium)

The dose is two capsules immediately followed by one capsule after each further bout of diarrhoea. It has minimal CNS side-effects, although CNS depressant

Table 6.12
Practical prescribing: Summary of medicines for diarrhoea

Medicine	Use in children	Likely side-effects	Drug interactions of note	Patients in whom care should be exercised	Pregnancy
ORT	Infant upwards	None	None	None	OK
Loperamide	> 12 years	Abdominal cramps, nausea, vomiting, tiredness	None	None	OK
Bismuth	> 6 years	Black stools or tongue	Quinolone antibiotics	None	OK, but manufacturers state avoid
Morphine salts Kaolin and morphine	> 12 years	None	None	None	OK
Diocalm	> 6 years				

HINTS AND TIPS BOX 6.5: ORAL REHYDRATION THERAPY

Reconstitution of ORT	The volume of water required to make up sachets depends on the brand used. For example, Diorolyte requires 200 mL water per sachet whereas Rehidrat needs 250 mL water. Once reconstituted, ORT must be stored in the fridge and drunk within 24 h
Rough guidelines for referral for children	< 1 year old: refer if duration > 1 day < 3 years old: refer if duration > 2 days > 3 years old: refer if duration > 3 days
Kaolin and morphine	Subject to abuse. Store out of sight

effects and respiratory depression have been reported at high doses. OTC doses are therefore limited to 16 mg a day and cannot be used in children under 12. The excellent safety record of loperamide has seen it granted General Sales List status, although abdominal cramps, nausea, vomiting, tiredness, drowsiness, dizziness and dry mouth have been reported. Loperamide is also available as dispersible tablets, melt-tabs and liquid (the Imodium range of products).

Bismuth (Pepto–Bismol)

Adults and children over 14 should take 30 mL, repeated every 30 to 60 min if needed, to a maximum of 240 mL in 24 h. Children aged between 10 and 14 should take 20 mL, to a maximum of 160 mL, and children between the ages of 6 and 10 should take 10 mL, to a maximum of 80 mL in 24 h. Bismuth subsalicylate is well tolerated and has a favourable side-effect profile, although black stools are commonly observed (caused by unabsorbed bismuth compound). Occasional use is not known to cause problems during pregnancy but the manufacturers state it should not be taken during pregnancy. Bismuth can decrease the bioavailability of quinolone antibiotics and a minimum 2-h gap should therefore be left between doses of each medicine.

Morphine (e.g. Kaolin and morphine, Diocalm Dual Action)

Morphine is generally well tolerated at OTC doses, with no side-effects reported. The products can be given to all patient groups, including pregnant women. There are no drug interactions of note.

Kaolin and morphine

This can only be given to adults and children over the age of 12. The normal dose is 10 mL every 4 h.

Diocalm Dual Action

Adults and children over the age of 12 should take two tablets every 2 to 4 h, as required; children aged 6 to 12 years should take half the adult dose.

Further reading

American Academy of Pediatrics (AAP) Committee on Quality Improvement SoAG 1996 Practice parameter. The management of acute gastroenteritis in young children. Pediatrics 97:4224–4433

Amery W, Duyck F, Polak J et al 1975 A multicentre double-blind study in acute diarrhoea comparing loperamide (R 18553) with two common antidiarrhoeal agents and a placebo. Current Therapeutic Research, Clinical and Experimental 17:263–270

Cornett J W D, Aspeling R L, Mallegol D 1977 A double blind comparative evaluation of loperamide versus diphenoxylate with atropine in acute diarrhoea. Current Therapeutic Research, Clinical and Experimental 21:629–637

Farthing M J G 1994 Oral rehydration therapy. Pharmacology and Therapeutics 64:477–492

Gavin N, Merrick N, Davidson B 1996 Efficacy of glucose-based oral rehydration therapy. Pediatrics 98:45–51

Islam A, Molla A M, Ahmed M A et al 1994 Is rice based oral rehydration therapy effective in young infants? Archives of Diseases of Childhood 71:19–23

Kroser J A, Metz D C 1996 Evaluation of the adult patient with diarrhoea. Gastroenterology 23:629–647

Molla A M, Sarker S A, Hossain M et al 1982 Rice-powder electrolyte solution as oral-therapy in diarrhoea due to *Vibrio cholerae* and *Escherichia coli*. Lancet 1(8285):1317–1319

Nelemans F A, Zelvelder W G 1976 A double-blind placebo controlled trial of loperamide (Imodium) in acute diarrhoea. Journal of Drug Research 2:54–59

Patra F C, Mahalanabis D, Jalan K N et al 1982 Is oral rice electrolyte solution superior to glucose electrolyte solution in infantile diarrhoea? Archives of Diseases of Childhood 57:910–912

Powell D W, Szauter K E 1993 Non-antibiotic therapy and pharmacotherapy of acute infectious diarrhoea. Gastroenterology Clinics of North America 22:683–707

Selby W 1990 Diarrhoea-differential diagnosis. Australian Family Physician 19:1683–1686

Steffen R 1990 Worldwide efficacy of bismuth subsalicylate in the treatment of travelers' diarrhea. Review of Infectious Diseases 12:S80–S86

Web sites
General information on diarrhoea: www.diarrhoea.org/index.html
National Association for Colitis and Crohn's disease (NACC): www.nacc.org.uk
Proctor and Gamble product site: www.pepto-bismol.com/

Constipation

Background

Constipation, like diarrhoea, means different things to different people. Constipation arises when the patient experiences a reduction in their normal bowel habit accompanied with more difficult defecation and/or hard stools. However, many people still believe that anything other than one bowel movement a day is abnormal.

Prevalence and epidemiology

Constipation is extremely common. It occurs in all age groups but is especially prevalent in the elderly. It has been estimated that 25 to 40% of all people over the age of 65 have constipation. The majority of the elderly have normal frequency of bowel movements but strain at stool. This is probably a result of sedentary lifestyle, a decreased fluid intake, poor nutrition, avoidance of fibrous foods and chronic illness. Women are three times more likely to suffer from constipation than men.

Aetiology

Intestinal transit time is increased, which allows greater water resorption from the large bowel leading to harder stools that are more difficult to pass. This is most frequently caused by a deficiency in dietary fibre, a change in lifestyle and/or environment and medication. Occasionally, patients ignore the defecatory reflex because it might be inconvenient for them to defecate.

Arriving at a differential diagnosis

The first thing a pharmacist should do is confirm that the patient is suffering from constipation. Questioning should then concentrate on establishing the cause. Constipation does not usually have sinister pathology and the most common cause in the vast majority of non-elderly adults will be a lack of dietary fibre, although in the elderly the cause might be multifactorial. A number of constipation-specific questions should be asked of the patient to aid in diagnosis (Table 6.13).

Clinical features of constipation

Besides the inability to defecate, patients might also have abdominal discomfort and bloating. In children, parents might also notice that the child is more irritable and has a decreased appetite. Specks of blood in the toilet pan might be present and are usually due to straining at stool. In the vast majority of cases, blood in the stool does not indicate sinister pathology. Those patients presenting with acute constipation with no other symptoms apart from very small amounts of bright red blood can be managed in the pharmacy, however, if blood loss is substantial (stools appear tarry, red or black) or the patient has other associated symptoms, such as malaise or abdominal distension, and is over 40 years old then referral is needed.

Conditions to eliminate

Medicine-induced constipation

A detailed medication history should always be sought from the patient because many medicines can cause constipation. Table 6.14 lists some of the more commonly implicated medicines that cause constipation.

Table 6.13
Specific questions to ask the patient: Constipation

Question	Relevance
Change of diet or routine	● Constipation usually has a social or behavioural cause. There will usually be some event that has precipitated the onset of symptoms
Pain on defecation	● Associated pain when going to the toilet is usually due to a local anorectal problem. Constipation is often secondary to the suppression of defecation because it induces pain. These cases are best referred for physical examination
Presence of blood	● Bright red specks in the toilet or smears on toilet tissue suggest haemorrhoids or a tear in the anal canal (fissure). However, if blood is mixed in the stool (melaena) then referral to the GP is necessary. A stool that appears black and tarry is suggestive of an upper GI bleed
Duration (chronic or recent?)	● Constipation lasting 6 weeks or more is said to be chronic. If a patient suffers from longstanding constipation and has been previously seen by the GP then treatment could be given. However, cases of more than 14 days with no identifiable cause or previous investigation by the GP should be referred
Lifestyle changes	● Changes in job or marital status can precipitate depressive illness that can manifest with physiological symptoms such as constipation

Table 6.14
Medicines known to cause constipation

Anticholinergics, e.g. TCAs, antiparkinsonian drugs, antipsychotics
Antihypertensives, e.g. verapamil
Opiate analgesics
Aluminium-containing antacids
Iron
Sucralfate (contains aluminium)

Irritable bowel syndrome

Patients younger than 45 with lower abdominal pain and a history of alternating diarrhoea and constipation are likely to have IBS. For further details on IBS see page 124.

Pregnancy

Constipation is common in pregnancy, especially in the third trimester. A combination of increased circulating progestogen, displacement of the uterus against the colon by the fetus, decreased mobility and iron supplementation all contribute to an increased incidence of constipation when pregnant. Most patients complain of hard stools rather than a decrease in bowel movements. If a laxative is used, a bulk-forming laxative should be recommended.

Functional causes in children

Constipation in children is common and the cause can be varied. Constipation is not normally a result of organic disease but stems from a traumatic experience associated with defecation, for example, unwillingness to defecate due to association of prior pain on defecation.

Depression

Upwards of 20% of the population will suffer from depression at some time. Many will present with physical rather than emotional symptoms. It has been reported that a third of all patients suffering from depression present with gastrointestinal complaints in a primary care setting.

Colorectal cancer

Colorectal carcinomas are rare in patients under the age of 40. However, the incidence of carcinoma increases with increasing age and any patient over the age of 40 presenting for the first time with a marked change in bowel habit should be referred. The patient might complain of abdominal pain, rectal bleeding and tenesmus. Weight loss – a classic textbook sign of colon cancer – is common but observed only in the latter stages of the disease. Therefore a patient is unlikely to have noticed marked weight loss when visiting a pharmacy early in disease progression.

Hypothyroidism

Hypothyroidism affects ten times more women than men. The signs and symptoms of hypothyroidism are often subtle and insidious in onset. Patients can experience weight gain, lethargy, coarse hair and dry skin as well as constipation. Because of the nature of the changes involved, patients might present with constipation because this is the symptom that causes them the most inconvenience.

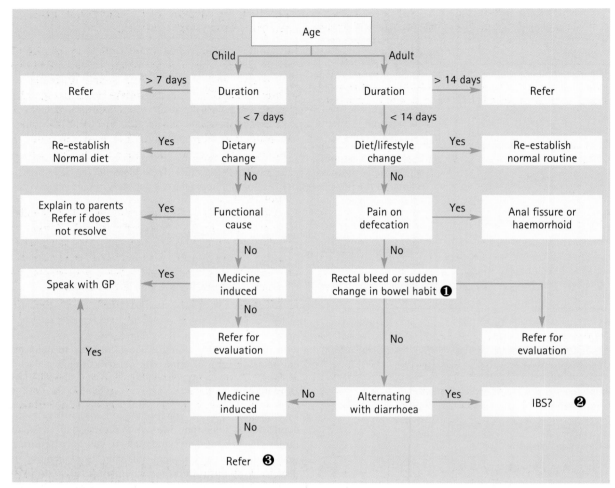

Fig. 6.10 Primer for differential diagnosis of constipation

❶ Patients with unexplained constipation of recent onset accompanied with rectal bleeding should be referred for further investigation; most likely a colonoscopy or sigmoidoscopy and stool culture to eliminate carcinoma

❷ See Fig. 6.11 for primer for differential diagnosis of IBS.

❸ If no obvious cause of constipation can be found referral to the GP is needed for further evaluation.

Figure 6.10 will aid differentiation between common causes of constipation and more serious causes.

> **TRIGGER POINTS indicative of referral: Constipation**
>
> - Blood in stool
> - Greater than 7 days duration with no identifiable cause
> - Pain on defecation causing patient to suppress defecatory reflex
> - Patients aged over 40 years old with sudden change in bowel habits with no obvious cause
> - Suspected depression

Evidence base for over-the-counter medication

Simple dietary and lifestyle modifications, such as increasing fruit and vegetables in the diet, fluid intake and exercise, will relieve the majority of acute cases of constipation.

If medication is required, four classes of OTC laxatives are available: bulk-forming agents, stimulants, osmotic laxatives and stool softeners. Despite their widespread use surprisingly few well-designed trials have substantiated clinical efficacy.

A recent systematic review by Tramonte et al (1997) identified 36 trials that met their inclusion criteria; these involved 25 different laxatives representing all four classes of laxative. Twenty of the trials compared laxative against placebo or regular diet, 13 of which demonstrated statistically significant increases in bowel movement. The remaining 16 trials compared different types of laxatives with each other. The review concluded that laxatives do increase the number of bowel movements and, in 9 of 11 trials studying overall symptom control, laxatives did perform significantly better than placebo. Unfortunately, because of a lack of comparative trial data, the review could not conclude which laxative was most efficacious.

A further review of laxative effect in elderly patients suffering with chronic constipation also failed to determine superior clinical effect between laxative classes. (See Petticrew et al, 1999.)

Summary

It appears from the evidence that laxatives do work, but deciding on which laxative to give a patient cannot be made on an evidence-based approach. Other factors will need to be considered such as the patient's status, the side-effect profile of the medicine and its cost.

Practical prescribing and product selection

Prescribing information relating to the medicines used for constipation reviewed in the section 'Evidence base for over-the-counter medication' is discussed and summarised in Table 6.15; useful tips relating to these medicines are given in Hints and Tips Box 6.6.

Bulk-forming laxatives (e.g. ispaghula husk, methylcellulose and sterculia)

Bulk-forming laxatives exert their effect by mimicking increased fibre consumption swelling in the bowel and increasing faecal mass. Patients should therefore be advised to increase their fluid intake when taking bulk-forming medicines. The laxative effect can take up to 72 h and commonly causes flatulence and abdominal distension. Bulk-forming laxatives are well tolerated in pregnancy and have no teratogenic effects. They appear to have no drug interactions of any note.

Ispaghula husk

Ispaghula husk is widely available as either granules (Fybogel and Isogel) or powder (Ispagel, Konsyl or Regulan). All have to be reconstituted with water prior to taking. The dose for adults and children over 12 years old can range from one to three sachets a day, depending on the brand used and the severity of the condition.

The dose for Isogel is two teaspoonfuls once or twice daily. For children over 6 the dose is half the adult dose.

Methylcellulose (Celevac)

Methylcellulose is only available as Celevac tablets. The product is recommended only for adults and the dose is three to six tablets twice daily. Each dose should be taken with at least 300 mL of liquid.

Table 6.15
Practical prescribing: Summary of medicines for constipation

Medicine	Use in children	Likely side-effects	Drug interactions of note	Patients in whom care should be exercised	Pregnancy
Bulk-forming laxatives					
Ispaghula husk	> 6 years	Flatulence and abdominal bloating	None	None	OK
Methylcellulose	Not recommended				
Sterculia	> 6 years				
Stimulant laxatives					
Senna	> 2 years	Abdominal pain	None	None	OK
Glycerol	Infant upwards				
Sodium picosulfate	> 4 years				
Bisacodyl	Infant upwards				
Osmotic laxatives					
Lactulose	Infant upwards	Flatulence, abdominal pain and colic	None	None	OK
Lactitol	> 1 year				
Magnesium hydroxide	Not recommended				
Stool softeners					
Docusate	> 6 months	None reported	None	None	OK

HINTS AND TIPS BOX 6.6: CONSTIPATION

Administration of suppositories	1. Wash your hands 2. Lie on one side with your knees pulled up towards your chest 3. Gently push the suppository, pointed end first, into your back passage with your finger 4. Push the suppository in as far as possible 5. Lower your legs, roll over onto your stomach and remain still for a few minutes 6. If you feel your body trying to expel the suppository, try to resist this. Lie still and press your buttocks together 7. Wash your hands
Sachets containing ispaghula husk	Once the granules have been mixed with water the drink should be taken as soon as the effervescence subsides because the drink 'sets' and becomes undrinkable
Prolonged use of lactulose	In children this can contribute to the development of dental caries. Patients should be instructed to pay careful attention to dental hygiene
Lactulose taste	The taste is unpalatable to many patients, especially if high doses need to be taken
Bisacodyl	Bisacodyl tablets are enterically coated and therefore patients should be told to avoid taking antacids and milk at the same time because the coating could be broken down, leading to dyspepsia and gastric irritation
Laxative abuse	Some people, especially young women, use laxatives as a slimming aid. Any very slim person who is purchasing laxatives regularly should be asked politely about why they are taking the laxatives. An opening question could be phrased 'We've noticed that you have been buying quite a lot of these and we are concerned that you should be better by now, is there anything we can do for you to help?'
Onset of action	Stimulants are the quickest-acting laxative, usually within 6 to 12 h. Lactulose and bulk-forming laxatives can take 48 to 72 h before an effect is seen

Sterculia (Normacol and Normacol Plus granules or sachets)

Both products contain 62% sterculia but Normacol Plus also contains 8% frangula. The dose for both products is the same. Adults and children over 12 should take either one or two sachets or heaped 5 mL spoonfuls, once or twice daily after meals. For children aged between 6 and 12 the dose is half that of the adult dose.

The granules should be placed dry on the tongue and swallowed immediately with plenty of water or a cool drink. They can also be sprinkled onto and taken with soft food such as yoghurt.

Stimulant laxatives (e.g. bisacodyl, glycerol, senna, sodium picosulfate)

Stimulant laxatives increase GI motility. It is this action that, presumably, causes the abdominal pain that is the main side-effect associated with stimulant laxatives. Additionally, stimulant laxatives are associated with the possibility of nerve damage with long-term use and are the most commonly abused laxatives. Their onset of action is quicker than other laxative classes, with patients experiencing a bowel movement in 6 to 12 h. They can be taken by all patient groups, have no drug interactions and are safe in pregnancy.

Bisacodyl (Dulco-Lax)

Bisacodyl is available as either tablets or suppositories and can be given to patients of all ages. The dose should be taken at bedtime. Children under 4 should use paediatric suppositories (5 mg). For children aged between 4 and 10 years the dose is 5 mg (one tablet) and for adults and children over 10 years the dose is 5 to 10 mg (one to two tablets).

Glycerol suppositories

Glycerol suppositories are normally used when a bowel movement is needed quickly. The patient should experience a bowel movement in 15 to 30 min. Varying sizes are made and can be used by all ages. The 1-g suppositories are designed for infants, the 2-g for children and the 4-g for adults.

Senna (e.g. Senokot, Nylax)

Senna is available as either syrup or tablets; both formulations deliver 7.5 mg of sennoside per dose. Adults and children over 12 should take 15 to 30 mg (two to four 5-mL spoonfuls or two to four tablets) each day. For children over 6 the dose is half that of the adult dose and for children over the age of 2 the dose is 3.75 to 7.5 mg (half to one 5-mL spoonful) each day.

Sodium picosulfate (Laxoberal Liquid)

Adults and children over 10 years old should take one to two 5-mL spoonfuls (5 to 10 mg) at night. Children aged between 4 and 10 years old can take half the adult dose (half to one 5-mL spoonful (2.5 to 5 mg) at night. Children aged under 4 can take Laxoberal but the dose must be based on the child's weight (250 µg per kg).

Osmotic laxatives (e.g. Lactulose, magnesium salts)

These act by retaining fluid in the bowel by osmosis or by changing the pattern of water distribution in the faeces. Flatulence, abdominal pain and colic are frequently reported. They can be taken by all patient groups, have no drug interactions and can be safely used in pregnancy.

Lactulose

Lactulose is given twice daily for all ages. The dose for adults is 15 mL, for children aged between 5 and 10 the dose is 10 mL, for those aged between 1 and 5 the dose is 5 mL and children under 1 year of age 2.5 mL. The dose for all ages can be reduced according to the need of the patient after 2 to 3 days. It has been reported that up to 20% of patients experience troublesome flatulence and cramps, although these often settle after a few days.

Lactitol is chemically very similar to lactulose and is taken in sachet form. It has the advantage of only being taken once daily compared to twice daily dosing for lactulose.

Magnesium salts

Magnesium when used as a laxative is usually given as magnesium hydroxide. The adult dose ranges between 20 to 50 mL when needed. It is generally not recommended for use in children but is commonly prescribed in the elderly.

Stool softeners (liquid paraffin and docusate sodium)

Liquid paraffin

Liquid paraffin has been traditionally used to treat constipation. However, the adverse side-effect profile of liquid paraffin now means it should never be recommended because other, safer and more effective medications are now available. There are also case reports of death caused by aspiration of liquid paraffin leading to lipid pneumonia.

Docusate sodium

Docusate acts as both a softening agent and a stimulant. Docusate is available as either capsules (Dioctyl) or solution (Docusal). It can be given to children aged 6 months and over. Children between the age of 6 months and 2 years should take 12.5 mg (5 mL of Docusal Paediatric solution) three times a day. For children aged between 2 and 12 the dose is 12.5 mg to 25 mg (5 to 10 mL) three times a day. Adults and children over 12 years old should take up to 500 mg daily in divided doses. In contrast to liquid paraffin, docusate sodium seems to be almost free of any side-effects. Docusate sodium can be given to all patients, including pregnant women.

Further reading

Elliot D, Glover G R 1983 Large bowel perforation due to excessive bran ingestion. British Journal of Clinical Practice 37:32–33

Gattuso J M, Kamm M A 1994 Adverse effects of drugs used in the management of constipation and diarrhoea. Drug Safety 10:47–65

Gerber P D, Barrett J E, Barrett J A et al 1992 The relationship of presenting physical complaints to depressive symptoms in primary care patients. Journal of General Internal Medicine 170–173

Herz M J, Kahan E, Zalevski S et al 1996 Constipation: a different entity for patients and doctors. Family Practice 13:156–159

Johanson J F, Sonnenberg A, Koch T R 1989 Clinical epidemiology of chronic constipation. Journal of Clinical Gastroenterology 11:525–536

Lederle F A 1995 Epidemiology of constipation in elderly patients. Drug utilisation and cost-containment strategies. Drugs and Ageing 6:465–469

Leng-Peschlow E 1992 Senna and its rational use. Pharmacology 44:S1–S52

Marshall J B 1990 Chronic constipation in adults. How far should evaluation and treatment go? Postgraduate Medicine 88:49–51, 54, 57–59, 63

Murray F E, Bliss C M 1991 Geriatric constipation: brief update on a common problem. Geriatrics 46:64–68

Paraskevaides E C 1990 Fatal lipid pneumonia and liquid paraffin. British Journal of General Practice 44:509–510

Petticrew M, Watt I, Brand M 1999 What's the 'best buy' for treatment of constipation? Results of a systematic review of the efficacy and comparative efficacy of laxatives in the elderly. British Journal of General Practice 49:387–393

Sarner M 1976 Problems caused by laxatives. Practitioner 216:661–664

Talley N J, Fleming K C, Evans J M et al 1996 Constipation in an elderly community: a study of prevalence and potential risk factors. American Journal of Gastroenterology 9:19–25

Tramonte S M, Brand M B, Mulrow C D et al 1997 The treatment of chronic constipation in adults. A systematic review. Journal of General Internal Medicine 12:15–24

Watson J S, Ebert W R 1969 Lactulose: a new bowel regulator. Clinical Medicine July:24–26

Web sites

Charity for research and information on digestive disorders including constipation: www.digestivedisorders.org.uk/index.htm

Irritable bowel syndrome

Background

Irritable bowel syndrome (IBS) is one of the most common GI tract conditions seen in primary care. Approximately 25% of GP consultations for GI conditions are finally diagnosed as IBS. It can be defined as a functional bowel disorder in which abdominal pain is associated with a change in bowel habit. The diagnosis is suggested by the presence of longstanding colonic symptoms without any deterioration in the patient's general condition.

Prevalence and epidemiology

Irritable bowel syndrome occurs in 10 to 20% of people worldwide and is twice as common in females than males. It is most commonly diagnosed in young adults.

Aetiology

No anatomic cause can be found to explain the aetiology of IBS but it is almost certainly multifactorial, with emotional, dietary and hormonal theories suggested. Psychological factors strongly influence symptom reporting and consultation and some studies have shown that patients who suffer from higher levels of stress or depression experience worse symptoms than other patients. Flare-up of symptoms has also been associated with periods of increased stress. Symptoms of diarrhoea and constipation appear to be linked with hyperactivity of the small intestine and colon in response to food ingestion and parasympathomimetic drugs. Excessive parasympathomimetic activity might account for mucous associated with the stool.

Arriving at a differential diagnosis

IBS is essentially a diagnosis of exclusion and a careful and thorough history of the patient is essential. Diagnostic aids, such as rectal examination and biopsy, that can be used by GPs are of limited use. A number of IBS-specific questions should always be asked of the patient to aid in diagnosis (Table 6.16).

Clinical features of IBS

IBS is characterised by abdominal pain, located especially in the left lower quadrant of the abdomen, which is sometimes relieved by defecation or the passage of wind. Altered defecation, either constipation or diarrhoea, with associated bloating is also normally present. During bouts of diarrhoea, mucus tends to be visible on the stools. Patients might also complain of increased stool frequency but pass normal or pellet-like stools. Diarrhoea on wakening and shortly after meals is also observed in many patients.

Conditions to eliminate

Constipation and diarrhoea

Because the major presenting symptom of IBS is an alteration in defecation, it is necessary to differentiate IBS from acute and chronic causes of constipation and

Table 6.16
Specific questions to ask the patient: IBS

Question	Relevance
Age	● IBS usually affects people under the age of 40 ● Particular care is required in labelling middle-aged and elderly patients with IBS when presenting with bowel symptoms for the first time. Such patients are best referred for further evaluation to eliminate organic bowel disease
Periodicity	● IBS tends to be episodic. The patient might have a history of being well for a number of weeks or months in between bouts of symptoms
Presence of abdominal pain	● The nature of pain experienced with IBS can be very varied, ranging from localised and sharp to diffuse and aching. It is therefore not very discriminatory, however, the patient will probably have experienced similar abdominal pain in the past. Any change in the nature and severity of the pain is best referred for further evaluation
Location of pain	● Pain from IBS is normally located in the left lower quadrant. For further information on other conditions that cause pain in the lower abdomen see page 131
Associated symptoms	● Patients with IBS experience altered defecation. They do not have textbook definitions of constipation or diarrhoea but bowel function will be different from normal ● The presence of blood in the stool is not usual in IBS and can suggest inflammatory bowel disease

diarrhoea. For further information on differentiating these conditions from IBS please refer to page 124 (for constipation) and 113 (for diarrhoea).

Figure 6.11 will aid differentiation of IBS from other abdominal conditions.

> **❗ TRIGGER POINTS indicative of referral: Irritable bowel syndrome**
>
> - Blood in the stool
> - Children under 16
> - Patients over 40 with recent change to bowel habit
> - Patients with no previous history of IBS and have no precipitating factors

Evidence base for over-the-counter medication

A number of OTC medicines are marketed specifically for the treatment of IBS symptoms. These include mebeverine, alverine, hyoscine and peppermint oil. In addition, medicines to treat specific symptoms associated with IBS (e.g. loperamide to relieve diarrhoea) can be used. This text concentrates only on those products specifically marketed for the treatment of IBS.

Hyoscine

A number of trials have investigated the effectiveness of hyoscine in the treatment of IBS. However, only three trials of sufficient methodological quality allow conclusions to be drawn regarding its effectiveness. Each of the three trials demonstrated partial symptomatic improvement in some of the patients, although no trial proved hyoscine to be significantly better than placebo. A recent meta-analysis conducted by Poynard et al (2001) confirmed these findings and suggested that hyoscine was the least effective of the six smooth-muscle relaxant medicines reviewed.

Antispasmodics (mebeverine, alverine and peppermint oil)

Mebeverine has been available as a POM for many years and as a pharmacy medicine since 1996, yet trial data to support its effectiveness is mixed. Conclusions drawn from five well-designed trials (two conducted outside the

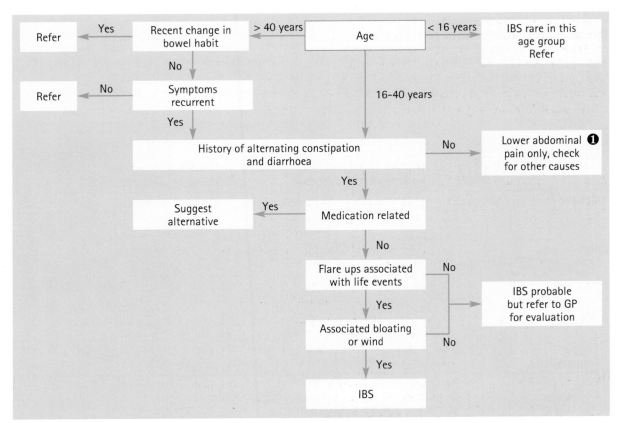

Fig. 6.11 Primer for differential diagnosis of irritable bowel syndrome (IBS)

❶ **Lower abdominal pain**
See Fig 6.27 for primer for differential diagnosis of abdominal pain.

UK) are conflicting. Of the three UK papers, two studies appear to show a significant effect and one no effect. The meta-analysis by Poynard et al suggests that a significant difference exists between mebeverine and placebo when data from all trials (including the two non-UK trials) are combined.

Even fewer trials appear to have been conducted with alverine than mebeverine. One study by Tudor (1986) compared alverine to mebeverine in 45 patients; the authors concluded that alverine had similar efficacy to mebeverine. However, no placebo group was included in this study and it is therefore unclear to what extent alverine is effective.

Peppermint oil is the major constituent of several OTC remedies yet it has little evidence to support its effectiveness. Pittler & Ernst (1998) evaluated eight randomised, controlled trials involving peppermint oil. Collectively, they indicate that peppermint oil could be efficacious for symptom relief in IBS but study design limitations meant that definitive judgement about efficacy was not possible.

Summary

On the basis of evidence, mebeverine should be the first-line choice.

Practical prescribing and product selection

Prescribing information relating to the medicines used for IBS reviewed in the section 'Evidence base for over-the-counter medication' is discussed and summarised in Table 6.17; useful tips relating to the treatment of patients presenting with IBS are given in Hints and Tips Box 6.7.

All marketed products can be given to children (see individual entries) but anyone aged under 16 suspected of having IBS for the first time should be referred to a GP.

Hyoscine butylbromide (Buscopan)

The recommended starting dose for adults is one tablet three times a day, although this can be increased to two tablets four times a day if necessary. It can be given to children over the age of 6 (one tablet three times a day). Buscopan is a quaternary derivative of hyoscine so it does not readily cross the blood–brain barrier and therefore sedation is not normally encountered, although it might cause dry mouth and constipation. Because of its anticholinergic effects it is best avoided with other medicines that also have anticholinergic effects, for example, antihistamines, tricyclic antidepressants, neuroleptics, and disopyramide. It can be given during pregnancy but patients with glaucoma, myasthenia gravis and prostate enlargement should not take Buscopan.

Mebeverine (e.g. Colofac IBS)

Adults and children 10 years and over should take one tablet three times a day, preferably 20 min before meals. Mebeverine is not known to interact with other medicines, has no cautions in its use and can be given in pregnancy. It is associated with very few side-effects although allergic reactions have been reported.

Table 6.17
Practical Prescribing: Summary of IBS Medicines

Medicine	Use in children	Likely side-effects	Drug interactions of note	Patients in whom care should be exercised	Pregnancy
Hyoscine (Buscopan)	> 6 years	Constipation and dry mouth	TCAs, neuroleptics, antihistamines and disopyramide	Glaucoma, myasthenia gravis and prostate enlargement	OK
Mebeverine Colofac IBS	> 10 years	None	None	None	OK
Peppermint oil Colpermin	> 15 years	Heartburn	None	None	OK
Mintec	Not recommended				
Alverine (Spasmonal)	> 12 years	Rash	None	None	OK

HINTS AND TIPS BOX 6.7: IRRITABLE BOWEL SYNDROME

Non-drug treatment	Hypnotherapy has been reported as being effective for some patients. A register of IBS therapists specialising in hypnotherapy can be found at www.ibs-register.co.uk

Alverine (Spasmonal)

Adults and children over 12 should take one or two capsules three times a day. It is suitable for pregnant women, has no interactions with other medicines and can be used by all patient groups. It can cause nausea, headache, dizziness, itching, rash and allergic reactions.

Peppermint oil (e.g. Mintec, Colpermin)

Adults and children aged over 15 can take peppermint oil. The dose is one capsule three times a day before food. It often causes heartburn and rarely allergic rashes have been reported. It is safe to use in pregnancy, has no drug interactions and can be used by all patient groups.

Further reading

Connell A M 1965 Physiological and clinical assessment of the effect of the musculotropic agent mebeverine on the human colon. British Medical Journal 5466:848–851

Farthing M J 1995 Irritable bowel, irritable body, or irritable brain? British Medical Journal 310:171–175

Jamieson D J, Steege J F 1996 The prevalence of dysmenorrhea, dyspareunia, pelvic pain, and irritable bowel syndrome in primary care practices. Obstetrics and Gynecology 87:55–58

Jones J, Spiller R 2001 IBS: current approaches to management. The Prescriber 5 November:93–100

Kruis W, Weinzierl M, Schussler P, Holl J 1986 Comparison of the therapeutic effect of wheat bran, mebeverine and placebo in patients with the irritable bowel syndrome. Digestion 34:196–201

Pittler M H, Ernst E 1998 Peppermint oil for irritable bowel syndrome: a critical review and metaanalysis. American Journal of Gastroenterology 93:1131–1135

Poynard T, Regimbeau C, Benhamou Y 2001 Meta-analysis of smooth muscle relaxants in the treatment of irritable bowel syndrome. Alimentary Pharmacology and Therapeutics 15:355–361

Ritchie J A, Truelove S C 1979 Treatment of irritable bowel syndrome with lorazepam, hyoscine butylbromide, and ispaghula husk. British Medical Journal 1979 1(6160):376–378

Tasmin-Jones C 1973 Mebeverine in patients with the irritable colon syndrome: double blind study. New Zealand Medical Journal 77:232–235

Tudor G J 1986 A general practice study to compare alverine citrate with mebeverine hydrochloride in the treatment of irritable bowel syndrome. British Journal of Clinical Practice 40:276–278

Whitehead W E, Crowell M D, Robinson J C et al 1992 Effects of stressful life events on bowel symptoms: subjects with irritable bowel syndrome compared with subjects without bowel dysfunction. Gut 33:825–830

Web sites

IBS Self-help groups: www.ibsgroup.org and www.ibsnetwork.org.uk

Haemorrhoids

Background

Haemorrhoids (piles) are a common complaint. Patients might feel embarrassed talking about symptoms and it is therefore important that any requests for advice are treated sympathetically and away from others to avoid embarrassment.

Prevalence and epidemiology

Haemorrhoids can occur at any age but are rare in children and adults under the age of 20. It has been estimated that up to 80% of all people will experience haemorrhoids at some point in their lifetime. Prevalence appears to increase with increasing age and is most common in patients aged between 40 and 65. There is a high incidence of haemorrhoids in pregnant women.

Aetiology

The cause of haemorrhoids is probably multifactorial with anatomical (degeneration of elastic tissue), physiological (increased anal canal pressure) and mechanical (straining at stool) processes implicated. Haemorrhoids have been traditionally described as engorged veins of the haemorrhoidal plexus. The analogy of varicose veins of the anal canal is often used but is misleading. Current thinking favours the theory of prolapsed anal cushions. Anal cushions are submucosal vascular structures attached to the anal mucosal wall. When sphincters relax veins in these cushions fill with blood and dilate; conversely, when the sphincter contracts blood empties out of the veins. Persistent straining against a relaxed sphincter causes the cushions – with their veins – to prolapse. Constipation and associated straining at stool are contributory factors in developing haemorrhoids.

Haemorrhoids can be classified as either external or internal. The differentiation is drawn from the anatomical location of the haemorrhoid. Superior to the anal sphincter there is an area known as the dentate line. At this junction epithelial cells change from squamous to columnar epithelial tissue. Above the dentate line haemorrhoids are classed as internal and below, external.

Arriving at a differential diagnosis

Patients who seek advice and help for haemorrhoids should be questioned carefully. Bleeding tends to cause the greatest concern and often instigates the patient to seek help. Invariably, rectal bleeding is of little consequence but should be investigated thoroughly to exclude sinister pathology. A number of haemorrhoid-specific questions should always be asked (Table 6.18).

Table 6.18
Specific questions to ask the patient: Haemorrhoids

Question	Relevance
Duration	• Patients with haemorrhoids tend to have had symptoms for some time before requesting advice. However, patients with symptoms that have been present for more than 3 weeks should be referred
Pain	• Pain associated with haemorrhoids tends to occur on defecation and at times other than defecation, for example when sitting. It is usually described as a dull ache • Sharp or stabbing pain at the time of defecation can suggest an anal fissure or tear
Rectal bleeding	• Slight rectal bleeding is often associated with haemorrhoids. Blood appears bright red and might be visible in the toilet bowl or on the surface of the stool. The presence of blood is usually a direct referral sign but if the cause is haemorrhoids this could be treated unless the patient is unduly anxious, in which case referral is appropriate • Blood mixed in the stool has to be referred to eliminate a GI bleed • Large volumes of blood or blood loss not associated with defecation must be referred to eliminate possible carcinoma
Associated symptoms	• Symptoms associated with haemorrhoids are usually localised, for example anal itching. Other symptoms such as nausea, vomiting, loss of appetite and altered bowel habit should be viewed with caution and underlying pathology suspected. Referral would be needed

Clinical features of haemorrhoids

Bleeding, pain and perianal itching can all occur. Often, patients are asymptomatic until the haemorrhoid prolapses. After defecation the haemorrhoids might return to their normal position spontaneously or be reduced manually. Any blood associated is bright red and is most commonly seen as spotting around the toilet pan, streaking on toilet tissue or visible on the surface of the stool.

Pain is experienced when the patient has external haemorrhoids that have become thrombosed. The pain is often described as a 'dull ache' that increases in severity when the patient defecates. Patients might therefore ignore the urge to defecate, which can lead to constipation that, in turn, will lead to more difficulty in passing stools and increase the pain associated with defecation.

Conditions to eliminate

Dermatitis

If pruritus is the chief presenting complaint and the patient does not complain of bleeding or prolapse then the most likely cause of their condition is contact dermatitis caused by toiletries.

Conditions causing rectal bleeding

A number of conditions can present with varying degrees of rectal bleeding. However, other symptoms should be present to allow them to be excluded.

Anal fissure

Anal fissures are common and are normally caused by straining at stool. Pain can be intense on defecation and

the blood is bright red. Non-urgent referral is necessary for confirmation of the diagnosis. In the meantime the patient should be instructed to eat more fibre and increase fluid intake.

Ulcerative colitis and Crohn's disease

Other symptoms besides blood in the stool are usually present with ulcerative colitis and Crohn's disease. These tend to be stools that are watery, abdominal pain and fever. Patients will appear unwell and also find that they have urgency, nocturnal diarrhoea and early morning rushes. In the acute phase patients will have malaise.

Upper GI bleeds

Erosion of the stomach wall or upper intestine is normally responsible for GI bleeds and is often associated with NSAID intake. The colour of the stool is related to the rate of bleeding. Stools from GI bleeds can be tarry (indicating a bleed of 100 to 200 mL of blood) or black (indicating a bleed of 400 to 500 mL of blood). Urgent referral is needed.

Colorectal cancer

Any middle-aged patient presenting with a change of bowel habit, especially if long established, must be viewed with suspicion. Colorectal bleeds depend on the site of tumour, for example sigmoid tumours lead to bright red blood in or around the stool. Rectal bleeding tends to be persistent and steady though slight for all tumours.

Figure 6.12 will aid the differentiation of haemorrhoids.

Evidence base for over-the-counter medication

Numerous products are marketed for the relief and treatment of haemorrhoids. These include a wide range of

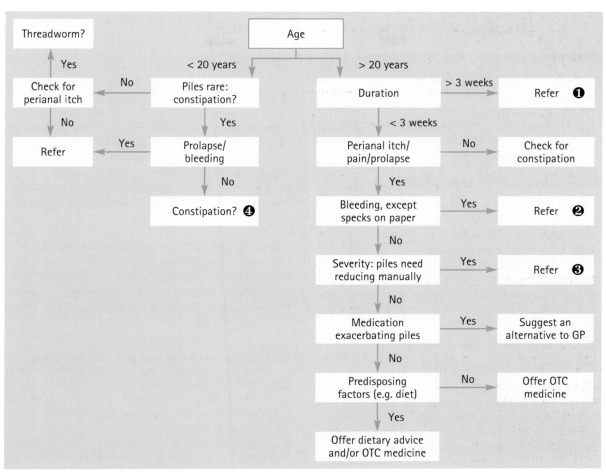

Fig. 6.12 Primer for differential diagnosis of haemorrhoids

❶ Duration
Patients with long-standing symptoms that have not been seen previously by the GP should be referred to eliminate any underlying pathology. In the vast majority of cases no sinister findings will result.

❷ Rectal bleeding
In the majority of cases rectal bleeding is a sign of referral. However, in cases where sinister pathology has been excluded and only mild local bleeding has occurred the pharmacist could instigate treatment.

❸ Severity
Medication is unlikely to help any patient who has to manually reduce haemorrhoids. Referral for other treatments is recommended.

❹ Constipation See Fig. 6.10

> **TRIGGER POINTS indicative of referral: Haemorrhoids**
>
> - Abdominal pain
> - Blood in the stool
> - Fever
> - Patients who have to reduce their haemorrhoids manually
> - Persistent change in bowel habit in middle-aged patients
> - Unexplained rectal bleeding

The inclusion of such a diverse range of chemical entities appears to be based largely on theoretical grounds rather than on any evidence base. Extensive literature searching found only one published trial regarding the efficacy of any marketed product. However, this trial suffered from serious methodological flaws.

Anaesthetics (lidocaine, benzocaine and cinchocaine)

No trials appear to have been conducted using local anaesthetics in the treatment and relief of symptoms for haemorrhoids. However, anaesthetics have proven efficacy when used on other mucosal surfaces; their use could therefore be justifiably recommended. Their action is short lived and will produce temporary relief from

therapeutic agents and commonly include anaesthetics, astringents, anti-inflammatories and protectorants. Most products contain a combination of these agents, with some having three or more different agents included.

perianal itching and pain. They require frequent application and might therefore cause skin sensitisation.

Astringents (bismuth, zinc, Peru balsam)

Astringents are included in haemorrhoid preparations on the theoretical basis that they precipitate surface proteins thus producing a protective coat over the haemorrhoid. There appears to be no evidence to support this theory. Certain proprietary products only contain astringents and at best will provide a placebo effect.

Anti-inflammatories (hydrocortisone)

Products containing hydrocortisone were deregulated to pharmacy sale in 1995. Steroids have proven effectiveness in reducing inflammation and would therefore be useful in reducing haemorrhoidal swelling. Trials with OTC products containing hydrocortisone appear not to have taken place. It must be assumed that manufacturers have incorporated hydrocortisone into haemorrhoid products on the assumption that it will have an effect. Recommendation of a steroid-containing product is probably justified.

Protectorants (e.g. shark liver oil)

Protectorants are claimed to provide a protective coating over the skin and thus producing temporary relief from pain and perianal itch. These claims cannot be substantiated and, as with astringents, any benefit conveyed by a protectorant is probably a placebo effect.

Other agents

Sclerosing agents (lauromacrogol) and wound-healing agents (yeast cell extract) can also be found in some products. There is no evidence supporting their effectiveness.

Summary

With so little data available on their effectiveness it is impossible to say whether any product is a credible treatment for haemorrhoids, and many medical authorities regard them as little more than placebos. However, products containing a local anaesthetic or hydrocortisone will probably confer some benefit, and they do have proven effectiveness in other similar conditions. It would therefore seem most prudent, if recommending a product, that it should contain one or both of these chemical entities.

Treatment should only be recommended to patients with mild haemorrhoids. Any person complaining of prolapsing haemorrhoids, which need reducing by the patient, should be referred because these patients require non-surgical intervention with sclerotherapy or rubber-band ligation. If these fail to cure the problem then a haemorrhoidectomy might be performed.

Practical prescribing and product selection

Prescribing information relating to the medicines used for haemorrhoids reviewed in the section 'Evidence base for over-the-counter medication' is discussed and summarised in Table 6.19.

All patient groups, except children under 12, can use haemorrhoidal products. They do not interact with any other medicines and can be used in pregnancy. The standard dose for any formulation is twice daily, plus application after each bowel movement. Minimal side-effects have been reported and are usually limited to

Table 6.19
Practical prescribing: Summary of haemorrhoid products

	Form	Anaesthetics	Astringents	Steroids	Protectorants
Anacal*	Cream or suppository	No	No	No	No
Anodesyn	Ointment or suppository	Yes	No	No	No
Anusol	Cream, ointment or suppository	No	Yes	No	No
Anusol Plus HC	Ointment or suppository	No	Yes	Yes	No
Germoloids	Cream, ointment or suppository	Yes	Yes	No	No
Germoloids HC	Spray	Yes	No	Yes	No
Hemocane	Cream	Yes	No	No	No
Nupercainal	Ointment	Yes	No	No	No
Perinal	Spray	Yes	No	Yes	No
Preparation H	Ointment, gel or suppository	No	No	No	Yes

* Contains a sclerosing agent.

slight irritation. Products that contain hydrocortisone are restricted to use in patients aged over 14 (e.g. Perinal and Germoloids spray) and 18 for Anusol Plus products.

Further reading
Dennison A R, Whiston R J, Rooney S, Morris D L 1989 The management of hemorrhoids. American Journal of Gastroenterology 84:475–481
Haas P A, Fox T A, Haas G P 1984 The pathogenesis of hemorrhoids. Diseases of the Colon and Rectum 27:442–450
Ledward R S 1980 The management of puerperal haemorrhoids: a double blind clinical trial of Anacal rectal ointment. Practitioner 224:660–661
Norman D A, Newton R, Nicholas G V 1989 Direct current electrotherapy of internal hemorrhoids: an effective, safe, and painless outpatient approach. American Journal of Gastroenterology 84:482–487
Smith L E 1990 Anal hemorrhoids. Netherlands Journal of Medicine 37:S22–S32

Web sites
General site on health information: www.omni.ac.uk/browse/mesh/detail/C0019112L0019112.html

Abdominal pain

Background

Abdominal pain is a symptom of many different conditions, ranging from acute self-limiting problems to life-threatening conditions such as ruptured appendix and bowel obstruction. However, the overwhelming majority of cases will be of a non-serious nature, self-limiting and not require medical referral. The most common conditions that present to community pharmacies are dyspepsia affecting the upper abdomen and IBS affecting the lower abdomen. These are covered in more detail on pages 108 and 124. However, other conditions will present with abdominal pain (Fig. 6.13) and these are covered in this chapter.

Prevalence and epidemiology

The prevalence and epidemiology of abdominal pain within the population is determined by those conditions that cause it. As so many conditions can give rise to abdominal pain it is likely that the majority of the population will, at some point, suffer from abdominal pain. For example, one study found that 40% of the UK population had suffered from dyspepsia during the previous 12 months and gastroenteritis, which is commonly associated with abdominal pain, is extremely common.

Aetiology

Abdominal pain does not arise only from the GI tract but also from the cardiovascular and musculoskeletal systems. Therefore the aetiology of abdominal pain is dependent on its cause. For example, GI tract causes include poor muscle tone leading to reflux (e.g. lower oesophageal sphincter incompetence), infections that cause peptic ulcers (from *H. pylori*) and mechanical blockages causing biliary colic. Cardiovascular causes include angina and myocardial infarction whereas musculoskeletal problems often involve tearing of abdominal muscles.

Arriving at a differential diagnosis

The main role of the community pharmacist is to identify patients in whom symptoms suggest more serious pathology, so that they can be further evaluated. This is not easy, as many abdominal conditions do not present with classic textbook symptoms in a primary care setting. Patients tend to present to the pharmacist early in the course of the disease, often before the presenting symptoms have assumed the more usual description. The low prevalence of serious disease and overlapping symptoms with minor illness makes the task even more difficult. Single symptoms are poor predictors of final diagnosis (except for reflux oesophagitis, in which the presence of heartburn is highly suggestive). It is therefore important to look for 'symptom clusters' and to use knowledge of the incidence and prevalence of conditions to determine if referral is needed. This necessitates taking a very careful history and not relying on a single symptom to label a patient with a particular problem. Specific questions relating to abdominal pain should be asked (Table 6.20).

Structures located in the RUQ
Liver
Gall bladder
Duodenum
Head of the pancreas
Right adrenal gland
Portion of the right kidney
Portions of the ascending
and transverse colon

Conditions arising from the RUQ
Biliary colic
Hepatitis
Peptic ulcer
Pancreatitis
Renal colic
Herpes zoster
Myocardial ischaemia

Structures located in the LUQ
Left lobe of liver
Stomach
Spleen
Body of the pancreas
Left adrenal gland
Portion of the left kidney
Portions of the transverse and
descending colon

Conditions arising from the LUQ
Gastritis
Splenic enlargement or rupture
Pancreatitis
Renal colic
Herpes zoster
Myocardial ischaemia

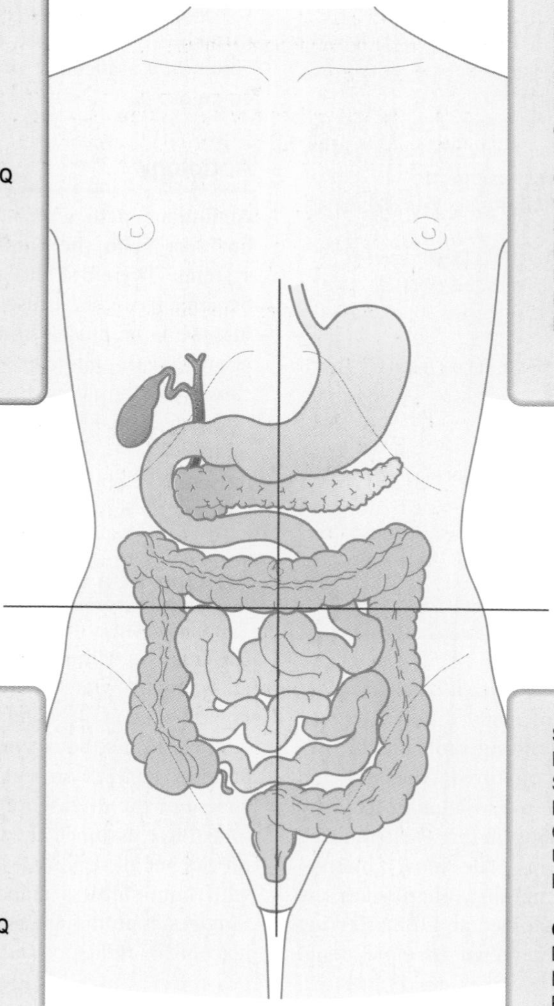

Structures located in the RLQ
Lower portion of the right kidney
Caecum and appendix
Portion of the ascending colon
Ovary and salpinx
Uterus if enlarged
Right ureter

Conditions arising from the RLQ
Appendicitis
Diverticulitis
Intestinal obstruction
Renal colic
Ectopic pregnancy
Ovarian cyst
Salpingitis
Endometriosis

Structures located in the LLQ
Lower portion of the left kidney
Sigmoid colon
Portion of the descending colon
Ovary and salpinx
Uterus if enlarged
Left ureter

Conditions arising from the LLQ
Diverticulitis
Intestinal obstruction
Renal colic
Irritable bowel syndrome
Ectopic pregnancy
Ovarian cyst
Salpingitis
Endometriosis

Fig. 6.13 Anatomical location of organs and conditions arising from the abdomen

Table 6.20
Specific questions to ask the patient: Abdominal pain

Question	Relevance
Location of pain	• Knowing the anatomical location of abdominal structures is helpful in differential diagnosis of abdominal pain (Fig. 6.14). It is therefore important to know the location of these structures
Presence only of abdominal pain/discomfort	• In general, patients without other symptoms rarely have serious pathology. The symptoms are usually self-limiting and often no cause can be determined
Nature of the pain	• Heartburn is classically associated with a burning sensation • Cramp-like pain is seen in diverticulitis, IBS, salpingitis and gastroenteritis • Colicky pain has been used to describe the pain of appendicitis, biliary and renal colic and intestinal obstruction
Radiating pain	• Abdominal pain that moves from its original site should be viewed with caution • Pain that radiates to the jaw, face and arm could be cardiovascular in origin • Pain that moves from a central location to the right lower quadrant could suggest appendicitis • Pain radiating to the back may suggest peptic ulcer or pancreatitis
Severity of pain	• Non-serious causes of abdominal pain generally do not give rise to severe pain. Pain associated with pancreatitis, biliary and renal colic and peritonitis tends to be severe
Age of patient	• With increasing age, abdominal pain is more likely to have an identifiable and serious organic cause. Appendicitis is the only serious abdominal condition that is much more common in the young than older patients
Onset	• Onset can be gradual or sudden. In general, if no identifiable cause can be found, abdominal pain with sudden onset is generally a symptom of more serious conditions. For example, peritonitis, appendicitis, ectopic pregnancy, renal and biliary colic
Aggravating or ameliorating factors	• The presence of food can aggravate gastric ulcers and antacids can relieve symptoms • Biliary colic can be aggravated by fatty foods • Pain in salpingitis, pancreatitis and appendicitis is often made worse by movement
Associated symptoms	• Vomiting, weight loss, melaena, altered bowel habit and haematemesis are all symptoms that suggest more serious pathology and require referral

Conditions affecting the upper abdomen

Left upper quadrant pain

Dyspepsia/gastritis

Patients with dyspepsia present with a range of symptoms that commonly involve vague abdominal discomfort (aching) above the umbilicus (Fig. 6.14) associated with belching, bloating, flatulence, a feeling of fullness and heartburn. It is normally relieved by antacids and aggravated by spicy foods or excessive caffeine. Vomiting is unusual. For further information on dyspepsia, see page 107.

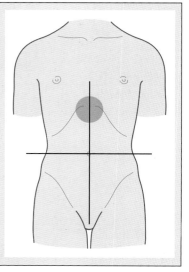

Fig. 6.14 The position of pain in gastritis and dyspepsia

Splenic enlargement or rupture

If the spleen is enlarged, generalised left upper quadrant pain associated with abdominal fullness and early feeding satiety is observed (Fig. 6.15). The condition is rare and is nearly always secondary to another primary cause, which might be an infection, a result of inflammation or haematological in origin.

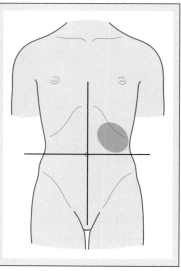

Fig. 6.15 The position of pain associated with splenic enlargement

Right upper quadrant pain

Acute cholecystitis and cholelithiasis

Acute cholecystitis (inflammation of the gall bladder) and cholelithiasis (presence of gallstones in the bile ducts, also called biliary colic) are characterised by persistent, steady, severe aching pain in the right upper quadrant (Fig. 6.16). Classically, the onset is sudden and starts a few hours after a meal, frequently waking the patient in the early hours of the morning. The pain can radiate to the tip of the right scapula in cholelithiasis. Fatty foods often aggravate the pain. The incidence increases with increasing age and is most common in people aged over 50. It is also more prevalent in women than men.

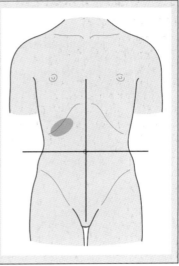

Fig. 6.16 The position of pain associated with acute cholecystitis and cholelithiasis

Hepatitis

Liver enlargement from any type of hepatitis will cause discomfort or dull pain (Fig. 6.17). Associated symptoms of nausea, vomiting, jaundice and pruritus should be present.

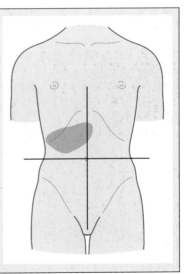

Fig. 6.17 The position of pain associated with hepatitis

Ulcers

Ulcers are classed as either gastric or duodenal. They occur most commonly in patients aged 30 to 50 years old. Typically, the patient will have well localised mid-epigastric pain (Fig. 6.18) described as 'constant', 'annoying' or 'gnawing'.

With gastric ulcers, symptoms are inconsistent but the pain usually comes on whenever the stomach is empty – usually an hour or so after eating – and is generally relieved by antacids or food and aggravated by alcohol and caffeine.

Duodenal ulcers tend to be more consistent in symptom presentation. Pain that wakes a person at night is highly suggestive of duodenal ulcer, especially if symptoms are mild or absent on awakening but return mid morning.

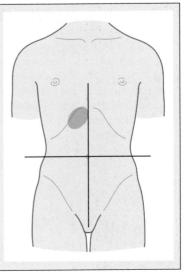

Fig. 6.18 The position of pain associated with ulcers

Pain affecting both right and left upper quadrants

Pancreatitis

The pain of pancreatitis develops suddenly and is described as agonising, with the focus being centrally located and often radiating into the back (Fig. 6.19). Pain reaches its maximum intensity within minutes and can last hours or days. Vomiting is common but does not relieve the pain. Pancreatitis is commonly seen in alcoholics and it is likely that the patient will have a history of long-term heavy drinking. Patients are very unlikely to present in a community pharmacy because of the severity of the pain but a mild attack could present with steady epigastric pain sometimes centred close to the umbilicus and can be difficult to distinguish from other causes of upper quadrant pain.

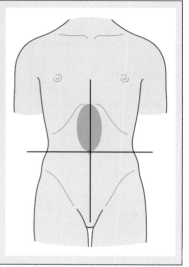

Fig. 6.19 The position of pain associated with pancreatitis

Renal colic

Urinary calculi (stones) can occur anywhere in the urinary tract, although most frequently stones get lodged in the **ureter**. Pain begins in the loin radiating round the flank into the groin and sometimes down the inner side of the thigh (Fig. 6.20). Pain is severe and colicky in nature. Attacks tend to last hours and often leave the person prostrate with pain. Symptoms of nausea and vomiting might also be present.

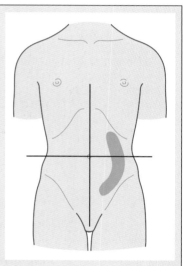

Fig. 6.20 The position of pain in renal colic

Myocardial ischaemia

Angina and myocardial infarction (MI) cause chest pain that can be difficult to distinguish initially from epigastric/retrosternal pain caused by dyspepsia (Fig. 6.21). However, pain of cardiovascular origin often radiates to the neck, jaw and inner aspect of the left arm. Typically, angina pain is precipitated by exertion and subsides after a few minutes once at rest. Pain associated with MI will present with a characteristic deep crushing pain. The patient will appear pale, display weakness and be tachycardic.

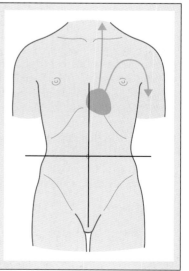

Fig. 6.21 The position of pain associated in myocardial ischaemia

Herpes zoster (shingles)

Pain associated with herpes zoster typically occurs once the rash has erupted, although it can occasionally precede the rash. Pain that precedes the rash and is right sided can be confused with appendicitis (Fig. 6.22).

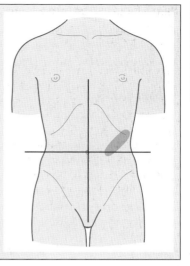

Fig. 6.22 The position of pain in herpes zoster

Conditions affecting the lower abdomen

The most common causes of lower abdominal pain are muscle strains, IBS, appendicitis and salpingitis in women. Apart from appendicitis, all these conditions can present in either quadrant.

Irritable bowel syndrome

Pain is most often observed in the left lower quadrant (Fig. 6.23), however, the discomfort can be vague and diffuse and about one-third of patients exhibit upper abdominal pain. The pain is described as 'cramp-like' and is recurrent. Alternating diarrhoea and constipation, with mucus coating the stools, is also often present.

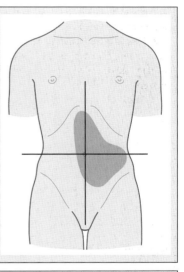

Fig. 6.23 The position of pain associated with irritable bowel syndrome

Diverticulitis

The incidence of **diverticulitis** increases with increasing age. It is most prevalent in the elderly and is characterised by pain and local tenderness. Pain is more commonly seen in the left lower quadrant (Fig. 6.24) but can be **suprapubic** and occasionally in the right lower quadrant. Pain tends to be cramp-like in nature. Fever is a prominent feature. The patient generally has a history of alternating constipation and diarrhoea.

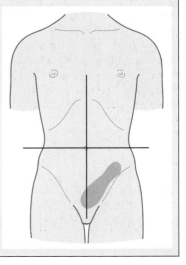

Fig. 6.24 The position of pain associated with diverticulitis

Intestinal obstruction

Intestinal obstruction is most prevalent in people over the age of 50. It has sudden and acute onset. The pain is described as colicky and can be experienced anywhere in the lower abdomen. Constipation and vomiting are prominent features. A patient with lower abdominal pain in the absence of constipation and vomiting is very unlikely to have an intestinal obstruction.

Appendicitis

Classically, the pain starts in the mid-abdomen region, around the umbilicus, before migrating to the right lower quadrant after a few hours (Fig. 6.25), although right-sided pain is experienced from the outset in about 50% of patients. The pain of appendicitis is described as colicky or cramp-like but after a few hours becomes constant. Movement tends to aggravate the pain and vomiting might also be present. Appendicitis is most common in young adults, especially young men. The absence of right lower quadrant pain and a history of the person suffering similar pain previously should eliminate appendicitis from any differential diagnosis.

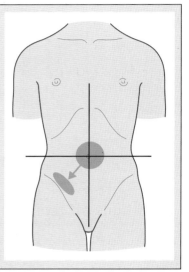

Fig. 6.25 The position of pain associated with appendicitis

Conditions affecting women

Generalised lower abdominal pain can be experienced in a number of gynaecological conditions:

- Ectopic pregnancy: patients suffer persistent moderate to severe pain that is sudden in onset. A menstrual history will reveal that the patient's last period is late. Additionally, the patient might be experiencing spotting. Any patient who is sexually active, with abdominal pain and whose period is late should be referred.
- Salpingitis (inflammation of the fallopian tubes): occurs predominantly in young, sexually active women, especially those fitted with an IUCD. Pain is usually bilateral and cramping. Pain starts shortly after menstruation and can worsen with movement.
- Endometriosis: patients experience lower abdominal aching pain that usually starts 5 to 7 days before menstruation begins and can be constant and severe. The pain often worsens at the onset of menstruation. Referred pain into the back and down the thighs is also possible.

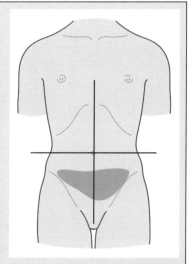

Fig. 6.26 The position of pain associated with women's conditions

Diffuse abdominal pain

A number of conditions will present with diffuse abdominal pain over the four quadrants. The most common cause of diffuse pain that will be seen by the pharmacist is gastroenteritis. Other causes include peritonitis and pancreatitis.

Gastroenteritis

Other symptoms of nausea, vomiting and diarrhoea will be more prominent in gastroenteritis than abdominal pain. The patient might also have a fever and suffer from general malaise.

Peritonitis

Although the pain of acute peritonitis can be diffuse, severe pain in the upper abdomen is often present. This is accompanied by intense rigidity of the abdominal wall producing a 'board-like' appearance; vomiting might also be present.

Figure 6.27 will aid in the differentiation of the different types of abdominal pain.

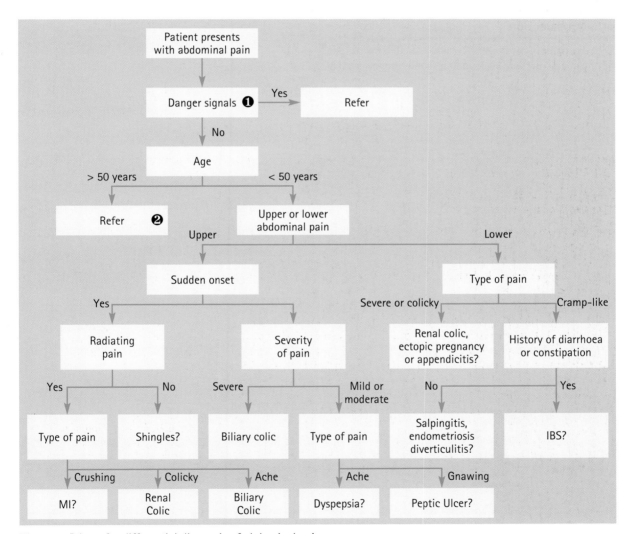

Fig. 6.27 Primer for differential diagnosis of abdominal pain

❶ Danger signals are significant bleeding, vomiting and fever.

❷ Organic disease is more likely to be the cause of abdominal pain in patients aged over 50, especially if symptoms are new or more severe than normal.

TRIGGER POINTS indicative of referral: Abdominal pain

- Abdominal pain with fever
- Elderly
- Melaena
- Pregnancy
- Trauma
- Severe pain or pain that radiates
- Vomiting

Evidence base for over-the-counter medication and practical prescribing and product selection

The two conditions that have abdominal pain as one of the major presenting symptoms and can be treated OTC are dyspepsia and IBS. For further information on products used to treat these conditions, please refer to pages 109 and 126.

Further reading

Bagshaw E J 1999 Abdominal pain protocol: right upper quadrant pain. Lippincott's Primary Care Practice 3:486–492

Guthrie E, Thompson D 2002 Abdominal pain and functional gastrointestinal disorders. British Medical Journal 325:701–703

Kalloo A N, Kantsevoy S V 2001 Gallstones and biliary disease. Primary Care 28:591–606

Lucenti M J, Nadel E S, Brown D F 2001 Right lower quadrant pain. Journal of Emergency Medicine 21:431–434

Self-assessment questions

The following questions are intended to supplement the text. Two levels of question are provided; multiple choice questions and case studies. The multiple choice questions are designed to test factual recall and the case studies allow knowledge to be applied to a practice setting.

6.1. Which one of the following statements about gastric ulcers is *not* true?

a. The pain is often aggravated by caffeine
b. The pain is localised
c. Nausea and vomiting are not associated with gastric ulcers
d. Endoscopical findings are usually positive for *H. pylori*
e. Weight loss is common

6.2. In the treatment of constipation which one of the following statements is true?

a. Bulk-forming laxatives usually act within 12 to 24 h
b. Senna tablets should be avoided in nursing mothers
c. Fybogel is not suitable for a patient with coeliac disease
d. Lactulose cannot be taken by diabetics
e. Liquid paraffin has been linked with causing lipid pneumonia

6.3. A man asks for the best thing to stop diarrhoea because he is going on holiday and he doesn't want to be caught short. Which of the following is the first-line treatment to be recommended?

a. Kaolin and morphine
b. Rehydration solution
c. Antibiotics
d. Antispasmodics
e. Loperamide

6.4. Antacids that contain aluminium, calcium or magnesium salts inhibit the intestinal absorption of which of the following?

a. Chloramphenicol
b. Cephalexin
c. Erythromycin
d. Tetracycline
e. Phenoxymethylpenicillin

6.5. What condition predisposes patients to oral thrush?

a. Heart failure
b. Asthma
c. Diabetes mellitus
d. Hyperlipidaemia
e. Parkinson's disease

6.6. Abdominal pain that starts centrally then moves to the right lower quadrant is indicative of?

a. Irritable bowel syndrome
b. Pancreatitis
c. Pyelonephritis
d. Appendicitis
e. Renal colic

6.7. Which condition is least likely to cause rectal bleeding?

a. Haemorrhoids
b. Crohn's disease
c. Colorectal cancer
d. Irritable bowel syndrome
e. Anal fissure

6.8. Which one of the following preparations would not be used for the treatment of pain-free gingivitis?

a. Corsodyl mouthwash
b. Eludril mouthwash
c. Corsodyl gel
d. Bocasan
e. Difflam mouthwash

Questions 6.9 to 6.11 concern the following conditions:

A. Irritable bowel syndrome
B. Constipation
C. Diarrhoea
D. Haemorrhoids
E. Dyspepsia

Select, from A to E, which of the above statements relate to the following conditions:

6.9. Is characterised with epigastric pain

6.10. Can be treated with antispasmodics

6.11. Is associated with left lower quadrant pain

Questions 6.12 to 6.14 concern the following OTC medications:

A. Gaviscon liquid
B. Asilone suspension
C. Milk of magnesia
D. Sodium bicarbonate powder
E. Aludrox liquid

6.12. Is most suitable for treating heartburn, which tends to get worse when lying down

6.13. Is most suitable to treat abdominal discomfort caused by trapped gas

6.14. Could be used to relieve constipation, as well as indigestion

Questions 6.15 to 6.17: for each of the questions below, *one* or *more* of the responses is (are) correct. Decide which of the responses is (are) correct. Then choose:

A. If a, b and c are correct.
B. If a and b only are correct.
C. If b and c only are correct.
D. If a only is correct.
E. If c only is correct.

Directions summarised

A	B	C	D	E
a, b and c	a and b only	b and c only	a only	c only

6.15. When questioning a client seeking advice for nausea and gastrointestinal upset, which of the following symptoms would indicate the need for direct referral to the general practitioner?

    a. Feeling of impending vomiting
    b. Loss of appetite over the last 24 h
    c. Dark brown coloured vomit

6.16. A common presentation of minor aphthous ulcers is:

    a. Pain
    b. Ulcers on the buccal mucosa and tongue
    c. They occur in crops of between 1 and 5

6.17. Which symptoms in a patient presenting with constipation should be referred?

    a. Melaena
    b. Greater than 7 days duration
    c. Abdominal pain

Questions 6.18 to 6.20: these questions consist of a statement in the left-hand column followed by a statement in the right-hand column. You need to:

● decide whether the first statement is true or false
● decide whether the second statement is true or false

Then choose:

A. If both statements are true and the second statement is a correct explanation of the first statement
B. If both statements are true but the second statement is not a correct explanation of the first statement
C. If the first statement is true but the second statement is false
D. If the first statement is false but the second statement is true
E. If both statements are false

Directions summarised

	First statement	Second statement	
A	True	True	Second explanation is a correct explanation of the first
B	True	True	Second statement is not a correct explanation of the first
C	True	False	
D	False	True	
E	False	False	

	First statement	*Second statement*
6.18.	IBS is common in people under the age of 40	It is caused by stress
6.19.	Gingivitis is caused by plaque build up	It is characterised by red and swollen gums
6.20.	Heartburn causes retrosternal pain	Sphincter incompetence is responsible for symptoms

Case study

CASE STUDY 6.1

Mrs SJ, a 28-year-old woman, asks to speak to the pharmacist because she wants something for stomach ache. You find out that the pain is located in the upper and lower left quadrants, but mainly the upper quadrant.

a. From which conditions might she be suffering?

Possible conditions are: reflux, non-ulcer dyspepsia, gastritis, primary dysmenorrhoea, endometriosis, IBS, pancreatitis, renal colic, MI and herpes zoster.

Further questioning reveals Mrs SJ to be suffering with pain she describes as 'an ache'.

b. From which likely conditions could she now be suffering?

The use of the word 'ache' means you can rule out those conditions that present with severe, stabbing, burning or gnawing pain:

- *pancreatitis, renal colic: severe*
- *reflux: burning*
- *herpes zoster: severe, lancing.*

But it could still be any of: non-ulcer dyspepsia, gastritis, primary dysmenorrhoea, IBS, endometriosis and, possibly, MI.

c. What symptom-specific questions are you now going to ask to differentially diagnose her condition?

The symptom-specific questions you would now ask relate to:

- *periodicity*
- *aggravation/relieving factors*
- *radiation*
- *associated symptoms*
- *previous episodes*
- *lifestyle*
- *timing of pain in relation to period.*

d. From which body systems can abdominal pain originate? For each system state what conditions could present with centrally located upper quadrant pain?

The body systems and relevant cause of pain are:

- *GI tract: reflux, non-ulcer dyspepsia, gastritis, primary dysmenorrhoea, endometriosis, IBS, pancreatitis, renal colic, MI and herpes zoster*
- *CVS: myocardial ischaemia*
- *musculcoskeletal: muscle strain*
- *reproductive: ectopic pregnancy, ovarian cyst.*

Before any course of action is taken you ask if she takes any medication from the GP, her response is as follows:

- Paracetamol prn: she has taken this for 6 months for knee pain.
- Atorvastatin 40 mg od: she has taken for the last 3 years for familial hyperlipidaemia.
- Naproxen 500 mg bd prn: she has taken this for 6 months for knee pain.

e. Which of these medications, if any, do you consider is contributing to Mrs SJ's pain? Explain your rationale.

Of the three medicines that Mrs SJ is taking, the one most likely to cause GI irritation is Naproxen. However, she has been taking this for the last 6 months and you would expect that dyspepsia symptoms would have been experienced already if she was going to have a reaction to Naproxen. It is therefore unlikely that Naproxen has caused the problem, unless the dose has been changed recently. Atorvastatin can also cause GI side-effects but has been taken for the last 3 years and is therefore almost definitely not the cause of the symptoms. Paracetamol is not known to cause GI irritation so can also be ruled out. In conclusion, it is likely that none of the medicines have caused Mrs SJ's symptoms.

CASE STUDY 6.2

A 37-year-old male – Mr PA – asks for a quick-acting medicine for constipation. The counter assistant finds out that he:

- Has had the constipation for about 10 days
- Has tried no medication
- Takes no medicines from the GP on a regular basis

a. What further information do you need to make a correct differential diagnosis?

Further information needed to make a diagnosis is:

- *Exact nature of bowel movement*
- *Consistency of stool*
- *Number of bowel movements now in comparison to normal*
- *Associated symptoms*
- *Previous history*
- *Social history*
- *Diet and lifestyle*

You find out that:

- He is going to the toilet about once every 2 days (usually once or twice a day).
- The stools are hard but otherwise normal.

- He suffers from aching pains in the lower quadrants.
- His lifestyle is busy but no different than normal.
- He returned from holiday about 3 weeks ago.
- His diet is fairly balanced, although he doesn't eat many vegetables.
- He has had the pain before, but not for quite some time.

b. What do you think is the likely cause of his symptoms?

It appears Mr PA is suffering from a simple case of constipation, possibly caused by a change in diet when he was on holiday. There appear to be no symptoms indicative of other medical conditions or sinister pathology.

c. What course of action are you going to recommend?

Conservative treatment with an increased fluid intake and more fibre (vegetables and fruit). If this fails to rectify the problem, or the patient is unwilling to try it, then a laxative could be given. Any agent could be tried although patient acceptability probably dictates the use of a stimulant, because he wants something to work quickly.

Answers to multiple choice questions

6.1 = a   6.2 = a   6.3 = b   6.4 = d   6.5 = c   6.6 = d   6.7 = d   6.8 = e   6.9 = e   6.10 = a,
6.11= a   6.12 = a   6.13 = b   6.14 = c   6.15 = e   6.16 = a   6.17 = d   6.18 = c   6.19 = b   6.20 = a.

Dermatology

Background

The skin is the largest organ of the body. It has a complex structure and performs many important functions. These include protecting underlying tissues from external injury, overexposure to ultraviolet light, barring entry to microorganisms and harmful chemicals, acting as a sensory organ for pressure, touch, temperature, pain and vibration and maintaining the homeostatic balance of body temperature.

It has been reported that dermatological disorders account for up to 15% of the workload of UK GPs, with similar findings reported from community pharmacy. It is therefore important that community pharmacists are able to differentiate between common dermatological conditions that can be managed appropriately without referral to the GP and those that require further investigation or treatment with a prescription-only medicine.

General overview of skin anatomy

Principally the skin consists of two parts, the outer and thinner layer called the epidermis and an inner, thicker layer named the dermis. Beneath the dermis lies a subcutaneous layer, known as the hypodermis (Fig. 7.1).

The epidermis

The epidermis is the major protective layer of the skin and has four distinct layers when viewed under the microscope. The basal layer actively undergoes cell division, forcing new cells to move up through the epidermis and form the outer keratinised horny layer. This process is continual and takes approximately 35 days. Pathological changes that affect this process lead to dermatological disorders.

The dermis

The dermis is the layer below the epidermis. It provides support to the epidermis as well as its blood and nerve supply. Also located in the dermis are the hair follicle, sebaceous and sweat glands and the arrector pili muscle. Under cold conditions the arrector pili muscle contracts, pulling the hair in to a vertical position and causing 'goosebumps'.

The hair

The primary function of hair is one of protection. Each hair consists of a shaft, the visible part of the hair, and a root. Surrounding the root is the hair follicle, the base of which is enlarged into a bulb structure. A sebaceous

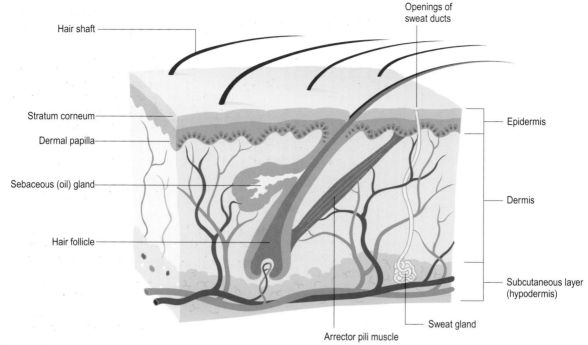

Fig. 7.1 The epidermis, dermis and associated structures

gland secretes sebum in to each hair follicle and this lubricates the hair and protects it from damage. Also associated with the hair follicle is the the arrector pili muscle, which is composed of smooth muscle.

Sebaceous glands

Sebaceous glands are found in large numbers on the face, chest and upper back. During puberty these glands become large and active due to hormonal changes.

Sweat glands

These are the most numerous of the skin glands and are classed as apocrine or eccrine. Eccrine glands are located all over the body and play a role in elimination of waste products and maintaining a constant core temperature. Apocrine sweat glands are mainly located in the axilla and begin to function at puberty.

History taking

Unlike internal medicine, the majority of dermatological complaints presenting in community pharmacy can be seen. This affords community pharmacists an excellent opportunity to base their differential diagnosis not only on questioning but also on physical examination. General questions that should be considered when dealing with a dermatological condition are listed in Table 7.1.

Physical examination

A more accurate differential diagnosis will be made if the pharmacist actually sees the person's athlete's foot or 'rash' on the back. Providing adequate privacy can be obtained there is no reason why the majority of skin complaints cannot be seen. Pharmacies with specific private areas or counselling rooms should be able to perform such exams relatively easily. It is worth remembering that many patients will be embarrassed by skin conditions and might be ashamed of their appearance. When performing an examination of the skin, a number of things should be looked for (Table 7.2).

Hyperproliferative disorders

Background

Hyperproliferative disorders are characterised by a combination of increased cell turnover rate and a shortening of the time it takes for cells to migrate from the basal layer to the outer horny layer. Typically, cell turnover rate is ten times faster than normal and cell migration takes 3 or 4 days rather than 35 days.

Psoriasis

Background

Psoriasis is very rarely life threatening but does cause considerable suffering and affects the patient's quality

Table 7.1
Questions to consider when taking a dermatological history

Question	Relevance
Where did the problem first appear?	● Certain skin problems start in one particular location before spreading to other parts of the body, e.g. impetigo usually starts on the face before spreading to the limbs ● Patients might need prompting to tell you where the problem started as they are likely to want help for the most obvious or large skin lesion but neglect to tell you about smaller lesions that appeared first but are now not the main cause for concern
Are there any other symptoms?	● These are generally itch and/or pain ● Mild itch is associated with many skin conditions including, psoriasis and medicine eruptions ● Severe itch is associated with conditions such as, scabies, atopic and contact dermatitis
Occupational history (relevant to adults only)	● This is particularly pertinent for contact dermatitis
General medical history	● Many skin signs can be the first marker of internal disease, e.g. diabetes can manifest with pruritus; fungal or bacterial infection and thyroid disease can present with hair loss and pruritus
Travel	● More people are taking long-haul holidays and therefore exposing themselves to tropical diseases that can manifest as skin lesions
Family and household contact history	● Infections such as scabies can infect relatives and others with whom the patient is in close contact
The patient's thoughts on the cause of the problem	● Ask for the patient's opinion. This might help with the diagnosis or alternatively shed light on anxieties and theories as to the cause of the condition

Table 7.2
Things to consider when performing a dermatological examination

Lesions	Relevance
Temperature	Use the backs of your fingers to make the assessment. This should enable you to identify generalised warmth or coolness of the skin and note the temperature of any red areas, e.g. generalised warmth can indicate fever whereas local warmth might indicate inflammation or cellulitis
Lesions	Assess the location and distribution over the body. For example, do they involve the exposed surfaces or intertriginous areas? Look at the pattern of involvement of the skin. Many skin diseases have a 'typical' or 'classic' distribution
Lesion arrangement	Check to see if the lesions are arciform (in an arc), linear, annular (in a ring) or clustered, e.g. tinea corporis (ringworm) infection usually presents as an annular rash
Recent trauma	Is there any sign that individual lesions have developed on a site of trauma or injury such as a scratch? This is seen in a number of conditions such as psoriasis and viral warts
Touching the skin	Remember that very few skin conditions are infectious, so do not be afraid to touch the patient's skin

of life. It is a chronic relapsing inflammatory disorder characterised by a variety of morphological lesions that present in a number of forms. The most common form of psoriasis is plaque psoriasis; this will be the form most familiar to pharmacists.

Prevalence and epidemiology

Psoriasis is a common skin disorder with an estimated worldwide prevalence between 1 and 3%. In the UK it has been reported to affect 2% of the population. However, this is probably a substantial underestimate, as many patients with mild psoriasis do not present to their GP.

Psoriasis can present at any time in life, although it appears to be more prevalent in the second and fifth decades. It is rare in infants and uncommon in children. The sexes are equally affected but it is more common in Caucasians.

Aetiology

The exact aetiology of psoriasis still remains unclear but it is known that inherited and environmental factors are implicated. If one parent has psoriasis then each sibling will have a 1 in 4 chance of psoriasis, and if both parents suffer from psoriasis the rate rises to 1 in 2. Studies in twins also suggest that environmental factors might be needed for clinical expression of the disease. Psoriasis lesions often develop at sites of skin trauma, such as sunburn and cuts (known as the Koebner phenomenon), following strepto-coccal throat infection and during periods of stress.

Arriving at a differential diagnosis

Psoriasis can be located on various parts of the body (Fig. 7.2) and presents in a variety of different forms. As plaque and scalp psoriasis are the only forms of the condition that can be managed by the community phar-macist, it is necessary that other forms of psoriasis, and conditions that look like psoriasis, can be distinguished. Asking symptom-specific questions will help the pharmacist to determine if referral is needed (Table 7.3).

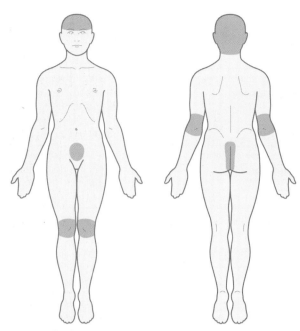

Fig. 7.2 Typical distribution of psoriatic plaques

Clinical features of plaque psoriasis

Plaque psoriasis classically presents with characteristic salmon-pink lesions with silvery-white scales and well defined boundaries (Fig. 7.3). Lesions vary in size from pinpoint to covering extensive areas. If the scales on the surface of the plaque are gently removed and the lesion is then rubbed, it reveals pinpoint bleeding from the superficial dilated capillaries. This is known as the Auspitz' sign and is diagnostic.

Table 7.3
Specific questions to ask the patient: Psoriasis

Question	Relevance
Onset	• Psoriasis usually occurs in early adult life, although a person of any age can develop psoriasis. However, in young and elderly patients the lesions tend to be atypical, which can complicate the diagnosis
Distribution of rash	• Psoriasis often presents in a symmetrical distribution and most commonly involves the scalp, extensor aspects of the elbows and knees. However the gluteal cleft and umbilicus can also be affected (Fig. 7.2) • Conditions such as lichen planus (often inside of the wrists) and pityriasis rosea (thighs and trunk) have a different distribution to psoriasis
Other symptoms	• Itch is not a normal feature of psoriasis, unlike other conditions such as dermatitis and fungal infections • Nail involvement in the form of pitting and onycholysis (separation of the nail plate from the nail bed) is often seen and can involve one or more of the nails. However, this is normally only observed in patients with longstanding psoriasis and is therefore of no value in patients presenting with rash of recent onset
Look of rash	• Scalp and plaque psoriasis usually show scaling as a predominant feature. This is not seen with other common skin conditions or other forms of psoriasis • When scalp involvement is mild psoriasis can be impossible to distinguish from seborrhoeic dermatitis
Previous history of lesions	• Psoriasis is a chronic relapsing and remitting disease and it is likely that the patient will have had lesions in the past. Other skin diseases, such as fungal infections, are acute and patients do not normally have a history of the problem

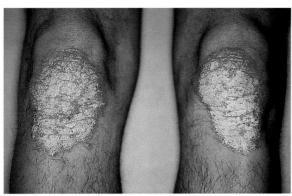

Fig. 7.3 Typical psoriatic plaques. Reproduced from *Dermatology: An Illustrated Colour Text* by D Gawkrodger, 2002, Mosby, with permission

Clinical features of scalp psoriasis

Scalp psoriasis can be mild, exhibiting slight redness of the scalp through to severe cases with marked inflammation and thick scaling. The redness often extends beyond the hair margin and is commonly seen behind the ears.

Conditions to eliminate for plaque psoriasis

Pustular psoriasis

In this form of psoriasis sterile **pustules** are an obvious clinical feature. The pustules tend to be located on the advancing edge of the lesions and typically occur on the palms of the hands and soles of the feet.

Seborrhoeic psoriasis (also known as flexural psoriasis)

Seborrhoeic psoriasis refers to classic lesions that affect the scalp but with less typical lesions in the body folds, especially the groins and axillae. Often, in mild cases the scalp might be the only part of the body involved and impossible to distinguish from seborrhoeic dermatitis.

Guttate psoriasis (also known as rain–drop psoriasis)

Guttate psoriasis is characterised by crops of scattered small lesions covered with light flaky scales that often affects the trunk and proximal part of the limbs. This form of psoriasis usually occurs in adolescents and often follows a streptococcal throat infection.

Erythrodermic psoriasis

Erythrodermic psoriasis presents as an extensive **erythema** and shows very few classic lesions. It is therefore difficult to diagnose. The condition is serious and even life threatening. Systemic symptoms can be severe and include fever, joint pain and diarrhoea. Patients are extremely unlikely to present at a community pharmacy with such symptoms.

Lichen planus

Lichen planus is an uncommon condition and is reported to only account for 0.2 to 0.8% of dermatological outpatient consultations. The lesions are similar in appearance to plaque psoriasis but are usually itchy and are normally located on the inner surfaces of the wrists and on the shins, an atypical distribution for psoriasis. Additionally, oral mucous membranes are normally affected with white, slightly raised lesions that look a little like a spider's web. The person will not have a family history of psoriasis.

Pityriasis rosea

The condition is characterised by erythematous scaling mainly on the trunk, but also on the thighs and upper arms. A 'target' disc lesion, often misdiagnosed as ringworm, is followed one week later with an extensive rash. It most commonly affects young adults. The condition usually remits spontaneously after 4 to 8 weeks. An accurate history will normally eliminate pityriasis rosea from psoriasis, as the condition is acute in onset and the patient can often identify the initial 'target' lesion.

Medication that can trigger or aggravate psoriasis

A number of medicines can cause rashes that look like psoriasis or aggravate existing psoriasis. These include, lithium, beta-blockers, chloroquine and terbinafine; withdrawal from steroids might also cause these symptoms.

Conditions to eliminate for scalp psoriasis

Seborrhoeic dermatitis

Mild scalp psoriasis can be very difficult to distinguish from seborrhoeic dermatitis. However, in practice this is rarely a problem because treatment for both conditions is often the same. For further information on seborrhoeic dermatitis see page 155.

Tinea capitis (fungal infection of the scalp)

Tinea capitis is an uncommon infection but if the patient has scaling skin, broken hairs and a patch of alopecia then a tinea infection should be considered. For further information on fungal infections see page 157.

Figure 7.4 will aid in the differentiation of plaque psoriasis.

Evidence base for over-the-counter medication

Before any treatment is offered to the patient it is worth noting that simple OTC remedies should be limited to

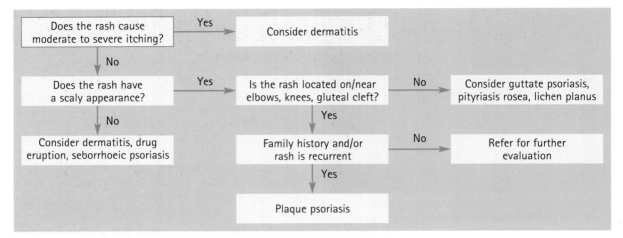

Fig. 7.4 Primer for differential diagnosis of plaque psoriasis

> ❗ **TRIGGER POINTS indicative of referral: Psoriasis**
>
> - Lesions that are extensive, follow recent infection or cause moderate to severe itching
> - Patients with no family history or past personal history of psoriasis
> - Pustular psoriatic lesions

mild to moderate plaque psoriasis and scalp psoriasis, as these are most likely to respond to such measures. A patient who presents with severe plaque psoriasis or another form of psoriasis should be referred.

Treatment OTC is limited to the use of emollients, keratolytics, coal tar or dithranol. There is limited published literature supporting efficacy of topical treatment, however systemic agents are available on prescription if topical therapy is ineffective.

Emollients

No published literature appears to have addressed either emollient efficacy or whether one emollient is superior to another in treating psoriasis. However, emollients are frequently prescribed and used to help soften and soothe the skin so reducing cracking and dryness. Subjective evidence over a long period of time has shown that emollients are useful for mild psoriasis and are an important aspect of psoriasis treatment. Unfortunately, on current evidence there is no way of knowing if one emollient is superior to another. Patients might have to try several emollients before finding one that is most effective for their skin.

Keratolytics

Keratolytics, such as salicylic acid and lactic acid have been incorporated into emollients to aid clearing scale and are often used for scalp psoriasis where very thick

scaling can occur. Although there appears to be no published evidence for their efficacy in clearing scale clinical practice suggests that they have a role to play.

Coal tar

Goeckerman demonstrated the effectiveness of coal tar as early as 1925. This remained the mainstay of treatment until the introduction of dithranol, corticosteroids and, more recently, vitamin D analogues. A number of clinical studies have confirmed the beneficial effect of coal tar on psoriasis, although a major drawback in assessing the effectiveness of coal tar preparations is the variability in their composition making meaningful comparisons between studies difficult. Comparisons between coal tar and other treatment regimens have been conducted. Tham et al (1994) compared the effectiveness of calcipotriol 50 μg twice daily versus 15% coal tar solution each day. Both treatments were shown to be effective, although calcipotriol was significantly better than the coal tar solution. Harrington (1989) compared two pharmacy-only products, Psorin and Alphosyl. Findings showed that both helped in the treatment of psoriasis but that Psorin (which includes 0.11% dithranol) was significantly more effective. Testament to coal tar's effectiveness is that it still features in the current *British National Formulary* (edition 46).

Dithranol

Dithranol was first used in the 1950s and has become an established treatment option as clinical trials have established its efficacy. There appears to be no definitive answer as to which strength is most appropriate, however, current practice dictates starting on the lowest possible concentration and gradually increasing the concentration until improvement is noticed. In addition, short-contact regimens are advocated. However, one review of published studies involving short-contact dithranol therapy concluded that methodological flaws

Table 7.4
Practical prescribing: Summary of tar-based products

	Scalp, skin or both	Salicylic acid	Sulphur	Other entities	Children	Application
Alphosyl 2 in 1 Shampoo	Scalp	No	No	No	All ages	Every 2 to 3 days
Alphosyl cream	Both	No	No	No	All ages	Two to four times daily
Capasal	Scalp	Yes	No	No	All ages	Daily
Carbo-Dome	Skin	No	No	No	All ages	Two or three times a day
Clinitar	Skin	No	No	No	All ages	Three times a week
Cocois	Scalp	Yes	Yes	No	> 6 years	Weekly
Denorex Shampoo	Scalp	No	No	No	> 12 years	Alternate days
Exorex	Scalp	No	No	No	> 2 years	Two or three times a day
Polytar & Polytar Plus	Scalp	No	No	No	All ages	Once or twice weekly
Polytar AF	Scalp	No	No	Zinc pyrithione 1%	All ages	Once or twice weekly
Pragmatar	Scalp	Yes	Yes	No	All ages	Once daily
Psoriderm	Both	No	No	No	All ages	Once or twice a day
Psorin	Both	Yes	No	Dithranol	All ages	Twice daily
T/Gel	Scalp	No	No	No	All ages	When needed

HINTS AND TIPS BOX 7.1: PSORIASIS

Problems with tar and dithranol products	Coal tar and dithranol share common problems of patient compliance. Both are messy to use, have an unpleasant odour and can stain skin and clothing
UV light	90% of patients with psoriasis improve when exposed to sunlight and most patients notice an improvement when they go on holiday
Emollient bath additives	Some bath additives, for example oilatum, will make the bath slippery and patients should be warned to exercise care when getting out of the bath

in many of the trials made it impossible to objectively determine the efficacy of this regimen.

Practical prescribing and product selection

Prescribing information relating to the medicines used to treat psoriasis discussed in the section 'Evidence base for over-the-counter medication' is summarised in Table 7.4; useful tips relating to patients presenting with psoriasis are given in Hints and Tips Box 7.1.

Emollients

There is a huge number of emollient products. All emollients should be regularly and liberally applied with no upper limit on how often they can be used. All are chemically inert and can therefore be safely used from birth onwards by all patients. They do not have any

interactions with other medicines. For a summary of marketed emollient products see Table 7.25 (page 184).

Tar-based products

Most non-emollient OTC products are based on coal tar but some are combinations of coal tar and salicylic acid or dithranol. All patient groups, including pregnant women, can use the majority of products on either the skin or scalp. They can cause local skin or scalp irritation and stain skin and clothes. They have no drug interactions.

Dithranol (Dithrocream)

Dithranol preparations are pharmacy-only medicines so long as the strength does not exceed a maximum of 1.0%.

Short-contact therapy is often advocated for dithranol because prolonged exposure can lead to irritation and burning skin. This involves using the lowest strength available (0.1%) for 30 min, which is then washed off. The concentration of dithranol is increased gradually to 1%. If psoriasis fails to respond with 1% treatment then referral to the GP is needed for higher strength treatment.

The patient might experience burning, even at low concentrations and if this becomes apparent therapy should either be discontinued or the concentration and/or the contact time reduced. Dithranol will stain skin a purple–brown colour but does clear in time.

Further reading

Dodd W A 1993 Tars. Their role in the treatment of psoriasis. Dermatological Clinics 11:131–135

Goeckerman W H 1925 The treatment of psoriasis. Northwest Medicine 24:229–231

Greaves M W, Weinstein G D 1995 Treatment of psoriasis. New England Journal of Medicine 332:581–588

Griffiths C, Kirby B 1999 Psoriasis management within primary care. The Prescriber 10:47–74

Harrington C I 1989 Low concentration dithranol and coal tar (Psorin) in psoriasis: a comparison with alcoholic coal tar extract and allantoin (Alphosyl). British Journal of Clinical Practice 43:27–29

Henseler T 1998 Genetics of psoriasis. Archives of Dermatological Research 290:463–476

Leary M R, Rapp S R, Herbst K C et al 1998 Interpersonal concerns and psychological difficulties of psoriasis patients: effects of disease severity and fear of negative evaluation. Health Psychology 17:530–536

Livingstone C 1997 Skin problems in pharmacy practice. Psoriasis. Pharmaceutical Journal 259:890–892

MacKie R M 1999 Clinical dermatology. Oxford University Press, Hong Kong

Naldi L, Carrel C F, Parazzini F et al 1992 Development of anthralin short-contact therapy in psoriasis: survey of published clinical trials. International Journal of Dermatology 31:126–130

Tham S N, Lun K C, Cheong W K 1994 A comparative study of calcipotriol ointment and tar in chronic plaque psoriasis. British Journal of Dermatology 131:673–677

Tristani-Firouzi P, Kruegger C G 1998 Efficacy and safety of treatment modalities for psoriasis. Cutis 61:11–21

Swanbeck G, Inerot A, Martinsson T et al 1995 Age at onset and different types of psoriasis. British Journal of Dermatology 133:768–773

Young E 1970 The external treatment of psoriasis. A controlled investigation of the effects of coal tar. British Journal of Dermatology 82:510–515

Web sites

The Psoriasis Association: www.timewarp.demon.co.uk/psoriasis.html

Australian Psoriasis Association: www.psoriasis.org.au/

Dandruff (pityriasis capitis)

Background

Dandruff is a chronic relapsing non-inflammatory hyperproliferative skin condition that is often seen as socially unsightly and is a source of embarrassment. Consequently, there are many products marketed to help with the problem.

Prevalence and epidemiology

Dandruff is very common and affects both sexes and all age groups, although it is unusual in prepubescent children. It has been estimated that 50% of Caucasians will experience dandruff at some time.

Aetiology

Increased cell turnover rate is responsible for dandruff but the reason cell turnover increases is unknown. Increasingly, research has focused on the role that micro-organisms have on the pathogenesis of dandruff, and in particular the yeast *Pityrosporum ovale*, although the evidence is inconclusive as to whether *P. ovale* is the primary cause of dandruff or is a contributory factor. It has been shown that *P. ovale* makes up more of the scalp flora of dandruff sufferers and might explain why dandruff improves in the summer months (fungal organisms thrive in the warm, moist environments that are encouraged in winter by the wearing of hats and caps). Further evidence to support a role of *P. ovale* in the aetiology of dandruff is the positive effect that antifungal therapy has on the resolution of dandruff.

Arriving at a differential diagnosis

Most patients will diagnose and treat dandruff without seeking medical help. However, for those patients that do ask for help and advice it is important to differentiate dandruff from other scalp conditions. Asking symptom-specific questions will help the pharmacist to determine if referral is needed (Table 7.5).

Clinical features of dandruff

The scalp will be dry, itchy and flaky. Visible dead cells can often be seen on the patient's clothing.

Conditions to eliminate

Seborrhoeic dermatitis

Typically, seborrhoeic dermatitis will affect areas other than the scalp. In adults, the trunk is commonly involved, as are the eyebrows, eyelashes and external ear. If only scalp involvement is present then the patient might complain of severe and persistent dandruff and the skin of the scalp will be red. For further information on seborrhoeic dermatitis see page 155.

Contact dermatitis

Enquiry should be made to the use of new hair products such as dyes and perms. These can cause irritation and

Table 7.5
Specific questions to ask the patient: Dandruff

Question	Relevance
Presence of erythema	● Dandruff is not associated with scalp redness unless the person has been scratching. Redness is characteristic of psoriasis and is common in adult seborrhoeic dermatitis
Itch	● Dandruff tends to cause itching of the scalp unlike psoriasis and seborrhoeic dermatitis
Presence of other skin lesions	● An adult with scalp involvement only is likely to have dandruff, especially in the absence of erythema

scaling. Avoidance of the irritant should see an improvement in the condition. If improvement is not observed after avoidance of 1 to 2 weeks then a re-assessment of the condition is needed.

Tinea capitis

If the problem is persistent and associated with hair loss then fungal infection of the scalp should be considered. For further information see page 149.

Figure 7.5 will aid the differentiation of dandruff from other scalp disorders.

TRIGGER POINTS indicative of referral: Dandruff

- OTC treatment failure with a 'medicated shampoo'
- Suspected fungal infection

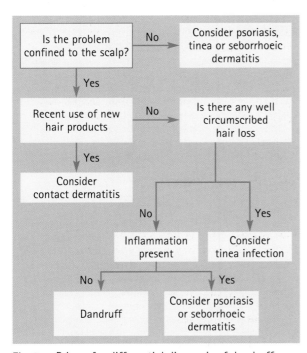

Fig. 7.5 Primer for differential diagnosis of dandruff

Evidence base for over-the-counter medication

The use of a hypoallergenic shampoo on a daily basis will usually control mild symptoms. In more persistent and severe cases a 'medicated' shampoo can be used to control the symptoms. Treatment options include coal tar, selenium sulphide, zinc pyrithione and ketoconazole.

Coal tar

The mechanism of action for crude coal tar in the management of dandruff is unclear, although it appears that tars affect DNA synthesis and have an antimitotic effect. There are virtually no published studies in the literature to assess the efficacy of coal tars in the treatment of dandruff. One study compared the efficacy between a tar and a non-tar shampoo (containing salicylic acid) but found no statistical difference between the two shampoos. Despite the lack of evidence, tar derivatives are found in a plethora of OTC-medicated shampoos and have been granted FDA approval in the US as an antidandruff agent.

Selenium sulphide

It is accepted that selenium is effective as an antidandruff agent. Studies have shown it to be significantly better than placebo and non-medicated shampoos.

Zinc pyrithione

Zinc pyrithione has been shown to exhibit antifungal properties and reduce cell turnover rates. It is believed that one or both of these properties confers its effectiveness in treating dandruff, however, very few trials have been published.

Ketoconazole

Ketoconazole was deregulated from POM to P status in 1995 and is available as a 2% shampoo. It helps in controlling the itching and flaking associated with dandruff. Studies have shown it to be effective and better tolerated than selenium sulphide. Ketoconazole has also been shown to act as a prophylactic agent in preventing relapse.

Table 7.6
Practical prescribing: Summary of medicines for dandruff

Medicine	Use in children	Likely side-effects	Drug interactions of note	Patients in whom care should be exercised	Pregnancy
Coal tar products	All ages	Local irritation and dermatitis reported but rare	None	None	OK
Selenium	> 5 years				OK but manufacturers state to avoid in first trimester
Zinc pyrithione	No lower age limit				OK
Ketoconazole	All ages				

Practical prescribing and product selection

Prescribing information relating to the specific products used to treat dandruff and discussed in the section 'Evidence base for over-the-counter medication' is discussed and summarised in Table 7.6; useful tips relating to dandruff shampoo are given in Hints and Tips Box 7.2.

All antidandruff shampoos can cause local scalp irritation. If this is severe the product should be discontinued. Any patient group can use them, although some manufacturers state products should be avoided during the first three months of pregnancy. However, there appear to be no data to substantiate this precaution during pregnancy. They have no drug interactions.

Coal tar products

Products containing coal tar are discussed under practical prescribing for psoriasis. For further information on coal tar products see page 151.

Selenium sulphide (e.g. Selsun)

Adults and children over the age of 5 should use the product twice a week for the first 2 weeks and then once a week for the next 2 weeks. Selenium should be avoided if the patient has inflamed or broken skin because irritation can occur. Selenium can also cause discoloration of the hair and alter the colour of hair dyes.

Zinc pyrithione (e.g. Head and Shoulders)

Zinc-based products can be used by all patients and at any age. They should be used on a daily basis until dandruff clears. Dermatitis has been reported with zinc pyrithione and should be borne in mind when treating patients with pre-existing dermatitis.

Ketoconazole (e.g. Nizoral Dandruff Shampoo)

Nizoral can either be used to treat acute flare-ups of dandruff or as prophylaxis. To treat acute cases adults and children should wash the hair thoroughly, leaving the shampoo on for 3 to 5 min before rinsing it off. This should be repeated every 3 or 4 days for between 2 and 4 weeks. If used for prophylaxis, the shampoo should be used once every 1 to 2 weeks. It can cause local itching or a burning sensation on application and may occasionally discolour hair.

Further reading

Arrese J E, Pierard-Franchimont C, De-Doncker P et al 1996 Effect of ketoconazole-medicated shampoos on squamometry and *Malassezia ovalis* load in pityriasis capitis. Cutis 58:235–237

Danby F W, Maddin W S, Margesson L J et al 1993 A randomized double-blind controlled trial of ketoconazole 2% shampoo versus selenium sulfide 2.5% shampoo in the treatment of moderate to severe dandruff. Journal of the American Academy of Dermatology 29:1008–1012

Nigam P K, Tyagi S, Saxena A K et al 1988 Dermatitis from zinc pyrithione. Contact Dermatitis 19:219

Orentreich N 1969 Comparative study of two antidandruff preparations. Journal of Pharmaceutical Sciences 58:1279–1284

Pereira F, Fernandes C, Dias M et al 1995 Allergic contact dermatitis from zinc pyrithione. Contact Dermatitis 33:131

Peter R U, Richarz-Barthauer U 1995 Successful treatment and prophylaxis of scalp seborrheic dermatitis and dandruff with 2% ketoconazole shampoo: results of a multicentre, double blind, placebo-controlled trial. British Journal of Dermatology 132:441–445

Rigoni C, Toffolo P, Cantu A et al 1989 1% econazole hair shampoo in the treatment of pityriasis capitis; a comparative study versus zinc pyrithione shampoo. Giornale Italiano di Dermatologia e Venereologia 124:67–70

Van Custem J, Van Gerven F, Fransen J et al 1990 The in vitro antifungal activity of ketoconazole, zinc pyrithione and selenium sulfide against *Pityrosporum* and their efficacy as a shampoo in the treatment of experimental pityrosporosis in guinea pigs. Journal of the American Academy of Dermatology 22:993–998

Seborrhoeic dermatitis

Background

There are two distinct types of seborrhoeic dermatitis, an infantile form, often referred to as cradle cap and an adult form. Seborrhoeic dermatitis can present with varying degrees of severity, ranging from mild dandruff to a severe and explosive form in AIDS patients.

Prevalence and epidemiology

Cradle cap is a relatively common disorder and is much more prevalent than the adult form. Cradle cap usually starts in infancy, before the age of 6 months and is usually self-limiting; the adult form tends to be chronic and persistent. In addition, men are six times more likely to suffer from the adult form than women.

Aetiology

Despite its name, there appears to be no changes in sebum secretion. Like psoriasis and dandruff, seborrhoeic dermatitis is characterised by an increased cell turnover rate. The precise cause of seborrhoeic dermatitis remains unknown and several theories have been put forward, ranging from hormonal to nutritional mechanisms. Like dandruff, *Pityrosporum ovale* has been implicated as an aetiological agent because a proportion of patients respond to antifungal therapy, however it has not yet been established whether it has a primary or secondary role in the clinical presentation of seborrhoeic dermatitis.

Arriving at a differential diagnosis

Infantile seborrhoeic dermatitis is relatively easy to recognise but can sometimes be confused with atopic dermatitis. Whereas seborrhoeic dermatitis can develop almost immediately in the newborn, atoptic dermatitis is rare before 3 months of age. Arriving at a differential diagnosis of the adult form can be more problematic because of confusion with allergic contact dermatitis, psoriasis, dandruff and pityriasis versicolor. Asking symptom-specific questions will help the pharmacist to determine if referral is needed (Table 7.7).

Clinical features of seborrhoeic dermatitis

The adult form of seborrhoeic dermatitis is characterised by a red, mildly itchy scaly rash that typically affects the

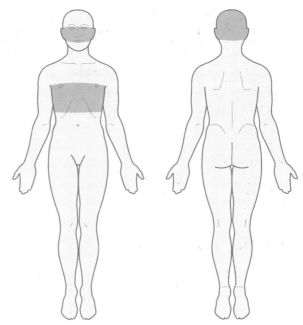

Fig. 7.6 Typical distribution of seborrhoeic dermatitis

central part of the face, scalp, eyebrows, eyelids, naso-labial folds and midchest. Blepharitis and otitis externa are also common secondary complications. Unlike cradle cap, the rash often itches. Cradle cap appears as large yellow scales and **crusts** on the scalp (Fig. 7.7, overleaf), face and napkin area.

Conditions to eliminate

Atopic dermatitis

In infants, atopic dermatitis usually presents as itchy lesions on the scalp, face and trunk. However, the nappy area is usually spared and most patients will have a positive family history of the atopic triad of dermatitis, asthma or hayfever. For further information on atopic dermatitis see page 212.

Psoriasis

Adults who suffer from scalp psoriasis could be confused with those patients who present with severe and persistent dandruff caused by seborrhoeic dermatitis. However, eyebrow and eyelid involvement is common in patients with seborrhoeic dermatitis.

Pityriasis versicolor

This condition usually develops after exposure to the sun. It can be mistaken for adult seborrhoeic dermatitis because the lesions exhibit fine superficial scale and are located on the trunk. However, the rash does not itch and the face is usually spared.

Table 7.7
Specific questions to ask the patient: Seborrhoeic dermatitis

Question	Relevance
Itching	● In cradle cap the rash does not itch. This is useful when differentiating atopic dermatitis from seborrhoeic dermatitis
Location	● Infantile and adult forms of seborrhoeic dermatitis do present in slightly different locations (Fig. 7.6). Additionally, the distribution of seborrhoeic dermatitis has a different location to other skin conditions
Positive family history	● Patients tend not to have a family history in seborrhoeic dermatitis but often patients suffering from atopic dermatitis usually have one or more parents who suffer from eczema, hayfever or asthma. Patients with psoriasis can have a positive family history of the disease
Other symptoms	● Ear and eye problems are associated with seborrhoeic dermatitis
	● The general health of a child with seborrhoeic dermatitis will be well and happy, a child who is fractious and miserable is more likely to have atopic dermatitis
	● Seborrhoeic dermatitis usually has yellow greasy scale, unlike psoriasis, which has a silvery scale
Physical signs	● If you run your fingers through the hair of someone with seborrhoeic dermatitis little is felt. In psoriasis, lumps are apparent

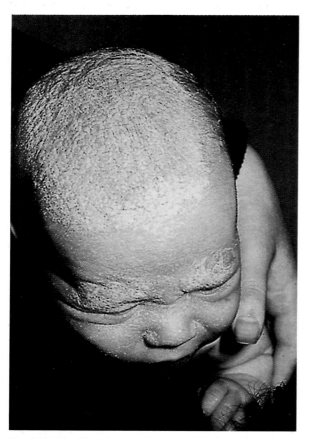

Fig. 7.7 Infantile seborrhoeic dermatitis. Reproduced from *Dermatology Colour Guide*, by J Wilkinson and S Shaw, 1998, Churchill Livingstone, with permission

 TRIGGER POINTS indicative of referral: Seborrhoeic dermatitis

● Treatment failure with OTC medicines
● Lesions that appear after exposure to sunlight

Evidence base for over-the-counter medication

Treatment options for seborrhoeic dermatitis are the same as dandruff. Unfortunately, seborrhoeic dermatitis tends to be more resistant to therapy and often recurs whatever treatment is chosen.

For infants with cradle cap, it might be possible to remove scales by applying olive oil to the scalp and leaving on overnight followed by using a non-medicated shampoo the next morning. If this fails, a medicated shampoo could be tried, used on alternate days until the condition is under control, at which point only twice weekly shampooing should be necessary. If this fails the child should be referred to the GP.

In adults, OTC preparations are often inadequate and topical steroid therapy may be required.

Practical prescribing and product selection

Prescribing information relating to specific products used to treat seborrhoeic dermatitis is discussed under 'Dandruff' on page 152. In addition, at least one product is marketed specifically for cradle cap and is discussed and summarised in Table 7.8.

Table 7.8 Practical prescribing: Summary of medicines for cradle cap					
Medicine	Use in children	Likely side-effects	Drug interactions of note	Patients in whom care should be exercised	Pregnancy
Dentinox Cradle Cap Shampoo	Birth onwards	None reported	None	None	Not applicable

Dentinox Cradle Cap Shampoo

This contains sodium lauryl ether sulpho-succinate 6% and sodium lauryl ether sulphate 2.7%. The shampoo should be applied twice during each bath time until the scalp clears, after which it can be used when needed.

Further reading

Bergbrant I M, Faergemann J 1990 The role of *Pityrosporum ovale* in seborrheic dermatitis. Seminars in Dermatology 9:262–268

Danby F W, Maddin W S, Margesson L J et al 1993 A randomized double-blind controlled trial of ketoconazole 2% shampoo versus selenium sulfide 2.5% shampoo in the treatment of moderate to severe dandruff. Journal of the American Academy of Dermatolgoy 29:1008–1812

Janniger C K, Schwartz R A 1995 Seborrheic dermatitis. American Family Physician 52:149–155, 159–160

Johnson B A, Nunley J R 2000 Treatment of seborrheic dermatitis. American Family Physician 61:2703–2710

Go I H, Wientjens D P, Koster M 1992 A double-blind trial of 1% ketoconazole shampoo versus placebo in the treatment of dandruff. Mycoses 35:103–105

McGrath J, Murphy G M 1991 The control of seborrhoeic dermatitis and dandruff by antipityrosporal drugs. Drugs 41:178–184

Web sites

Johnson and Johnson sponsored site: www.pediatricinstitute.com

Fungal infections

Background

Two main groups of fungi infect man: Candida yeasts and the dermatophytes. This text will consider only dermatophyte infections. Fungal infections are commonly referred to as ringworm, although this is inaccurate because a worm does not cause the infection and most variants are not observed as a ring. This terminology only serves to cause confusion and should, where possible be avoided.

Prevalence and epidemiology

Globally, dermatophytic fungi are more prevalent in tropical and subtropical areas because fungal organisms prefer high temperatures and high humidity. Having said this, dermatophyte infections are commonly met in UK practice. Tinea pedis (athlete's foot) is the most common dermatophyte infection and appears to be on the increase. Other tinea infections, such as tinea corporis (ringworm), tinea cruris (jock itch) and tinea unguium (nail infection) might present in the community pharmacy but are less common. Fungal infection affecting the scalp (tinea capitis), once common, has now declined in many nations and is very infrequently encountered.

Aetiology

Dermatophyte infections are contagious and transmitted directly from one host to another. They invade the stratum corneum of the skin, hair and nails but do not generally infiltrate living tissues. The fungus then begins to grow and proliferate in the non-living cornified layer of keratinised tissue of the epidermis.

Arriving at a differential diagnosis

Depending on the area affected (Fig. 7.8) the infection will manifest itself in a variety of clinical presentations. Recognition of symptoms for each site affected will facilitate recognition and accurate diagnosis. All forms of tinea infection should be easy to recognise, perhaps with the exception of isolated lesions on the body.

Patients with athlete's foot will often accurately self-diagnose the condition. However, the pharmacist should still confirm this self-diagnosis through a combination of questions (Table 7.9) and inspection of the feet. This is important because it also provides an opportunity to check for fungal nail involvement.

Clinical features of tinea infections

Athlete's foot

The usual site of infection is in the toe webs, especially the fourth web space (web space next to the little toe). The skin appears white and 'soggy' (Fig. 7.9). The area is normally itchy and the feet tend to smell. Occasionally, the infection can spread to involve the sole and instep of the foot. Cases of tinea infection where the plantar surface has become involved can be persistent and difficult to treat.

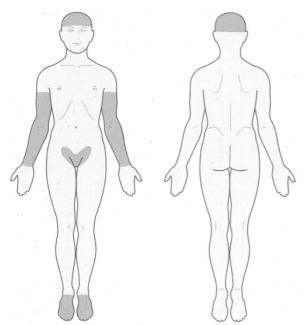

Fig. 7.8 Distribution of fungal infections

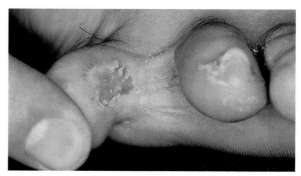

Fig. 7.9 Athlete's foot. Reproduced from *Color Atlas of Dermatology*, by G White, 2004, Churchill Livingstone, with permission

Tinea corporis

Tinea corporis is defined as an infection of the major skin surfaces that do not involve the face, hands, feet, groin or scalp. The usual clinical presentation is of itchy pink or red scaly patches with a well-defined inflamed border (Fig. 7.11). The lesions often show 'central clearing' as the central area is relatively resistant to colonisation. This appearance led to the term 'ringworm'. Lesions can occur singly, be numerous or overlap to produce a single large lesion and appear polycyclic (several overlapping circular lesions).

Tinea cruris

Tinea cruris is fungal infection of the groin, also known as 'jock itch'. The rash is usually isolated to the groin and inner thighs but can spread to the buttocks. The lesion is normally intensely itchy, reddish brown and has a well-defined edge.

The nail can become involved in severe and persistent cases of athlete's foot. The nail takes on a dull opaque and yellow appearance (Fig. 7.10). Over time, the nail thickens, becoming more brittle and prone to crumbling. This is most commonly seen in patients over 50 years old. Treatment must be systemic and hence referral is needed.

Table 7.9
Specific questions to ask the patient: Fungal infections

Question	Relevance
Location	● Fungal infections present in a number of body locations (Fig. 7.8). The clinical presentation varies according to which part of the body is affected
Age and sex of patient	● Athlete's foot is most prevalent in adolescents and young adults ● Nail involvement usually occurs in older adults ● Infection in the groin (jock itch) is much more common in men than women
Presence of itch	● Fungal infections usually itch. This usually eliminates conditions such as psoriasis but not dermatitis/eczema
Associated symptoms	● Fungal lesions tend to be dry and scaly (except athlete's foot) and have a sharp margin between infected and non-infected skin
Previous and family history	● Fungal infections are usually acute in onset with no previous episodes, although athlete's foot may become recurrent ● For lesions that do not show a classic textbook description, a positive family history of dermatitis or psoriasis might influence your differential diagnosis

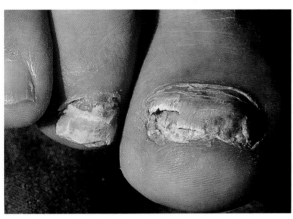

Fig. 7.10 Tinea unguium. Reproduced from *Dermatology: An Illustrated Colour Text* by D Gawkrodger, 2002, Mosby, with permission

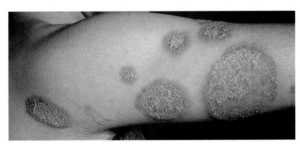

Fig. 7.11 Tinea corporis showing intense inflammation. Reproduced from *Dermatology: An Illustrated Colour Text* by D Gawkrodger, 2002, Mosby, with permission

Conditions to eliminate

Tinea faciei

Fungal infections on the face are rare. The lesions are similar in appearance to tinea corporis but are often mistaken for other facial skin conditions. In common with tinea corporis the lesions will normally have a sharp, well-defined border, show scaling and be itchy.

Tinea manuum

Tinea manuum (fungal infection of the hand) is often misdiagnosed as eczema or psoriasis because of its atypical tinea appearance. The patient usually suffers from chronic diffuse scaling of one palm. Athlete's foot will often be present and the infection will have spread to the hands from the feet due to the patient scratching the feet. The condition is not common and if no foot involvement is implicated then the diagnosis strongly points to dermatitis if it affects both palms.

Psoriasis

Isolated fungal body lesions can be difficult to distinguish from plaque psoriasis. However, if the patient has psoriasis there will normally be a family history of psoriasis and psoriatic lesions tend not to itch, exhibit more scaling and do not show central clearing.

Dermatitis

Both fungal infections and dermatitis exhibit red, itchy lesions and can therefore be difficult to distinguish from one another. Patients with dermatitis will often have a family and personal history of dermatitis or be able to describe an event that triggered the onset of the rash. Misdiagnosis of a fungal infection for dermatitis and subsequent treatment with a steroid-based cream will diminish the itch, redness and scaling but the infecting organism will proliferate. On withdrawal of the steroid cream the visible signs of the infection will return and be worse than before, often in a papular form (tinea incognito).

> **❗ TRIGGER POINTS indicative of referral: Tinea infections**
>
> - Nail involvement
> - OTC treatment failure
> - Suspected facial or scalp involvement

Evidence base for over-the-counter medication

All tinea infections, except nail and scalp involvement, can be treated effectively with topical OTC preparations. A plethora of topical antifungal preparations are marketed for the treatment of superficial fungal infections. Five classes of medicines have proven efficacy in the treatment of superficial dermatophyte infections.

Benzoic acid

Benzoic acid acts by lowering intracellular pH of dermatophytes and is combined with salicylic acid (Whitfield's Ointment). Although Whitfield's Ointment has been on the market for nearly a century it still has a role to play as an effective antifungal, although newer products – with higher cure rates, quicker resolution and more cosmetically acceptable formulations – have replaced its widespread use in Western society. However, it remains one of the essential drugs on the World Health Organization's model list.

Undecenoates

Undecenoates have been used to treat athlete's foot for over 30 years and feature in the most recent US Pharmacopoeia. In a recent Cochrane review, undecenoic acid was said to be efficacious in treating fungal infections for skin and nail infections of the foot.

Tolnaftate

Tolnaftate appears to have the least amount of trial data supporting its efficacy. Low patient numbers involved in the studies further compounds the difficulty in assessing its efficacy.

Imidazoles

Imidazoles have largely replaced benzoic acid, undecenoates and tolnaftate because they have greater efficacy and an excellent safety record. There appears to be no clinically significant differences in cure rates between the different imidazoles and treatment choice will probably be driven by patient acceptability and cost.

Allylamines

Recently, terbinafine has been exempt from POM control for external use in the treatment of tinea pedis and tinea cruris. This is an important step forward for OTC treatment of fungal infections as comparative trials between allylamines and imidazoles have shown allylamines to be more efficacious.

Summary

On current evidence, an imidazole derivative or terbina-fine would be first-line treatment choices for fungal infection. If treatment is refractory to imidazole therapy then terbinafine could be tried, although the higher cost of terbinafine might deter some patients from purchasing the product.

Practical prescribing and product selection

Prescribing information relating to specific products used to treat fungal infections and discussed in the section 'Evidence base for over-the-counter medication' is summarised in Table 7.10; useful tips relating to patients presenting with fungal infections are given in Hints and Tips Box 7.3.

Imidazoles (e.g. clotrimazole (Canesten), miconazole (Daktarin), ketoconazole (Daktarin Gold))

All topical imidazoles are very safe and can be used by all patient groups, including pregnant women. They do not have any drug interactions and the major side-effect associated with their use is irritation on application. To prevent reinfection, imidazoles should be used after the lesions have cleared, although the length of time varies from product to product.

Table 7.10
Practical prescribing: Summary of medicines for tinea infections

Medicine	Use in children	Likely side-effects	Drug interactions of note	Patients in whom care should be exercised	Pregnancy
Imidazoles Canesten and Canesten AF	All ages	Mild burning or itching	None	None	OK
Daktarin Dual Action					
Daktarin Gold					
Canesten Hydrocortisone	> 10 years				
Daktacort HC					
Tolnaftate Mycil	No lower age stated	None reported	None	None	OK
Tinaderm					
Undecenoates Mycota	No lower age stated	None reported	None	None	OK
Monphytol	> 12 years	Stinging			OK, but manufacturer states avoid
Benzoic acid Whitfield's Ointment	No lower age stated	None reported	None	None	OK
Terbinafine Lamisil AT	> 16 years	Redness, itching	None	None	OK

HINTS AND TIPS BOX 7.3: FUNGAL INFECTION

Practical advice to help prevent reinfection	1. Dry the skin thoroughly after showering or having a bath. Keep a personal towel and do not share it to prevent the infection spreading from person to person 2. Socks should be frequently changed 3. Avoid wearing occlusive, non-breathable shoes 4. Dust shoes and socks with antifungal powder
Canesten Hydrocortisone	The licence states that the maximum period of treatment is 7 days because this product contains hydrocortisone. This limits its usefulness because many fungal infections will take longer to clear than 7 days, especially if the product is used for 3 days once the lesions have cleared to prevent re-infection. The pharmacist has to either break the law or recommend the use of an imidazole-only product after the initial 7 days treatment with the product containing a steroid

Clotrimazole (e.g. Canesten, Canesten AF, Canesten Hydrocortisone)

Clotrimazole-containing products can be used for all dermatophyte and candidal infections, except Canesten Hydrocortisone, which is licensed for athlete's foot only. Canesten and Canesten AF cream should be applied two or three times a day, whereas Canesten Hydrocortisone can only be used twice a day.

Bifonazole (Canesten AF Once Daily)

Licensed for the treatment of *tinea pedis*, bifonazole should be applied once daily, preferably at night. Its only advantage over the other imidazoles is the dosing schedule, which may improve compliance.

Miconazole (e.g. Daktarin Dual Action Cream, Daktacort HC)

Products containing miconazole only are suitable for patients of all ages and should be used twice a day. Treatment should continue for 10 days after all lesions have disappeared to prevent relapse. Daktacort HC is suitable for children aged over 10 and is licensed for sweat rash and athlete's foot.

Ketoconazole (Daktarin Gold)

Ketoconazole has a licence for tinea pedis, cruris and candidal **intertrigo**. For athlete's foot the cream should be applied twice a day for 1 week. For tinea cruris and candidal intertrigo, the cream should be applied once or twice daily. If no improvement in symptoms is experienced after 4 weeks treatment then the patient should be referred to the GP. For all conditions treatment should be continued for 2 to 3 days after all signs of infection have disappeared to prevent relapse.

Tolnaftate (e.g. Mycil, Tinaderm)

Products containing tolnaftate have no interactions or side-effects and can be used by all patients, including pregnant women. They can be used for athlete's foot and infections of the groin and should be used twice a day with treatment continuing for at least 1 week after the infection has cleared up.

Undecenoates (e.g. Mycota, Monophytol)

Products containing undecenoates have no interactions and can be used by all patients, including pregnant women. They are licensed for athlete's foot and should be used twice a day and treatment continued for at least 1 week after the infection has cleared up. Local irritation has been reported.

Benzoic acid (e.g. Whitfield's ointment)

Benzoic acid in combination with salicylic acid (known as Whitfield's ointment) is now rarely used. However, it can be used by all patients. A proprietary product called Toepedo is available OTC.

Terbinafine (Lamisil AT cream and spray)

Terbinafine can be used to treat athlete's foot and jock itch (the spray can also be used for tinea corporis). The cream should be applied once or twice a day whereas the spray should be used only once daily. It has no interactions and can be used by all patients, including pregnant women. It has few reported side-effects.

Further reading

Crawford F, Hart R, Bell-Syer S et al 2000 Topical treatments for fungal infections of the skin and nails of the foot. Cochrane Review. In: The Cochrane Library, Issue 3. Update Software, Oxford

Drake L A, Dinehart S M, Farmer E R et al 1996 Guidelines of care for superficial mycotic infections of the skin: tinea corporis, tinea cruris, tinea faciei, tinea manuum, and tinea pedis. Guidelines/Outcomes Committee of the American Academy of Dermatology. Journal of the American Academy of Dermatology 34:282–286

Elewski B 1996 Tinea capitis. Dermatology Clinics 14:23–31

Pierard G E, Arrese J E, Pierard-Franchimont C 1996
Treatment and prophylaxis of tinea infections. Drugs
52:209–224

Web sites
General site on tinea infection: www.nlm.nih.gov/
medlineplus/ency/article/001439.htm

Hair loss

Background

Hair loss affects both men and women. It is associated
with strong emotional and psychological consequences.
People have been socialised to link a full head of hair with
youth and vitality, whereas baldness portrays a feeling of
unattractiveness and loss of youth. Hair loss can be due
to a number of aetiologies, however, this section concentrates on androgenetic alopecia (male-pattern baldness)
because it is the most common cause of hair loss.

Prevalence and epidemiology

Men are more susceptible than women to androgenetic
alopecia and usually experience more severe hair loss
than women. It is said that the prevalence of male-
pattern baldness in Caucasians who reach old age
approaches 100%.

Patients usually have a positive family history. The
nature and extent of hair loss will follow identical
patterns to those seen in the patient's immediate parents
and grandparents, which can be used as a predictor to the
patient's potential hair-loss pattern. In some male
patients, hair loss can occur as early as their teens.

Aetiology

Hair is classed as either terminal or vellus hair. Terminal
hair is longer and thicker and found on the scalp and
eyebrows. Vellus hair covers the remainder of the body
and is shorter and downy. In androgenetic alopecia
terminal hair follicles transform in to more vellus-like
hair follicles as a result of preferential binding by
dihydrotestosterone (produced from the conversion of
androgen by 5-alpha-reductase) to hair follicle receptors.
Eventually the follicle ceases activity completely with
resulting hair loss. It appears that there is a genetic
component determining the age of onset and the severity
of the problem.

Arriving at a differential diagnosis

It should not be too difficult to spot someone with hair
loss! Empathy and understanding towards the patient
needs to be exercised. Although androgenetic alopecia is
the most common form of hair loss, other causes need

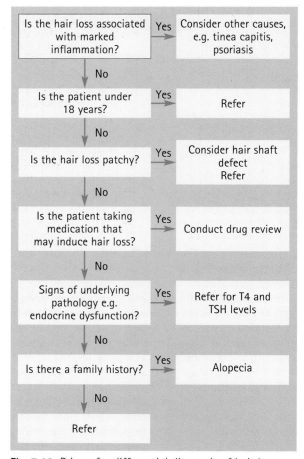

Fig. 7.12 Primer for differential diagnosis of hair loss

to be eliminated (Fig. 7.12). Asking symptom-specific
questions will help the pharmacist to determine if referral
is needed (Table 7.11).

Clinical features androgenetic alopecia

Men initially notice a thinning of the hair and a frontal
receding hairline that might or might not be accompanied with hair loss at the crown. In women the frontal
hairline is maintained with diffuse hair loss that is
somewhat accentuated at the crown.

Conditions to eliminate

Telogen effluvium

Telogen effluvium represents a shift of more hairs in to
the resting phase (telogen) of the hair cycle, which results
in shedding of hair. This can be caused by a number of
factors:

Postpartum

During pregnancy, circulating levels of oestrogen
increase, with a resulting rise in the number of follicles

Table 7.11
Specific questions to ask the patient: Hair loss

Question	Relevance
Hair loss accompanied by other symptoms	● Androgenetic alopecia is not associated with other symptoms. Itch and erythema are indicators that another cause, e.g. fungal scalp infection, psoriasis or seborrhoeic dermatitis, might be responsible for the hair loss
Pattern of hair loss	● In men, hair loss begins at the front of the head and recedes backwards or at the crown. In women, hair loss tends to generalised and diffuse. Presentations that differ to this or are sudden in onset suggest another cause of hair loss
Deficiency states	● There is now strong evidence that iron deficiency in women can cause hair loss
Underlying pathology	● A number of endocrine conditions can cause hair loss, most notably thyroid disorders
Medicine-induced hair loss	● A number of medicines can cause hair loss (see Table 7.12)
Hair loss triggered by a specific event	● Hair loss can be caused by a stressful event or following surgery or after childbirth

in anagen (growth phase); the hair therefore thickens. However, after delivery the hair follicles return to the resting phase and the hair is shed. Women might believe that they are experiencing hair loss when in reality the hair is returning to the normal prepregnancy state. Reassurance should be given that this is a temporary and self-limiting problem.

Stress

Stress is known to induce hair loss. The reason behind this is poorly understood. Enquiry to ascertain lifestyle factors that might have caused recent stress and anxiety to the patient should be explored.

Nutritional factors

Iron deficiency is associated with female hair loss. If iron deficiency is the cause, a 2-month course of iron supplementation should result in thickening of the hair. If the patient fails to respond to treatment then the patient should be reassessed.

Underlying endocrine disorder

Diabetes mellitus, hypopituitarism and hypothyroidism can result in poor hair growth. In hypothyroidism the hair is thin and brittle and the patient might be lethargic and have a history of recent weight gain. If the patient is currently taking levothyroxine then T4 measurements should be performed to ensure the condition is not being treated sub-therapeutically.

Fungal scalp infection (tinea capitis)

The first signs of infection are the appearance of a well-circumscribed round patch of alopecia that is associated with itch and scaling. Common areas of involvement include the occipital, parietal and crown region. Inspection of the area might reveal 'black dots' on the scalp as a result of infected hairs. It is an uncommon infection and unlikely to be seen in practice.

Alopecia areata

Refers to hair loss of unknown origin, although there is often an association with **atopy** and autoimmune disease. Unlike androgenetic alopecia the hair loss is sudden and mainly affects children and adolescents. It might involve only small patches of hair loss or the whole scalp could be affected. The condition is usually self-limiting and regrowth of hair is often observed but repeated episodes are not unusual.

Traction alopecia

Most commonly seen in women, traction alopecia refers to hair loss due to excess and sustained tension on the hair, usually as a result of styling hair with rollers or a particular type of hairstyle.

Medicine-induced causes

Many medicines can interfere with the hair cycle and cause transient hair loss, cytotoxic medicines being one of the most obvious examples. However, many medicines have been associated with hair loss. Table 7.12 lists some of the more commonly implicated medicines. If medicines other than cytotoxics are suspected of causing hair loss, the prescriber should be contacted to discuss other possible treatment options.

Trichotillomania

This refers to patients who have an impulsive desire to twist and pull scalp hair. The patient usually has some form of psychiatric illness and it would be very unusual for such patients, or their carers, to present in a pharmacy with hair loss as the presenting symptom.

Table 7.12
Medicines known to cause hair loss

Medicine or medicine class	Incidence of hair loss
Antineoplastics	Almost 100% (to varying degrees)
Anticoagulants	Telogen effluvium in approximately 50%
Lithium carbonate	Telogen effluvium in approximately 10%
Interferons	Telogen effluvium in 20 to 30%
Oral contraceptives	Seen 2 to 3 months after stopping
Retinoids	Approximately 20% of patients

❗ TRIGGER POINTS indicative of referral: Hair loss

- Fungal infection of the scalp
- Patients under 18 years old
- Possible endocrine cause
- Suspected iron deficiency for blood test
- Trichotillomania

Evidence base for over-the-counter medication

Currently, minoxidil is the only product marketed for androgenetic alopecia. It is available as either a 2% or a 5% solution.

A number of clinical trials have investigated the efficacy and safety of minoxidil at 2% and 5% concentrations. The majority of these have been conducted on precisely the population that would respond the best to treatment; men aged between 18 to 50, with mild to moderate thinning of the hair at the vertex. Despite this, trial results are not totally convincing. Minoxidil is superior to placebo (although placebo does invoke a large initial response) and promotes a small increase in regrowth of vellus hair and increases the diameter of the hair shaft. However, longitudinal studies show that less than half of patients treated experience moderate to marked hair growth. Hair counts appear to be greatest after 12 months of treatment but, by 30 months, hair counts will have decreased (although they are still above baseline) and the bald area increases in size to its initial diameter.

Minoxidil therefore appears to delay and slow down hair loss in less than half of its target patient population. Furthermore, if treatment is stopped any hair growth achieved is lost within 6 to 8 weeks on discontinuation of therapy and baldness returns to pretreatment levels.

The situation in women is not dissimilar, although the 5% solution offers no advantage over the 2% solution and therefore has not been granted a product licence at that strength.

Summary

Minoxidil will not significantly help the majority of balding individuals. It will promote hair growth in approximately 50% of minimally balding young men but, over time, the effect tails off. After 30 months the effect is still greater than baseline but, on the whole, will not achieve cosmetically acceptable hair growth. In other words, the use of minoxidil is useful for specific patients who want to 'buy' themselves time from the inevitable balding process.

Oral finasteride (1 mg per day) is used to treat androgenetic alopecia in men because it has shown to promote hair growth and prevent further loss in a significant proportion of men with male pattern baldness. Comparison trials with minoxidil have not yet been conducted, although when used in an animal model the combination was reported to have a synergistic effect. If treatment with minoxidil is unsatisfactory then the patient could be referred for evaluation by the GP and potentially be given finasteride.

Practical prescribing and product selection

Prescribing information relating to minoxidil is discussed and summarised in Table 7.13; useful tips relating to the treatment of patients with minoxidil are given in Hints and Tips Box 7.4.

Minoxidil (e.g. Regaine Regular (2%) and Extra (5%) Strength)

The dose for minoxidil is 1 mL applied to dry hair to the total affected areas of the scalp twice daily. If fingertips are used to facilitate drug application, hands should be washed afterwards. Although minoxidil is applied topically, absorption into the systemic circulation can occur and can result in chest pain, rapid heart beat, faintness or dizziness. If these occur the patient should stop using the product immediately. Other less important adverse effects associated with topical minoxidil are local irritation, redness and itching but these appear to be related to the vehicle – propylene glycol – rather than minoxidil. Changes in blood pressure should not occur because the serum level of minoxidil after topical application is below that needed to cause changes to blood pressure, however as a precaution minoxidil should be avoided in hypertensive patients if possible. Some patients also report a temporary increase in hair shedding 2 to 6 weeks after beginning treatment. This subsides and is most likely due to the action of minoxidil, shifting hairs from the resting telogen phase to the growing anagen phase.

Table 7.13
Practical prescribing: Summary of medicines for hair loss

Medicine	Use in children	Likely side-effects	Drug interactions of note	Patients in whom care should be exercised	Pregnancy
Minoxidil (Regaine)	Not applicable	Skin irritation	None	Avoid in hypertensive patients	Avoid

---

HINTS AND TIPS BOX 7.4: HAIR LOSS

Changes to hair colour and texture	Some patients have experienced changes in hair colour and/or texture with Regaine use. Patients should be warned of this possible problem before using Regaine
How long should the patient use Regaine?	It can take 4 months or more before evidence of hair growth can be expected. Users should discontinue treatment if there is no improvement after 1 year

Further reading

Burke K E 1989 Hair loss. What causes it and what can be done about it. Postgraduate Medicine 85:52–58, 67–73, 77

Hong D, Hart L L 1990 Topical minoxidil for hair loss in women. DICP: the annals of pharmacotherapy 24:1062–1063

Katz H I, Hien N T, Prawer S E et al 1987 Long-term efficacy of topical minoxidil in male pattern baldness. Journal of the American Academy of Dermatology 16:711–718

Koperaki J A, Orenberg E K, Wilkinson D L 1987 Topical minoxidil therapy for androgenetic alopecia: a 30 month study. Archives of Dermatology 123:1483–1487

Price V H 1999 Treatment of hair loss. New England Journal of Medicine 1999; 341:964–973

Price V H, Menefee E, Strauss P C 1999 Changes in hair weight and hair count in men with androgenetic alopecia, after application of 5% and 2% topical minoxidil, placebo, or no treatment. Journal of the American Academy of Dermatology 41:717–721

Rietschel R L, Duncan S H 1987 Safety and efficacy of topical minoxidil in the management of androgenetic alopecia. Journal of the American Academy of Dermatology 16:677–685

Roberts J L 1997 Androgenetic alopecia in men and women: an overview of cause and treatment. Dermatology Nursing 9:379–388

Tosti A, Misciali C, Piraccini B M et al 1994 Drug-induced hair loss and hair growth: incidence, management and avoidance. Drug Safety 10:310–317

Web sites

General medical site containing information on hair loss: www.nlm.nih.gov/medlineplus/ency/article/003246.htm

Warts and verrucas

Background

Warts and verrucas are benign growths of the skin caused by the human papilloma virus (HPV). Certain types of HPV have an affinity for certain body locations, for example hands, face, anogenital region and feet. Although self-limiting, they are cosmetically unacceptable to many patients who frequently seek advice and treatment.

Prevalence and epidemiology

The prevalence of warts has not been accurately documented. However, they are more common in children, having been reported to affect between 2 and 20% of schoolchildren, with a peak incidence in children aged between 12 and 16 years old. Warts are uncommon in the elderly and caution should be exercised if an elderly patient presents to the pharmacy with a self-diagnosed wart.

Aetiology

HPV gain entry to the host by epithelial defects in the epidermis. It is transmitted by direct skin-to-skin contact, although contact with an infected person's shed skin can also transmit the virus. Once established in the epithelial cells, the virus stimulates basal cell division to produce the characteristic lesion.

Patients, especially children, should be warned not to pick, bite or scratch warts as this can allow viral particle shedding to penetrate skin breaks. This process is known as autoinoculation and is responsible for multiple lesions becoming established and transferred to other parts of the body.

Arriving at a differential diagnosis

Warts and verrucas are not difficult to diagnose. However, pharmacists must be able to recognise other similar conditions that superficially look like warts and verrucas. Asking symptom-specific questions will help the pharmacist to determine if referral is needed (Table 7.14). It is worth noting that HPV infections involving the anogenital area are outside the remit of community pharmacists and must be referred.

Clinical features of warts and verrucas

Warts

Warts occur on the hands and knees either singly or in crops. When examined, the wart appears as a raised, hyperkeratotic papule with thrombosed, black vessels visible as black dots within the wart (Fig. 7.13).

Verrucas

Verrucas are found on the sole of the foot, usually in weight-bearing areas, for example on the metatarsal heads or heel. Due to constant pressure imparted on the sole of the foot the normal outward expansion of the wart is thwarted and instead it grows inward. Pressure on nerves can then cause considerable pain and patients often complain of pain when walking. Inspection of the lesion will normally reveal tiny black dots on the surface

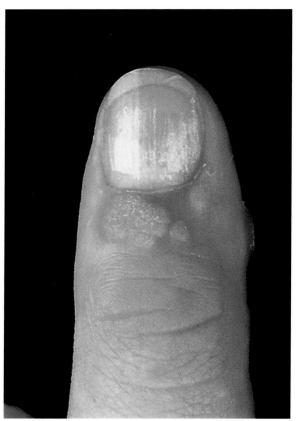

Fig. 7.13 Common wart. Reproduced from *Dermatology Colour Guide,* by J Wilkinson and S Shaw, 1998, Churchill Livingstone, with permission

Table 7.14
Specific questions to ask the patient: Human papilloma virus

Question	Relevance
Age of patient	• Warts are particularly common in children under the age of 10 • The likelihood that nodular lesions are caused by seborrhoeic warts or carcinoma increases with increasing age
Location	• Warts are common on the hands and knees; verrucas are usually on the weight-bearing parts of the sole • Warts can occur on the face but so too can plane warts and carcinoma. Referral is always needed as any OTC treatment can cause scarring
Associated symptoms	• Itching and bleeding is not associated with warts and verrucas and must be viewed with suspicion especially in older patients • Pain on walking is often associated with verruca
Colour/appearance	• Typically warts have a 'cauliflower' appearance and are raised and pale • Warts with a reddish hue or which change colour should be referred • Lesions that are raised, smooth and have a central 'dimple' suggests molluscum contagiosum

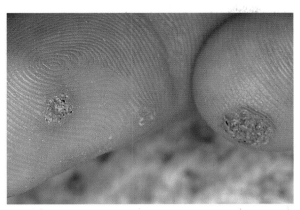

Fig. 7.14 Verruca. Reproduced from *Dermatology: An Illustrated Colour Text* by D Gawkrodger, 2002, Mosby, with permission

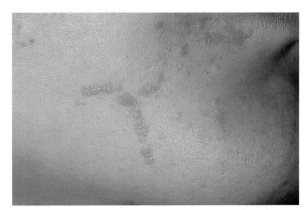

Fig. 7.15 Plane warts. Reproduced from *Dermatology: An Illustrated Colour Text* by D Gawkrodger, 2002, Mosby, with permission

(Fig. 7.14). Occasionally, a number of closely located plantar warts can coalesce to form a large single plaque, which is called a mosaic wart.

Conditions to eliminate

Plane warts (flat warts or verruca plana)

These most frequently occur in groups on the face and the back of the hands. They are small in size (1 to 5 mm in diameter), slightly raised and can take on the skin colour of the patient. (Fig. 7.15). As drug treatment is destructive in nature, plane warts located on the face should be referred to avoid the risk of scarring.

Molluscum contagiosum

Molluscum contagiosum primarily affects children under 5 years old. It is caused by a pox virus and patients present with multiple lesions usually on the face and neck, although the trunk can be involved. The lesions resemble common warts but each raised papule tends to be smooth and have a central dimple, the latter is a useful diagnostic point (see Fig. 9.5, page 219). The condition is self-limiting and will resolve without medical intervention. Patients should be told this, but if they believe treatment is necessary, referral to the GP is advisable. Cryotherapy or imiquimod might be considered.

Corns

Corns and plantar warts can be confused. The reader is referred to page 170 on corns and calluses for information on differentiating corns from verrucas.

Basal cell papilloma (seborrhoeic wart)

Basal cell papillomas are benign growths that are increasingly common with increasing age. They usually

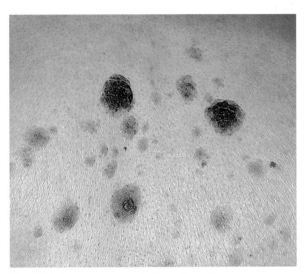

Fig. 7.16 Seborrhoeic wart. Reproduced from *Dermatology: An Illustrated Colour Text* by D Gawkrodger, 2002, Mosby, with permission

present as raised often multiple brown lesions and have a superficial 'stuck on' appearance (Fig. 7.16).

Basal cell carcinoma

Skin cancers typically occur in older age groups. Often there will be a history of prolonged skin exposure. Any wart like lesion that is itchy, has an irregular outline, prone to bleeding and exhibits colour change should be referred to eliminate serious pathology.

Evidence base for over-the-counter medication

A number of ingredients can be used to treat warts and verrucas, however, salicylic acid is the most commonly used agent and can be found in many OTC treatments

> ❗ **TRIGGER POINTS indicative of referral: Warts and verrucae**
>
> - Anogenital warts
> - Diabetic patients
> - Lesions on the face
> - Multiple and widespread warts
> - Patients aged over 50 presenting with a first-time wart
> - Warts that itch or bleed without provocation
> - Warts that have grown and changed colour

both alone and combined with lactic acid or podophyllum. The concentration of salicylic acid in proprietary preparations varies widely from 11 to 50%.

Salicylic acid preparations have been shown to heal 60 to 80% of lesions after 12 weeks, although there are no trials comparing different concentrations to determine if there is an optimum concentration. There is some evidence to show that common warts are more responsive to keratolytic therapy than plantar warts and resolution might be enhanced by soaking the wart or verruca prior to application and/or occlusion of the site (by use of plasters or collodion like vehicle) to aid penetration.

Compliance with treatment has been identified as a limiting factor in the cure rate for warts and verrucas. One study that investigated Occlusal reported an 80% cure rate after only 2 weeks of therapy. This might be an alternative option for patients whose compliance could be questioned. However, the study suffered from poor design and had only a small number of patients and the results must be viewed with caution.

Salicylic acid is often combined with other ingredients, in particular lactic acid. However, there is no evidence to support additionally efficacy when lactic acid is added. Monochloroacetic acid has also been combined with salicylic acid. Cure rates for this combination are comparable to cure rates of salicylic acid alone or when monochloroacetic acid is used singly. It therefore appears that the combination has no additional benefit than when active ingredients are used as monotherapy. As far as the author is aware, no commercially available preparation contains monochloroacetic acid.

Other agents available commercially include formaldehyde, gluteraldehyde, podophyllum resin and silver nitrate pencils. Information regarding their effectiveness stems either from small-scale or poorly designed studies, and they should therefore be relegated to second-line choices. However, it should be noted that cure rates reported with these agents, except silver nitrate, were equal if not better than those reported with salicylic acid.

Summary

Any salicylic-acid-based product should have modest success rates in clearing warts and verrucas after a 12-week treatment period, providing patient compliance is good. If treatment has been unsuccessful with salicylic acid then a second-line medicine such as glutaraldehyde, formaldehyde or podophyllum could be tried. Alternatively, referral to the GP for cryotherapy or imiquimod would be another option.

Practical prescribing and product selection

Prescribing information relating to the specific products used to treat warts and verrucas and discussed in the section 'Evidence base for over-the-counter medication' is summarised in Table 7.15; useful tips relating to patients presenting with warts and verrucas are given in Hints and Tips Box 7.5.

Over half of all common warts and verrucas will spontaneously resolve after 2 years, therefore treatment is not necessarily needed. Pharmacists should determine from the patient how much the wart or verruca affects day-to-day life and also what social impact the lesions have on the patient. It is also worth assessing patient motivation to comply with medication regimes because treatment is over a period of months not days or weeks.

Salicylic acid products (e.g. Compound W, Bazuka, Bazuka Extra Strength, Salactol, Salatac, Duofilm, Cuplex)

There is a wide choice of salicylic-acid-based products for the removal of warts, verrucas (and corns). Some of the more commonly prescribed and purchased products are listed but this is by no means an exhaustive list. Prior to using a salicylic-acid-based product the affected area should be soaked in warm water and towelled dry. The surface of the wart or verruca should be rubbed with a pumice stone or emery board to remove any hard skin. After which a few drops of the product should be applied to the lesion, taking care to localise the application to the affected area. The procedure should be repeated daily. Salicylic acid can be recommended to most patients, although diabetics are a notable exception. Salicylic acid does not interact with any medicines and can be used in pregnancy. It can cause local skin irritation and because of its destructive action should be kept away from unaffected skin.

Glutaraldehyde (Glutarol)

Application of glutaraldehyde is the same as salicylic acid but it should be used twice a day. It can cause skin irritation and stains the outer layer of the skin brown.

Formaldehyde (Veracur)

Veracur is marketed particularly for verrucas and, like glutaraldehyde, is applied twice a day. In all other respects it has same side-effects and precautions for use as salicyclic acid.

Table 7.15
Practical prescribing: Summary of medicines for warts and verrucas

Medicine	Use in children	Likely side-effects	Drug interactions of note	Patients in whom care should be exercised	Pregnancy
Salicylic acid					
Compound W	> 6 years	Local skin irritation	None	Avoid in diabetics	OK
Bazuka Extra Strength	No lower age stated				
Occlusal					
Verrugon					
Salicylic acid and lactic acid					
Bazuka	No lower age stated	Local skin irritation	None	Avoid in diabetics	OK
Cuplex					
Duofilm	> 2 years				
Salactol	No lower age stated				
Salatac					
Glutaraldehyde					
Glutarol	No lower age stated	Local skin irritation. Skin will be stained brown	None	Avoid in diabetics	OK
Formaldehyde					
Veracur	No lower age stated	No local effects reported	None	Avoid in diabetics	OK, but manufacturers advise avoidance
Podophyllum and salicylic acid					
Posalfilin	No lower age stated	Local skin irritation	None	Avoid in diabetics	Avoid

HINTS AND TIPS BOX 7.5: VERRUCAS AND WARTS

Is it a verruca or a corn?	If diagnosis is uncertain then removal of the top layer of skin from the lesion can be performed. If black spots (capillary blood supply of verruca) are not visible this implies the lesion is a corn and not a verruca
Length of treatment	Patients should be told that it is a slow process. Treatment commonly lasts 3 months. If OTC medication has been unsuccessful after this time then the patient could be referred to the GP for other treatment options such as cryotherapy
Salatac gel	The gel forms an elastic film after application. This has to be removed each time before the gel can be reapplied
Bazuka and Bazuka Extra Strength	Don't be fooled into thinking the extra strength has better cure rates. It has a higher concentration of salicylic acid (26% as opposed to 12%) but this does not necessarily equate to a more efficacious product

Posalfilin (Podophyllum Resin BP and 25% salicylic acid)

Posalfilin is licensed for verrucas only. As with all other products containing salicylic acid, it must not be used in diabetic patients, however, it is also contraindicated in pregnancy (and breast feeding) because podophyllum is cytotoxic and possesses teratogenic properties. To apply the ointment, a corn ring should be placed around the verruca and a minimal amount of ointment applied on to the verruca. The verruca and corn ring should be covered with a plaster and the treatment repeated daily.

Further reading

Ahmed I 2001 Management of viral warts in primary care. The Prescriber 5 May:43–54

Bunney M H, Nolan M W, Williams D A 1976 An assessment of methods of treating viral warts by comparative treatment trials based on a standard design. British Journal of Dermatology 94:667–679

Cobb M W 1990 Human papillomavirus infection. Journal of the American Academy of Dermatology 22:547–566

Esterly N B 1987 Management of warts in children. Pediatric Dermatology 4:36

Hirose R, Hori M, Shukuwa T et al 1994 Topical treatment of resistant warts with glutaraldehyde. Journal of Dermatology 21:248–253

Johnson L W 1995 Communal showers and the risk of plantar warts. Journal of Family Practice 40:136–138

Livingstone C 1998 Warts and cold sores. Pharmaceutical Journal 260:556–558

Steele K, Irwin W G 1988 Liquid nitrogen and salicylic/lactic acid paint in the treatment of cutaneous warts in general practice. Journal of the Royal College of General Practitioners 38:256–258

Steele K, Shirodaria P, O'Hare M et al 1988 Monochloroacetic acid and 60% salicylic acid as a treatment for simple plantar warts: effectiveness and mode of action. British Journal of Dermatology 118:537–543

Yazar S, Basaran E 1994 Efficacy of silver nitrate pencils in the treatment of common warts. Journal of Dermatology 21:329–333

Web sites

British Association of Dermatologists: www.bad.org.uk

Corns and calluses

Background

In general, people do not tend to give their feet the care they deserve. It is estimated that on average a person walks the equivalent of 1000 miles a year. It is therefore hardly surprising that people experience foot problems. Foot disorders can be broadly subdivided into those that result from opportunistic infection and those resulting from incorrect distribution of pressure. This section discusses the latter.

Prevalence and epidemiology

The exact prevalence of corns and calluses is not known. However, it has been reported that about 40% of people visiting podiatrists do so because of a corn problem. Corns and calluses tend to be seen more often in older patients and are probably due to the aetiology of the condition.

Aetiology

Corns form due to a combination of friction and pressure against one of the bony prominences of the feet. Inappropriate footwear is frequently the cause. Continued pressure and friction results in hyperkeratoses (excessive skin growth of the keratinised layer) leaving even less space between the shoe and the foot and therefore the corn is pressed even more firmly against the underlying soft tissues and bone.

Callus formation is also caused by constant friction and pressure. Calluses can be beneficial providing a natural barrier to objects and protects underlying tissues, however, when such thickened mass of skin occurs in abnormal places (e.g. border of the big toe) pain is experienced.

Arriving at a differential diagnosis

To assess the patient's particular problem accurately, the pharmacist needs to inspect the feet. Trying to take a description of what the problem looks like is very difficult. If the patient is present it is much more sensible to get them to take his or her shoes and socks off and have a look for yourself.

Differential diagnosis should be simple and is usually between corns, calluses and verruca. Most patients will accurately self-diagnose and seek advice and help to remedy the situation. The pharmacist's role will be to confirm the self-diagnosis and give advice and/or treatment where appropriate. Asking symptom-specific questions will help the pharmacist to determine the best course of action (Table 7.16).

Clinical features of corns

Corns (helomas) have been classified in to a number of types, although only soft and hard corns are commonly met in practice. Hard corns (heloma durum) are generally located on the top of the toes. Corns exhibit a central core of hard grey skin surrounded by a painful, raised, yellow ring of inflammatory skin. Any of the toes can be affected but it is most common on the second toe. Soft corns (heloma molle) form between the toes rather on the tops of toes and are due to pressure exerted by one toe against another. They have a whitened appearance and remain soft because of the moisture that is present between the toes, which causes maceration of the corn. Soft corns are most common in the fourth web space.

Clinical features of calluses

Calluses, depending on the cause and site involved, can range in size from a few millimetres to centimetres. They appear as flattened, yellow–white, thickened skin. In women, the balls of the feet are a common site as a result of prolonged wearing of ill-fitting high-heeled shoes.

Table 7.16
Specific questions to ask the patient: Corn/callus

Question	Relevance
Location	• Lesions on the tops or between the toes suggest a corn compared with verrucas, which are on the plantar surface of the foot
Aggravating or relieving factors	• Pain experienced with corns is a result of pressure between footwear and the toes. If footwear is taken off the pain is relieved • Pain associated with verrucas will be felt irrespective of whether footwear is worn
Appearance	• Corns and calluses appear as white or yellow hyperkeratinised areas of skin, unlike verrucas, which show black thrombosed capillaries seen as black dots on the surface of the verruca
Previous history	• Patients will often have a previous history of foot problems. The cause is usually due to poorly fitting shoes, such as high heels. Prolonged wear of such footwear can lead to calluses and permanent deformity of bunions

Other sites that can be affected are the heel and lower border of the big toe. Patients frequently complain of a burning sensation resulting from fissuring of the callus.

Conditions to eliminate

Verrucas

Verrucas can be mistaken for a corn or callus, although verrucas tend to have a spongy texture with the central area showing tiny black spots. They are also rarely located on or between the toes and more commonly occur in younger patients than corns and calluses.

Bunions

Bunions are 10 times more common in women than men and are directly related to the wearing of tight shoes. Initially, irritation of skin by ill-fitting shoes causes bursitis of the big toe. Over time the inflamed area begins to harden and subsequently bursal fluid solidifies into a gelatinous mass. The result will be a bunion joint. This will be seen as a lump on the instep of the foot just below the big toe. Referral to a podiatrist is recommended.

 TRIGGER POINTS indicative of referral: Corns and calluses

Initially a patient should be referred to a podiatrist if:

• Discomfort/pain is causing difficulty in walking
• Soft corns
• Treatment failure

Evidence base for over-the-counter medication

Corns and calluses caused by friction and pressure. Removal of the precipitating factors will result in resolution of the problem. Therefore preventive measures should form the mainstay of treatment. Correctly fitting shoes are essential to help prevent corn and callus formation. If pressure and friction still persist when correctly fitted shoes are worn then patients can obtain relief by shielding or padding. Moleskin or thin podiatry felt placed around the corn allows pressure to be transferred from the corn to the padding. Specific proprietary products are available for such purposes. In callus formation a 'shock-absorbing' insert such as a metatarsal pad is useful to relieve weight off the callus and so reduce stress on the plantar skin.

Treatment should be avoided if possible but, if deemed appropriate, keratolytics can be used, although there is no evidence to suggest that they are effective.

Practical prescribing and product selection

Products used to treat corns and calluses are exactly the same as those used for warts and verrucas. Prescribing information relating to specific products used to treat corns and calluses is therefore discussed in the section 'Evidence base for over-the-counter medication' for warts and verrucas on page 167. However, a number of proprietary products are marketed specifically for sufferers with corns and calluses, for example products in the Carnation and Scholl ranges (see Hints and Tips Box 7.6).

Further reading

Robbins J M 2000 Recognizing, treating and preventing common foot problems. Cleveland Clinic Journal of Medicine 67:45–56

Silfverskiold J P 1991 Common foot problems. Relieving the pain of bunions, keratoses, corns and calluses. Postgraduate Medicine 89:183–188

HINTS AND TIPS BOX 7.6: CORNS

Shoes to relieve pressure	Patients should be encouraged to wear open shoes such as sandals or thongs

Scabies

Background

Scabies is a pruritic skin condition caused by the mite *Sarcoptes scabiei*. It is easily missed or misdiagnosed as dermatitis. The diagnostic burrows are small and difficult to locate because they are often obscured by the effects of scratching.

Prevalence and epidemiology

Scabies is not gender or age specific. Infants to the elderly can acquire the infestation, although it is more common in the elderly. Outbreaks in care homes are not uncommon and can affect staff as well as patients. The incidence of scabies in the UK is low but epidemics seem to occur on a cyclical basis every 7 to 15 years.

Aetiology

The mite is transmitted by direct physical contact (e.g. holding hands, hugging or sexual contact). The female mite burrows into the stratum corneum to lay eggs. The faecal pellets she leaves in the burrow cause a local hypersensitivity reaction and is assumed to cause the release of the inflammatory mediators that trigger an allergic reaction invoking intense itching. However, this response can take up to 6 weeks to develop. During this asymptomatic period the mite can be passed onto others unknowingly. The eggs hatch and mature in 14 days, after which the cycle can begin again.

Arriving at a differential diagnosis

The diagnosis of scabies is confirmed by extraction of the mite from its burrow, although in primary care this is rarely performed and a differential diagnosis is made on clinical appearance, patient history and symptoms reported by close family. Confusion can arise from mistaking scabies for allergic contact dermatitis or dermatitis herpetiformis, especially when the condition is extensive. Asking symptom-specific questions will help the pharmacist to determine the best course of action (Table 7.17).

Clinical features of scabies

Severe pruritus is the hallmark symptom of scabies, although this is diffuse and not localised. It can be worse at night and after bathing. Besides classic location of lesions, in men the penile and scrotal skin and in women beneath the breasts and nipples can be affected. Infants who are not yet walking might have marked sole involvement.

Conditions to eliminate

Allergic contact dermatitis

This condition presents as an area of inflamed, itchy skin with either **papules** or **vesicles** being present. However, enquiry into the patient's history should reveal a past history of similar lesions in allergic contact dermatitis. For further information on dermatitis see page 180.

Table 7.17
Specific questions to ask the patient: Scabies

Question	Relevance
Visible signs of the mite	● Burrows, which are up to 1 cm long and blue–grey in colour, might be visible although in practice this characteristic is often not present. For the pharmacist, who will see a limited number of cases, it is probably best to concentrate on other clinical signs rather than attempt to look for signs of burrows
Location of rash	● Scabies classically affects the finger webs, the sides of the fingers and wrists. Hand involvement is rare in dermatitis herpetiformis
History of presenting complaint	● If contact dermatitis is suspected then questioning should reveal a past history of similar skin lesions ● Often people with scabies will be care workers looking after institutionalised people

Dermatitis herpetiformis

Dermatitis herpetiformis is a chronic condition characterised by intense itchy clusters of papules and vesicles; it also exhibits urticarial-type lesions. It commonly involves the elbows, knees and sacral region. The lesions usually exhibit a symmetrical distribution and hand involvement is rare. Therefore, differences in distribution of the lesions should allow it to be differentiated from scabies.

 TRIGGER POINTS indicative of referral: Scabies

- Severe and extensive symptoms
- Suspected dermatitis herpetiformis

Evidence base for over-the-counter medication

The efficacy and safety of scabicidal agents is difficult to determine. Benzyl benzoate, crotamiton, permethrin and malathion have all been used. The current edition of the *British National Formulary* (Edition 46) advocates the use of permethrin and malathion.

A Cochrane review conducted in 1999 found permethrin to have cure rates of approximately 90%. This review also compared permethrin against other scabicidal agents and concluded that it was superior to crotamiton and as effective as gamma-benzene hexachloride. The latter was withdrawn from the UK market in 1995 because of concern about possible adverse effects.

The efficacy of malathion is questionable as no random controlled trials appear to have been conducted. However, case reports have suggested malathion is effective in curing scabies, with a cure rate of over 80%.

Benzyl benzoate has been used to treat scabies for many years. However, its efficacy has not been demonstrated in randomised controlled trials. In uncontrolled trials benzyl benzoate has been shown to provide cure rates of approximately 50%. Unfortunately, up to 25% of patients experience side-effects such as burning, irritation and itching on application. Therefore its use has declined over time and it should now no longer be recommended as a first-line treatment.

Summary

On current evidence, permethrin (Lyclear Dermal Cream) is the medicine of choice because it has the highest cure rate, resistance appears rare and is associated with minimal side-effects.

Practical prescribing and product selection

Prescribing information relating to specific products used to treat scabies in the section 'Evidence base for over-the-counter medication' is discussed and summarised in Table 7.18; useful tips relating to patients presenting with scabies are given in Hints and Tips Box 7.7.

All products for scabies can be used by all patient groups and have no drug interactions.

Permethrin (Lyclear Dermal Cream)

Permethrin is suitable for use by adults and children over 2 months of age. General guidance for application of Lyclear is that adults and children over 12 should use up to a full tube as a single application. Some adults might need to use more than one tube to ensure total body coverage but a maximum of two tubes (60 g in total) is recommended for a single application. For children under 12 the manufacturers suggest the following: 2 months

Table 7.18
Practical prescribing: Summary of medicines for scabies

Medicine	Use in children	Likely side-effects	Drug interactions of note	Patients in whom care should be exercised	Pregnancy
Permethrin	> 2 months	Burning, stinging or tingling	None	None	OK
Benzyl benzoate	No lower age limit stated	Burning, irritation	None	None	OK
Crotamiton	> 3 years	Skin irritation reported	None	None	Manufacturer advises avoidance but no teratogenic reports could be found
Malathion Derbac M Quellada M	> 6 months	Skin irritation but rare	None	None	OK

HINTS AND TIPS BOX 7.7: SCABIES

Itching after treatment	Pruritus can persist for several weeks after treatment and the patient might benefit from crotamiton or antihistamines
Lyclear	If necessary, a second application can be given – not less than 7 days after the initial application – if there are no signs of the original lesions healing or if new lesions are present
Who to treat?	All close personal contacts should be treated

to 1 year should use up to $1/8$ of a tube; children aged between 1 and 5, up to $1/4$ of a tube and those aged between 6 and 12 years should use $1/2$ a tube.

Lyclear Dermal Cream should be applied to the whole body, excluding the head, of all patients over the age of 2. However, children between 2 months and 2 years should have the cream applied to the palms, soles, face, neck, scalp and ears. Care must be taken to avoid the vicinity of the mouth and eyes. The whole body should be washed thoroughly 8 to 12 h after treatment.

Benzyl benzoate (e.g. Ascabiol)

Benzyl benzoate can be used by adults and children. It is applied to the whole body except the head and face. If the application is thorough, one treatment should suffice but the possibility of failure is lessened if a second application is made within 5 days of the first. Alternatively, benzyl benzoate can be applied to the whole body, on three occasions, at 12-hourly intervals. When used in older children, benzyl benzoate should be diluted with an equal quantity of water and with three parts of water for babies.

It appears to be safe in pregnancy, although the manufacturers of Ascabiol recommend that it should be avoided wherever practicable. The main drawback with benzyl benzoate is its side-effect profile. It causes skin irritation and a transient burning sensation. This is usually mild but can occasionally be severe in sensitive individuals. In the event of a severe skin reaction the preparation should be washed off using soap and warm water. Ascabiol is also irritating to the eyes, which should be protected if it is applied to the scalp.

Crotamiton (Eurax)

Eurax should be rubbed into the entire body surface, apart from the face and scalp, once a day for between 3 and 5 consecutive days for adults and children over the age of 3. It can cause irritation on application. Treatment of scabies with Eurax is now no longer advocated although it is still used to control itch after scabies eradication.

Malathion (Derbac M and Quellada M liquid)

Of the malathion products marketed, only Derbac M and Quellada M have a licensed indication for the treatment of scabies.

The liquid can be used on adults and children over 6 months old. The liquid should be applied to the entire skin surface below the head for all patients aged over 2. For children younger than 2 years old a thin film of liquid should be applied to the scalp, face and ears. The liquid has to be left on for 24 h. If hands, or any other parts of the body must be washed during this period, the treatment must be reapplied to those areas immediately.

Further reading

Angarano D W, Parish L C 1994 Comparative dermatology: parasitic disorders. Clinics in Dermatology 12:543–550

Burgess I, Robinson R, Robinson J et al 1986 Aqueous malathion 0.5% as a scabicide: clinical trial. British Medical Journal 292:1172

Glaziou P, Cartel J L, Alzieu P et al 1993 Comparison of ivermectin and benzyl benzoate for treatment of scabies. Tropical Medicine and Parasitology 44:331–332

Hanna N F, Clay J C, Harris J R 1978 Sarcoptes scabiei infestation treated with malathion liquid. British Journal of Venereal Diseases 54:354

Walker G, Johnstone P 1999 Interventions from treating scabies. Cochrane Review, Issue 2. The Cochrane Library, Update Software, Oxford

Web sites

New York State Department of Health Communicable Disease Fact Sheet: www.health.state.ny.us/nysdoh/consumer/scabies.htm

Acne vulgaris

Background

Acne is a disorder of the pilosebaceous follicles causing **comedones**, papules and pustules on the face, chest and upper back. It affects virtually all adolescents, to varying degrees of severity, and usually appears at the time of puberty. Diagnosis is usually straightforward and most patients presenting in the community pharmacy will generally be seeking appropriate advice on correct product selection rather than wanting someone to put a name to their rash. The majority of cases seen in the pharmacy setting will be mild and can be managed appropriately without referral to the GP. However, more persistent and severe cases need referral for more potent topical or systemic treatment.

Prevalence and epidemiology

Acne lesions develop at the onset of puberty. Girls therefore tend to develop acne at an earlier age than boys. The peak incidence for girls is between the ages of 14 and 17, compared with 15 to 19 years of age for boys. There might be a familial tendency to acne and it is slightly more common in boys, who also experience more severe involvement. In addition, white patients are more likely to experience moderate to severe acne than black patients, although black skin is prone to worse scarring.

Acne usually resolves within 10 years of onset, although women in their 30s can have mild persistent acne.

Aetiology

At the onset of puberty a cascade of events takes place resulting in the formation of non-inflammatory and inflammatory lesions. In response to increased testosterone levels, the pilosebaceous gland begins to produce sebum (if the sebaceous glands become oversensitive to testosterone they produce excess oil and the skin becomes greasy; a hallmark of acne). At the same time epithelial cells lining the follicle undergo change. Prior to puberty dead cells are shed smoothly out of the ductal opening but at puberty this process is disrupted and in patients with acne these cells develop abnormal cohesion and partially block the opening and effectively reduce sebum outflow. Over time the opening of the duct becomes blocked trapping oil in the hair follicle. Bacteria, particularly *Propionibacterium acnes*, proliferate in the stagnant oil stimulating cytokine production, which in turn produces local inflammation leading to the appearance of a spot. In response to the proliferation of bacteria white blood cells infiltrate the area to kill the bacteria and in turn die leading to pus formation.

The pustule eventually bursts on the skin surface, carrying the plug away. The whole process then starts again.

Arriving at a differential diagnosis

Differential diagnosis of acne is routine and should not be difficult. The pharmacist will, however, need to assess the severity of the acne. Several rating scales have been developed with the aim of trying to grade the severity of an individual's condition. None has gained universal acceptance and most dermatology texts simply grade the severity of acne in to mild, moderate or severe. Asking symptom-specific questions will help the pharmacist to determine if referral is needed (Table 7.19).

Clinical features of mild acne vulgaris

Patients suffering from mild acne characteristically have predominatly open and closed comedones (blackheads and white heads) with a small number of active lesions normally confined to the face. Mild acne will not cause permanent scarring (Fig. 7.17).

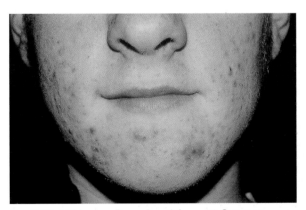

Fig. 7.17 Mild acne. Reproduced from *20 Common Problems in Dermatology* by A Fleischer et al, 2000, with permission of the McGraw-Hill Companies

Table 7.19 Specific Acne related questions to ask the patient	
Question	**Relevance**
Severity	● Moderate and severe acne should be referred because current OTC treatment is unlikely to help. ● A patient with moderate acne has many inflammatory spots that are not confined to the face Lesions are often painful and there is a real possibility of scarring ● Patients with severe acne will have all the characteristics of moderate acne plus the development of cysts. Lesions are often widespread involving the upper back and chest. Scarring will usually result
Age of onset	● Patients presenting with acne-type lesions who fall outside the normal age range should be questioned closely. Adverse drug reactions and rosacea should be considered
Occupation	● Certain jobs can predispose patients to acne-like lesions and acne is commonly associated with long-term contact with oils

Conditions to eliminate

Rosacea

Rosacea is an inflammatory disease of the skin follicles. It is uncertain what causes rosacea although successful treatment with antibiotics suggests that bacterial pathogens play a significant role in the disease. It is normally seen in patients over 40 years of age and is classically characterised by recurrent flushing and blushing of the central face especially the nose and medial cheeks. Crops of inflammatory papules and pustules are also a common feature. Comedones are not present in rosacea and eye irritation and blepharitis are present in about 20% of rosacea patients.

Medicines causing acne-like skin eruptions

A number of medicines can produce acne-like lesions, including lithium, oral contraceptives (especially those with high progestogen levels), phenytoin, azathioprine and rifampicin.

TRIGGER POINTS indicative of referral: Acne

- Moderate or severe acne
- Occupational acne
- OTC treatment failure
- Rosacea

Evidence base for over-the-counter medication

The aim of treatment must be to clear the lesions and prevent scarring. Mild acne can be managed OTC but it is important to show understanding and empathy when advising patients. Acne is predominantly a condition that affects adolescents, a time when appearance is very important. It is worth taking a few minutes to counsel patients about their condition and empower them to manage their condition.

OTC acne treatments contain benzoyl peroxide, salicylic acid, sulphur or an antibacterial.

Benzoyl peroxide

Benzoyl peroxide is now widely believed to exert its main effect by reducing the concentration of *Propionibacterium acnes*. Additionally, it has slight anti-inflammatory and very mild anticomedogenic effects. Many studies have investigated the efficacy of benzoyl peroxide. It has been proven to be effective, especially in mild to moderate acne. However, there is no evidence to suggest that 10% benzoyl peroxide is more effective than 5%. Therefore, because of its potential to cause erythema and irritation, concentrations of 10% should probably be avoided.

Various other agents have been compared against or in combination with benzoyl peroxide. None of these products has been shown to be significantly better than benzoyl peroxide alone.

The addition of miconazole 2% (Acnidazil) was shown to be no more effective than benzoyl peroxide alone, despite manufacturer claims to the contrary. Likewise, when Quinoderm was compared to Quinoderm HC (benzoyl peroxide and hydrocortisone) no significant differences in efficacy were observed. One trial comparing tea tree oil with benzoyl peroxide showed benzoyl peroxide to be significantly more effective. A further study, which compared gluconolactone and benzoyl peroxide found gluconolactone to be better than placebo but not significantly different than benzoyl peroxide.

Evidence of efficacy for salicylic acid and sulphur is poor. Both agents have been used for many years on the basis of their keratolytic action. On current evidence they are probably best avoided.

Summary

First-line treatment of acne should be benzoyl peroxide 2.5% or 5%. Patients should see an improvement in their symptoms after 8 to 12 weeks. Upwards of 60% of patients will visibly see an improvement in this time, however, if the patient fails to respond in this time then referral to the GP would be appropriate.

Practical prescribing and product selection

Prescribing information relating to benzoyl peroxide is discussed and summarised in Table 7.20; useful tips relating to patients presenting with acne are given in Hints and Tips Box 7.8.

Benzoyl peroxide (e.g. Brevoxyl, Oxy and Panoxyl range, Quinoderm)

Benzoyl peroxide can be used by adults and children. However, acne is very uncommon in children under 12 and should not be given to this age group. Benzoyl peroxide is usually applied once or twice daily depending on patient response. It can cause drying, burning and peeling on initial application. If this occurs the patient should be told to stop using the product for a day or two before starting again. Patients should therefore start on the lowest strength commercially available, especially if the patient suffers from sensitive or fair skin. Occasionally, patients will experience contact dermatitis, although this has been reported to affect only 1 to 2% of patients. Apart from local adverse effects benzoyl peroxide can be used by all patient groups, including pregnant women. It has no drug interactions, although it does bleach clothing.

Table 7.20
Practical prescribing: Summary of medicines for acne

Medicine	Use in children	Likely side-effects	Drug interactions of note	Patients in whom care should be exercised	Pregnancy
Benzoyl peroxide	Not appropriate	Skin irritation, burning or peeling	None	None	OK

HINTS AND TIPS BOX 7.8: ACNE

Myths surrounding acne	Only teenagers get acne. Acne is most prevalent in this age group but can persist into the third decade Chocolate causes spots. There is no proof that any food causes acne Stress causes acne. Stress cannot cause acne, although it can make it worse
Applying benzoyl peroxide	Benzoyl peroxide has a potent bleaching effect. It has the ability to permanently bleach clothing and bed linen. Patients should be advised to always wash their hands after applying the product

Further reading
Bassett I B, Pannowitz D L, Barnetson R S 1990 A comparative study of tea-tree oil versus benzoyl peroxide in the treatment of acne. Medical Journal of Australia 153:455–458

Burke B, Eady E A, Cunliffe W J 1983 Benzoyl peroxide versus topical erythromycin in the treatment of acne vulgaris. British Journal of Dermatology 108:199–204

Cunliffe B 2001 Acne. Pharmaceutical Journal 267:749–752

Cunliffe B 2001 Rosacea. Pharmaceutical Journal 267:782–783

Fluckiger R, Furrer H J Rufli T 1988 Efficacy and tolerance of a miconazole–benzoyl peroxide cream combination versus a benzoyl peroxide gel in the topical treatment of acne vulgaris. Dermatologica 177:109–114

Gollnick H, Schramm M 1998 Topical drug treatment in acne. Dermatology 196:119–125

Healy E, Simpson N 1994 Acne vulgaris. British Medical Journal 308:831–833

Hunt M J, Barnetson R S 1992 A comparative study of gluconolactone versus benzoyl peroxide in the treatment of acne. Australasian Journal of Dermatology 33:131–134

Johnson B A, Nunley J R 2002 Topical therapy for acne vulgaris. How do you choose the best drug for each patient? Postgraduate Medicine 107:69–70, 73–76, 79–80

Kligman A M 1995 Acne vulgaris: tricks and treatments. Part II: The benzoyl peroxide saga. Cutis 56:260–261

Nguyen Q H, Kim Y A, Schwartz R A 1994 Management of acne vulgaris. American Family Physician 50:89–96, 99–100

Zander E, Weisman S 1992 Treatment of acne vulgaris with salicylic acid pads. Clinical Therapeutics 14:247–253

Web sites
Acne Support Groups: www.m2w3.com/acne and www.stopspots.org

Cold sores

Background

A cold sore is an infection caused by the herpes simplex virus (HSV). There are two main subtypes of the virus: HSV1 and HSV2. Cold sores are caused by HSV1, whereas HSV2 is most commonly implicated in genital lesions.

Prevalence and epidemiology

Herpes simplex virus infection is one of the most commonly encountered human viral infections. It is estimated that up to 50% of adults in the Western world show serologic evidence of having been infected by HSV1, although this might not manifest as symptoms. When first contracted, the virus is known as the primary infection. This is often asymptomatic; it is most commonly contracted by preschool children.

Aetiology

Infection usually results from direct mucous membrane (e.g. kissing) contact at sites of abraded skin between an infected and an uninfected individual. The virus then infects epidermal and dermal cells, causing skin vesicles. At the same time, nerve endings are also infected with the virus, which travels to the sensory ganglia where it lies dormant until reactivation. During reactivation the virus actively replicates, leading to lesions in the distribution of the affected nerve. Once contracted the infection lasts the lifetime of the host.

Table 7.21
Specific questions to ask the patient: Cold sores

Question	Relevance
Appearance	● Patients with cold sores will often have symptoms prior to the skin eruption whereas no warning symptoms are present with impetigo
Location	● Cold sores typically occur around the mouth and for this reason are known as herpes simplex labialis. They can also occur around and inside the nose, but this is less common ● Impetigo also occurs in the same areas but is much more likely to spread to other areas of the face or move to other parts of the body, for example the arms ● Angular cheilitis occurs at the corners of the mouth and can be mistaken for cold sores due to their similar locations
Trigger factors	● Stress, ill health and sunlight are all implicated in triggering cold-sore attacks. These triggers are not seen with other similar conditions and the patient should be asked to identify what brought on the lesions if possible

Arriving at a differential diagnosis

Cold sores should not be too difficult to diagnose, although conditions such as impetigo can look similar to cold sores. Asking symptom-specific questions will help the pharmacist to determine if referral is needed (Table 7.21).

Clinical features of cold sores

Patients with cold sores typically experience itching, burning or tingling symptoms. These symptoms might be noticed from a few hours to a couple of days before the lesions develop. The lesions appear as blisters and vesicles with associated redness (Fig. 7.18). These crust over – usually within 24 h – and tend to itch and be painful. The lesions spontaneously resolve in 7 to 10 days, therefore most outbreaks last 14 days from the recognition of prodromal symptoms to the resolution of lesions.

Many patients can identify a cause of their cold sore, with sunlight (UV light) reported to induce cold sores in 20% of sufferers. Recurrence is common and patients will often experience two or three episodes each year.

Conditions to eliminate

Impetigo

Impetigo usually starts as a small, red, itchy patch of inflamed skin that quickly develops into vesicles that rupture and weep. The exudate dries to a brown, yellow sticky crust. Currently, referral is needed for either topical (e.g. fusidic acid) or systemic (flucloxacillin) therapy.

Angular cheilitis

Angular cheilitis can occur at any age but is more common in patients who wear dentures. The corners of

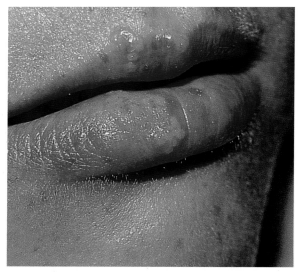

Fig. 7.18 Cold sore. Reproduced from *Color Atlas of Dermatology* by G White, 2004, Churchill Livingstone, with permission

the mouth become cracked, fissured and red. The lesions can become boggy and macerated and are slow to heal because movement of the mouth hinders healing of the lesions. It is painful but generally does not itch or crust over as is typical with cold sores.

 TRIGGER POINTS indicative of referral: Cold sores

- Duration of longer than 14 days
- Lesions that are located within the mouth
- Lesions that spread rapidly over the face
- Patients who take immunosuppressive medicines
- Severe and widespread lesions
- Systemic symptoms such as fever and malaise

Evidence base for over-the-counter medication

A number of products are marketed for the relief and treatment of cold sores. None has been shown conclusively to be effective in both its prevention and treatment. Products containing ammonia, zinc and povidone–iodine appear to have no evidence of efficacy. However, they might be useful in drying the lesions and preventing secondary bacterial infections.

Only aciclovir, a specific antiviral treatment that works by inhibiting the herpes virus DNA polymerase, has demonstrated clinical effectiveness against the herpes virus. Orally, it is a highly effective antiviral but the evidence for topical administration is less conclusive. Trial data have failed to show any significant effects on speeding the resolution of established cold sores when using aciclovir, although there is some data to support its use as a prophylactic agent. If applied in the prodromal stage the total healing time of subsequent lesions is reduced by a day or so.

Other non-specific products containing local anaesthetics and analgesics can be of value in reducing the pain and itching associated with cold sores. For information on these products see page 102.

Summary

Aciclovir is first-line therapy for the prevention of cold sores. However, it should be recommended only to patients who experience prodromal symptoms. If lesions have already appeared then no product is effective and patients, if they want to purchase a product, could be recommended any of the marketed products. The decision as to which product should be given will be made on symptomatic relief and cost of product.

Practical prescribing and product selection

Prescribing information relating to aciclovir is discussed and summarised in Table 7.22. For completeness, the table also contains some of the other commonly used cold-sore products; useful tips relating to patients presenting with cold sores are given in Hints and Tips Box 7.9.

Aciclovir (e.g. Soothelip, Virasorb, Zovirax)

Aciclovir can be used topically by all patient groups, including pregnant women, although the manufacturers advise caution because of limited data regarding the exposure of pregnant women to aciclovir. It has no drug

Table 7.22
Practical prescribing: Summary of medicines for cold sores

Medicine	Use in children	Likely side-effects	Drug interactions of note	Patients in whom care should be exercised	Pregnancy
Aciclovir Soothelip Virasorb Zovirax	Yes, but no lower age stated	Stinging	None	None	OK
Ammonia Blistex, Blistex relief cream (formerly Blisteze)	Yes, but no lower age stated	None	None	None	OK
Povidone iodine Brush Off	> 2 years	None	None	None	OK
Zinc & Lidocaine Lypsyl cold sore gel	> 12 years	Stinging	None	None	OK
Urea Cymex	Yes, but no lower age stated	None	None	None	OK

HINTS AND TIPS BOX 7.9: COLD SORES

Sun-induced cold sores	For those patients in whom the sun triggers cold sores, a sun block would be the most effective prophylactic measure
Applying products	Patients should be encouraged to use a separate towel and to wash their hands after applying products because viral particles are shed from the cold sore and can be transferred to others

interactions and causes only transient stinging after first application in the minority of patients. Aciclovir should be applied five times daily at approximately 4-hourly intervals and treatment should be continued for 5 days.

Further reading
Emmert D H 2000 Treatment of common cutaneous herpes simplex virus infections. American Family Physician 61:1697–1704

Livingstone C 1998 Warts and cold sores. Pharmaceutical Journal 260:556–558

Raborn Q W, McGaw W T, Grace M et al 1988 Treatment of herpes labialis with acyclovir. American Journal of Medicine 85:39–42

Whitley R J, Kimberlin D W, Roizman B 1998 Herpes simplex viruses. Clinical Infectious Diseases 26:541–555

Web sites
Mayo Foundation for Medical Education and Research: www.mayoclinic.com/invoke.cfm?id=DS00358

Eczema and dermatitis

Background

The terms 'eczema' and 'dermatitis' are often used interchangeably. Dermatitis simply means inflammation of the skin, whereas eczema has no universally agreed definition but in some countries indicates a more acute condition. Many authorities subdivide eczema and dermatitis into either exogenous (due to an obvious external cause) or endogenous (assumed to be of a genetic cause), however, the distinction is not clear. In this section, for consistency, the term 'dermatitis' will be used.

Dermatitis disorders are characterised by sore, red, itching skin that can be classed as acute, subacute or chronic in nature. However, the patient might present with lesions that are in more than one phase at the same time. A number of types of dermatitis are met commonly in primary care, including: atopic dermatitis (discussed in the Chapter 9, page 212), irritant, allergic and occupational dermatitis.

Irritant contact dermatitis is caused by direct exposure to a substance that has a damaging effect to the skin. Skin trauma associated with exposure to the substance is a result of direct toxicity, unlike allergic contact dermatitis, which is due to a sensitisation reaction.

Prevalence and epidemiology

Irritant contact dermatitis is the most common form of dermatitis to affect adults. It is said to account for 80% of all occupational skin disorders. The exact prevalence and incidence of allergic contact dermatitis is not known but it has been reported to affect 1 to 2% of the population. However, certain groups of patients are at higher risk of developing allergic contact dermatitis, for example patients with leg ulcers. In addition, women are more likely to develop nickel sensitivity than men.

Aetiology

Irritant dermatitis is more easily understood than allergic dermatitis. Dermatitis occurs soon after exposure and the severity varies with the type of irritant, the concentration and quantity involved, as well as the length of exposure. For example, strong acids and alkaline substances produce ulceration whereas others (e.g. zinc oxide tape, ultraviolet radiation) cause a prickly-heat-type of dermatitis. Lesions usually develop within 6 to 12 h of exposure to the irritant, although this will vary depending on the irritant involved and individual patient response.

Allergic contact dermatitis occurs only in patients whose skin has previously been sensitised by contact with an allergen. This results in specific cell-mediated sensitisation. Once the skin has become sensitised to an allergen, re-exposure to the allergen triggers memory T cells to initiate an inflammatory response. Re-exposure might occur days and sometimes years after initial exposure. This can be difficult to explain to a patient who has been working with the offending substance for many years, especially when your advice is now that they must avoid future contact.

Arriving at a differential diagnosis

Many patients will present in the pharmacy with an itchy red rash. Gaining an accurate diagnosis might be difficult because identification of the cause can be almost impossible. However, generally speaking treatment is the same regardless of the form of dermatitis the person might have, and this makes a definitive diagnosis less important. However, asking symptom-specific questions will help the pharmacist to determine if referral is needed (Table 7.23).

Clinical features of irritant contact dermatitis

The lesions appear red – and sometimes brown – in colour and will itch. Itching is a prominent feature and often causes the patient to scratch, which results in broken skin with subsequent weeping. The skin often exhibits scaling and dryness as the condition persists (Fig. 7.19).

Clinical features of allergic contact dermatitis

Allergic contact dermatitis presents in the same manner as irritant dermatitis. However, milder involvement might be noticed on skin areas distant from where the allergen

Table 7.23
Specific Dermatitis related questions to ask the patient

Question	Relevance
Location	● The distribution of rash for contact dermatitis is closely associated with clothing and jewellery (Fig. 7.20)
Work-related exposure	● Dermatitis is often occupational. A history of when the rash occurs gives a useful indication as to the cause, e.g. a construction worker might complain of sore hands when at work and when on holiday the condition improves, only for it to worsen when they go back to work
	● Commonly implicated substances that cause occupational dermatitis include chromate (found in cement and leather), rubber and hair-dressing chemicals

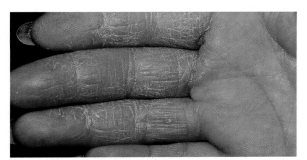

Fig. 7.19 Irritant dermatitis. Reproduced from *Color Atlas of Dermatology* by G White, 2004, Churchill Livingstone, with permission

was in direct contact with the skin. The site of involvement often provides a major clue as to the identity of the allergen. For example, ear lobes and neck (nickel in jewellery), wrist (leather or metal watchstraps) and the feet (dyes from the tanning process of leather) (Fig. 7.20). A small minority of patients (5%) on topical corticosteroid therapy can become sensitised to hydrocortisone.

Conditions to eliminate

Discoid dermatitis

This form of dermatitis usually presents in adults who have often had a past history of atopic dermatitis. As its name implies the lesions are circular, intensely itchy and are often distributed symmetrically on the limbs but sometimes the trunk as well.

Dishydrotic eczema (pompholyx)

Pompholyx, simply means 'bubble' and refers to the presence of intensely itchy vesicles or blisters on the palms of the hands and occasionally on the soles of the feet. Stress is known to precipitate the condition.

Occupational dermatitis

The clinical presentation of this form of dermatitis will be the same as for other forms of dermatitis. However, it is

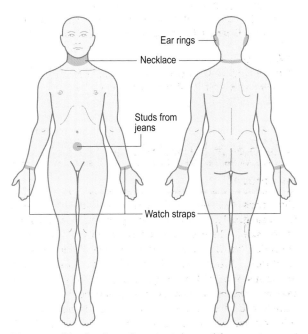

Fig. 7.20 Distribution of contact dermatitis

important to try and determine the cause of the problem because continued exposure to the substance will result in non-resolution of the condition. Careful enquiry about the type of work the person does and what products or equipment they come into contact with should be made. In most cases, if the substance can be identified a solution can usually be found, for example dermatitis of the hands caused by hair dyes and chemicals for the hair can be overcome by wearing gloves.

Urticaria

Urticarial rashes can result from many causes, most notably due to food allergies, food additives and medicines. The rash is itchy and red like dermatitis but resembles the rash seen when stung by a stinging nettle. In addition, the skin might be oedematous and blanch when pressed.

Figure 7.21 will aid the differentiation of dermatitis.

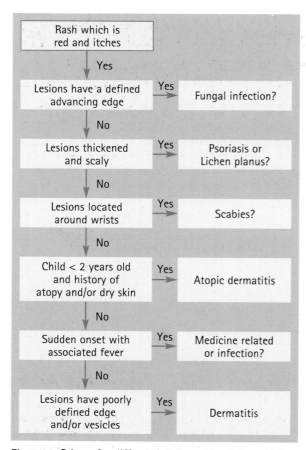

Fig. 7.21 Primer for differential diagnosis of dermatitis

> ❗ **TRIGGER POINTS indicative of referral: Eczema and dermatitis**
>
> - Children under 10 in need of corticosteroids
> - Lesions on the face unresponsive to emollients
> - OTC treatment failure
> - Suspected pompholyx
> - Widespread or severe dermatitis

Evidence base for over-the-counter medication

All forms of dermatitis cause redness, drying of the skin and irritation/pruritus to varying degrees. Treatment should include three steps: managing the itch, avoiding irritants and maintaining skin integrity.

Non-pharmacological interventions include avoidance of the causative agent, however determining the cause is often difficult and avoidance is sometimes impractical. Sweating intensifies the itching so strategies to keep the person cool will help; cotton and loose fitting clothing can be worn.

Pharmacological treatment of dermatitis should be managed with a combination of emollients and steroid based products.

Emollients

Emollients should be used on a regular basis to keep the condition under control and flare-ups can be treated with corticosteroids. Choosing the most efficacious emollient for an individual is difficult because of the lack of comparative trial data between products and the variable nature of patient response. In general, patients respond to a thicker emollient rather than an elegant cosmetic brand because these allow greater retention of water, for example 50% liquid paraffin and 50% white soft paraffin. However, patient acceptability of such products needs to be considered. Cream formulations rather than ointments tend to be more readily accepted by patients and these are easier and less messy to use.

Steroids

Two steroids are available OTC: hydrocortisone and clobetasone. Both have proven efficacy in treating dermatitis and should be considered first-line treatment for acute dermatitis. Once symptoms are controlled then the patient should be instructed to revert back to emollient therapy.

Practical prescribing and product selection

Prescribing information relating to the specific products used to treat dermatitis discussed in the section 'Evidence base for over-the-counter medication' is summarised in Table 7.24; useful tips relating to using products to treat dermatitis are given in Hints and Tips Box 7.10.

Emollients

The number of emollients on the market is truly staggering. They come in a range of formulations to suit all skin types and patient preference (Table 7.25). Their place in therapy is well known and patients should be instructed to apply emollients liberally and whenever needed. They are pharmacologically inactive and so can be used by all patients regardless of age or medical status. A number of ingredients incorporated into emollients do have the potential to sensitise skin and patients should be advised to patch test the product on the back of the hand before starting to routinely use it.

Corticosteroids

Although corticosteroids can be sold to patients OTC, there are a number of restrictions to their sale:

- the patient must be aged over 10 for hydrocortisone and 12 for clobetasone
- duration of treatment is limited to a maximum of 1 week
- a maximum of 15 g can be sold at any one time
- they cannot be used on facial skin, the anogenital region, broken or infected skin.

Table 7.24
Practical Prescribing: Summary of Medicines for Dermatitis

Medicine	Use in children	Likely side-effects	Drug interactions of note	Patients in whom care should be exercised	Pregnancy
Emollients	From birth	None	None	None	OK
Corticosteroids					
Hydrocortisone	> 10 years	None	None	None	OK
Clobetasone	> 12 years				

HINTS AND TIPS BOX 7.10: DERMATITIS

How much to apply?	Patients should be instructed to use a fingertip unit. This is the distance from the tip of the adult index finger to the first crease. One unit is sufficient to cover an area twice the size of an adult flat hand
Quantity required?	The *BNF* gives the following guidance for a weeks use: *Both hands:* 15 to 30g *Both arms:* 30 to 60g *Both legs or trunk:* 100 g

In the opinion of the author, these restrictions limit their usefulness and means that many patients, who could be otherwise treated successfully if the product licences were not so prohibitive, must be referred to a GP. For example, 1% hydrocortisone cream, if used short term, is an ideal steroid to use on the face with no adverse events; also, 15 g of product is often insufficient for surface areas such as limbs and the body even if used only for a week.

Despite these restrictions, corticosteroids can be used by many patients and, when used short term, have been shown to have minimal side-effects, no drug interactions and can be used by all patient groups, including pregnant women.

Hydrocortisone

Hydrocortisone can either be bought alone (e.g. Dermacort, HC45, Lanacort, Zenoxone) or in combination with other ingredients (e.g. Eurax HC, Canesten Hydrocortisone). It is prudent to use products containing only hydrocortisone for dermatitis, applying them twice a day for a maximum of 7 days. If secondary infection is suspected, for example with a fungal infection, then products such as Canesten Hydrocortisone should be used.

Clobetasone (Eumovate eczema and dermatitis cream)

Clobetasone was deregulated in 2002 and presents the pharmacist with a choice between two different-potency steroids for the first time. Clobetasone is classed as moderately potent, whereas hydrocortisone is classed as mild. It would therefore seem sensible to reserve clobetasone for more severe flare-ups of dermatitis or for those patients in whom hydrocortisone has in the past failed to control symptoms. Like hydrocortisone, clobetasone should be applied twice a day.

Further reading

Bellingham C 2001 Proper use of topical corticosteroids. Pharmaceutical Journal 267:377

Clark C 2002 Over-the-counter treatment of common skin complaints. Pharmaceutical Journal 269:284–286

Clark C, Hoare C 2001 Making the most of emollients. Pharmaceutical Journal 266:277–279

Cunliffe B 2001 Eczema. Pharmaceutical Journal 267:855–856

Web sites

National Eczema Society: www.eczema.org/
National Eczema Society for Science and Education: www.nationaleczema.org/

Table 7.25
Summary of proprietary emollient products

Product	Formulation	Combination product	Contains potential sensitising agents
Alpha Keri	Bath oil		No
Aveeno	Bath oil, cream and lotion		No
Aquadrate	Cream	Urea	No
Balneum	Bath oil		Yes
Balneum Plus	Bath oil, cream		Yes
Calmurid	Cream	Urea, lactic acid	No
Cetraben	Cream		Yes
Decubal	Cream		Yes
Dermamist	Spray		No
Dermalo	Bath oil		No
Dermol	Lotion, shower and bath emollient	Antimicrobials	Yes
Diprobase	Cream, ointment		No
Diprobath	Bath oil		No
Doublebase	Gel		No
E45	Cream, lotion, bath oil, emollient wash cream		Yes (cream and lotion only)
E45 Itch Relief	Cream	Urea	Yes
Emulsiderm	Bath emulsion	Antimicrobials	
Epaderm	Ointment		Yes
Eucerin	Cream, lotion	Urea	Yes
Eurax	Bath oil, cream		No
Gammaderm	Cream		Yes
Hydromol	Cream, ointment, bath oil		Yes (cream and ointment)
Imuderm	Bath oil		Yes
Keri	Lotion		Yes
LactiCare	Lotion	Lactic acid	Yes
Lipobase	Cream		Yes
Neutrogena	Cream		Yes
Nutraplus	Cream	Urea	Yes
Oilatum	Cream, shower emollient, bath oil		Yes
Oilatum Plus	Bath oil	Antimicrobials	Yes
Ultrabase	Cream		Yes
Unguentum M	Cream		Yes
Vaseline Dermacare	Cream, lotion		Yes

Self-assessment questions

The following questions are intended to supplement the text. Two levels of questions are provided; multiple choice questions and case studies. The multiple choice questions are designed to test factual recall and the case studies allow knowledge to be applied to a practice setting.

Multiple choice questions

7.1 Which medicine has *not* been proved to be efficacious in treating dandruff?

a. Coal tar
b. Cetrimide
c. Ketoconazole
d. Zinc pyrithione
e. Selenium sulphide

7.2. Which form of psoriasis can be managed OTC?

a. Guttate
b. Pustular
c. Plaque
d. Seborrhoeic
e. Erythrodermic

7.3. Which medicine is known to cause hair loss?

a. Nifedipine
b. Simvastatin
c. Ranitidine
d. Ibuprofen
e. Warfarin

7.4. What symptom is not associated with athlete's foot?

a. Itch
b. Redness
c. Involvement between the toes
d. Scaling
e. Odour

7.5. With which form of tinea infection are imidazoles ineffective?

a. Athlete's foot
b. Jock itch
c. Infection involving the body
d. Infection involving the nail
e. Infection on the hand

7.6. A corn is caused by?

a. Sweating feet
b. Too much pressure caused by ill-fitting shoes
c. Too little pressure caused by ill-fitting shoes

d. Secondary bacterial infection of a verruca
e. None of the above

7.7. Itching is not observed in which condition?

a. Allergic dermatitis
b. Scabies
c. Fungal infection
d. Acne vulgaris
e. Lichen planus

7.8. What skin condition is characterised by silvery-white scaly lesions of salmon-pink appearance with well defined boundaries?

a. Contact dermatitis
b. Rosacea
c. Plaque psoriasis
d. Seborrhoeic dermatitis
e. Pityriasis versicolor

Questions 7.9 to 7.11 concern the following conditions:

A. Dermatitis
B. Plaque psoriasis
C. Fungal infection
D. Acne
E. Cold sores

Select, from A to E, which of the above conditions:

7.9. Is characterised by itching and scaling

7.10. Often has prodromal symptoms prior to the rash appearing

7.11. Has a strong genetic link

Questions 7.12 to 7.14 concern the following medicines:

A. Hydrocortisone cream
B. Clotrimazole cream
C. Posalfilin ointment
D. Salicylic acid solution
E. E45 cream

Select, from A to E, which of the above medicines

7.12. Can be given to all patient groups

7.13. Is contraindicated in pregnancy

7.14. Should be used for no longer than 1 week

Questions 7.15 to 7.17: for each of these questions *one* or *more* of the responses is (are) correct. Decide which of the responses is (are) correct. Then choose:

A. If a, b and c are correct
B. If a and b only are correct
C. If b and c only are correct
D. If a only is correct
E. If c only is correct

Directions summarised

A	B	C	D	E
a, b and c	a and b only	b and c only	a only	c only

7.15. For the following statements about cradle cap which is/are true?

   a. There is normally no family history
   b. Ear and eye involvement is common
   c. The rash tends not to itch

7.16. Warts and verrucas are:

   a. Caused by the human papilloma virus
   b. Infections that never affect adults
   c. Precancerous growths

7.17. When supplying aciclovir, patients should be told to:

   a. Use the product 4 times a day
   b. Apply once the rash has appeared
   c. Wash their hands after application

Questions 7.18 to 7.20: these questions consist of a statement in the left-hand column followed by a statement in the right-hand column. You need to:

● decide whether the first statement is true or false
● decide whether the second statement is true or false

Then choose:

A. If both statements are true and the second statement is a correct explanation of the first statement
B. If both statements are true but the second statement is *not* a correct explanation of the first statement
C. If the first statement is true but the second statement is false
D. If the first statement is false but the second statement is true
E. If both statements are false

Directions summarised

	First statement	Second statement	
A	True	True	Second explanation is a correct explanation of the first
B	True	True	Second statement is *not* a correct explanation of the first
C	True	False	
D	False	True	
E	False	False	

	First statement	*Second statement*
7.18.	Benzoyl peroxide should be used to treat mild acne	It should be used for at least 6 weeks
7.19.	Scabies is intensely itchy	The mites faeces cause a hypersensitivity reaction
7.20.	Minoxidil is used to treat hair loss	It works on over 80% of patients

Case study

Mr RJ and his 9-year-old son Jimmy want to buy something for Jimmy's verruca. Mr RJ thinks that Jimmy has had the verruca for about 4 to 6 weeks. He describes it as a circular discoloured piece of skin that looks like the verrucas he used to get.

a. What course of action are you going to take?

Try and question Jimmy directly. See if Jimmy knows how long the suspected verruca has been there. Ask if the lesion is causing any pain when walking. Instead of asking for further descriptions of what the lesion looks like and where it is positioned ask if you can actually look at the lesion. Remember to wash your hands before and after inspecting the foot.

On further questioning and examination you concur with the self-diagnosis of a verruca. The lesion is small (less than 0.5 cm in diameter) and causes no pain when direct pressure is applied.

b. What are you going to recommend?

A salicylic-acid-based product is the most suitable product and you recommend Bazuka, after first making sure Jimmy is not diabetic.

Six weeks later Mrs J returns with Jimmy and demands to see the pharmacist. She says the stuff you recommended is rubbish and that Jimmy's verruca is bigger than it was before!

c. How are you going to respond?

First, you must stay calm and not be defensive. Ask open questions to find out why Mrs J is unhappy; this approach will generally reveal what the problem is. Second, if the reason is not obvious then you must find out about compliance. Who has been responsible for applying the product? If the parents have told Jimmy to use it, has he been using the product correctly and at the correct dosage frequency? In addition, many patients have unrealistic expectations on how quickly the verruca will resolve with therapy. Did you tell them how long it would take before an effect will be seen? This is a vital piece of information to ensure patients realise that treatment is not a quick cure.

You find out that Mrs J has been applying the Bazuka and doing everything the instruction leaflet says. You inspect Jimmy's feet again and from what you can remember the lesion does look slightly larger.

d. Why might this be the case?

Salicylic acid is destructive in nature and if the product comes in to contact with non-affected skin then it can damage skin and appear to the patient that the lesion has indeed got bigger.

Mrs J wants to try Bazuka Extra Strength because the normal Bazuka isn't helping.

e. What are you going to do?

You must try to stress to Mrs J that she continues with the normal Bazuka because 6 weeks of therapy is not long enough to make a decision to alter therapy.

Reluctantly, Mrs J accepts your advice and leaves the pharmacy promising she will try for a bit longer. One week later she presents a prescription for Cuplex gel for Jimmy.

f. What are you going to do?

It appears that Mrs J was not satisfied or convinced with your advice and has decided to see the GP. You do not know whether she told the GP about using an OTC product. You could ring the GP to tell him or her that Mrs J has been using a salicylic-acid-based product already, however, this is likely to have little bearing on the outcome of product selection as Jimmy will still need to continue treatment with something for a few more weeks. The prescription should be dispensed and Mrs J counselled appropriately. It would be unprofessional to point out to that Cuplex is unlikely to be any better than Bazuka.

When you hand Mrs J the Cuplex she mentions that the doctor said this was stronger than Bazuka and should do the trick.

CASE STUDY 7.1

g. How do you reply?

Be diplomatic and non-judgemental. It is likely that the GP knows that Cuplex is no better than Bazuka but if the patient is convinced that what she is now getting is superior to the previous product then her

motivation to comply with directions might be better and hence the outcome for Jimmy will be eradication of the verruca. It might be worth asking the GP, the next time you have a conversation, what his or her rationale for prescribing Cuplex was.

CASE STUDY 7.2

Case study 7.2

Ms AH is the mother of an infant son aged 4 months. She asks for your help in treating her son's flaky skin on his scalp. She says he has had the problem on and off for the last 6 weeks. She hasn't yet tried anything except baby shampoo, as recommended by the health visitor. However, she now wants a cream or something to get rid of the problem once and for all.

a. What further information do you require to be in a position to help her?

You need to know more about the severity of the problem, for example whether any other parts of the baby's skin is affected. Does the baby appear to scratch at the rash and what were the previous episodes like? Were they the same as this time or different? Also, is there a family history of atopy or other dermatological conditions in the family.

You decide the child has cradle cap.

b. What treatment are you going to recommend?

The use of a mild tar-based product every other day until the scalp clears would be appropriate. In between using the tar-based product Ms AH should be instructed to use the baby shampoo.

Ms AH returns to the pharmacy 2 weeks later with another of her children. Impressed that her son's scalp

is now clear she now wants some advice for her 7-year-old daughter. She has a sore on the corner of her mouth.

c. What further information do you require to be in a position to help her?

You need to know:

- *How long the sore has been present.*
- *How the sore first developed.*
- *What symptoms are associated with the sore.*
- *The progression of the sore. Has it spread?*
- *If the girl is taking any medicine.*
- *Family history.*

You find out the sore appeared overnight and is now itchy. On inspection the lesion appears to be weeping a clear exudate.

d. What is the most likely diagnosis?

Based on this information the likely diagnosis is a cold sore.

e. What treatment, if any, are you going to recommend?

No treatment necessary but if the parent insists on therapy then any product could be given, although antiviral therapy is expensive and the cost difficult to justify. In addition, advice on minimising transmission could be given, such as not sharing towels and trying to avoid kissing (e.g. mum and dad).

Answers to multiple choice questions

7.1 = b, 7.2 = c   7.3 = e   7.4 = e   7.5 = d   7.6 = b   7.7 = d   7.8 = c   7.9 = c   7.10 = e,
7.11 = b   7.12 = e   7.13 = d   7.14 = a   7.15 = c   7.16 = d   7.17 = e   7.18 = b   7.19 = a   7.20 = c.

Musculoskeletal conditions

Background

The musculoskeletal system comprises hard (bone and cartilage) and soft (muscles, tendons, ligaments) tissues. It is responsible for mobility and provides protection to vital structures. Most musculoskeletal problems occur as a result of injury or organic illness. The majority of patients presenting to a community pharmacist will have an acute and self-limiting problem, which will resolve spontaneously. Chronic conditions such as osteoarthritis will be encountered routinely when issuing prescriptions to patients.

The key role of the pharmacist when dealing with patients with a musculoskeletal problem is to establish the cause, its severity and whether it can be self-managed appropriately or requires further investigation.

General overview of musculoskeletal anatomy

The skeletal system of the human body is composed of 206 bones. At the point of contact between two or more bones an articulation (joint) is formed. This system of bones and joints maximises movement while maintaining stability. There are two basic types of joints:

- synovial joints: allow considerable movement (e.g. shoulder or knee)
- fibrocartilaginous joints: are completely immovable (e.g. the skull) or permit only limited motion (e.g. spinal vertebrae).

Bones and joints cannot move by themselves. The integrity of the musculoskeletal system depends on the interaction between skeletal muscle and bones, and coordinated movement is only possible because of the way muscle is attached to bone. Tendons attach the end of the muscle to the bone or to another structure upon which the muscle acts. To perform such a function, tendons are composed of very dense fibrous tissue.

Joints require additional stability and support. Strong bands of fibrous tissue known as ligaments bind together the bones entering a joint to provide this additional support and stability. It is often the integrity of the connecting structures that is damaged in a musculoskeletal injury. The simplified diagram of the medial aspect of the knee joint in Fig. 8.1 illustrates the relationship of the connective structures to the skeleton and musculature.

The knee joint is an example of a synovial joint. The femur, tibia and fibula do not touch each other because they are covered with **articular cartilage** and separated by the synovial cavity. The knee joint also contains bursae – small fluid-filled sacs – that provide protection at points in the joint where friction or pressure is great. These can become inflamed, leading to bursitis.

History taking

Gaining an accurate history from the patient should provide enough information to determine if their injury is within the scope of a community pharmacist. By the very nature of musculoskeletal injuries, if someone manages to come into the pharmacy then the injury is unlikely to be serious. Information gathering should con-

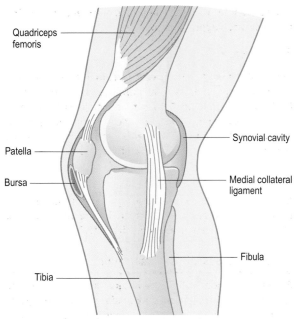

Fig. 8.1 The knee joint: medial view

centrate on when the injury occurred, what precipitated the injury, the level of discomfort, any restriction in range of motion and whether the injury appears to be worsening, and on finding out what expectations the patient has.

In general, any patient who presents with an injury that is causing extreme discomfort or if the pain is worsening, adversely affects mobility and has been present for more than a week would probably be better managed by a GP or physiotherapist/sports therapist and referral should be made.

Acute low back pain

Background

Back pain is very common; there were approximately 14 million GP consultations in the UK in 1993. Acute low back pain is self-limiting and over 90% of patients will get better within 6 weeks, although up to two-thirds will have a recurrence within 1 year of the initial onset and fewer than 5% of patients go on to develop chronic back pain. It is hardly surprising that the economic burden to society is huge.

Prevalence and epidemiology

Back pain is most common between the ages of 20 and 50 years and adults have a lifetime prevalence of approximately 80%. It is more common in people such as industrial workers, people who do heavy manual labour and people who play certain sports such as golf and gymnastics.

There is little difference in the prevalence between men and women, although between 50 to 90% of pregnant women develop low back pain.

Aetiology

In the majority of cases a cause cannot be determined for the patient's symptoms. Pain originates from the lumbosacral region and is often mechanical in origin (Fig. 8.2) and includes problems caused by muscles, tendons, ligaments and discs. Contributory factors in the cause of low back pain are a general lack of fitness, occupational and psychological factors. Rarely underlying pathology is implicated but if it is then the cause is usually from infection or malignancy.

Arriving at a differential diagnosis

The vast majority of patients (95%) who present in the pharmacy will have simple back pain that will, in time, resolve with conservative treatment. Bad posture when seated and poor lifting technique when performing day-to-day tasks such as cleaning or gardening are very common predisposing factors. The remaining cases will have back pain with associated nerve root compression. It is extremely unlikely that a pharmacist will encounter a patient with serious spinal pathology, such as malignancy. The principal diagnosis varies with age. It is important to begin questioning the patient with traditional questions regarding the pain: location, radiation, evidence of trauma, the effect pain has on mobility and factors that aggravate or relieve the pain. Asking a number of symptom-specific questions will aid differential diagnosis (Table 8.1).

Clinical features of acute low back pain

Pain in the lower lumbar or sacral area is usually described as aching or stiffness. Depending on the cause, pain might be localised (e.g. lumbosacral strains following physical activity) or more diffuse (e.g. from postural backache after sitting incorrectly for a prolonged period). In cases of acute injury the symptoms come on quickly and there will be a reduction in mobility.

Conditions to eliminate

Causes of low back pain not related to back pathophysiology

It must be remembered that acute illness, for example colds and influenza, can give rise to generalised aching or pain. Likewise, pre-rash pain associated with shingles and referred pain from abdominal organs (e.g. pyelonephritis) can present as low back pain. A careful history

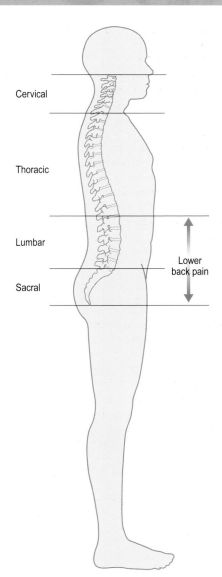

Cervical

Thoracic

Lumbar

Lower
back pain

Sacral

Fig. 8.2 Location and distribution of lower back pain:
L4/L5, pain radiates down outer calf and onto the top of
the foot; L5/S1, pain radiates to the outside and sole of
the foot

of the presenting symptoms should enable exclusion of
such conditions.

Sciatica

Pain is acute in onset and radiates to the leg. Pain starts
in the lower back and as it intensifies radiates into the
lower extremity. The most common sites of involvement
are between L4–L5 and L5–S1 vertebrae (see Fig. 8.2).
With **disc herniation**, pain is characterised as being dull,
deep and aching. It is usually felt in the upper part rather
than the lower part of the leg and spreads from the
lumbar spine. If the disc ruptures or herniates under
strain then the pain is usually lancinating in quality,
shooting down the leg like an electric shock. Valsalva

movements, for example coughing, sneezing or straining
at stool, often aggravate the pain.

Malignancy

Thankfully, malignancy is very rare. Malignancy is more
prevalent in patients over 50, although rates are still low;
0.14% in under 50 and 0.56% in patients over 50. History
of significant weight loss, presence of anaemia, general
malaise, night pain and failure to improve over a 4-week
period warrant referral for further evaluation.

Infection

Infection is a rare cause of back pain. Presence of fever
is the most suggestive historical feature for infection,
although pain tends to worsen with activity.

Chronic causes of low back pain

Patients in whom pain lasts longer than 3 months are
said to suffer from chronic back pain. Degenerative joint
disease is probably the most common cause of chronic
low back pain in people older than 50.

Degenerative joint disease (osteoarthritis)

Associated with advancing age osteoarthritis affects up
to one-third of people aged over 65. It might be localised
to a single joint or involve multiple joints. It is thought
that an imbalance of synthesis and degradation of
cartilage is responsible for the disease, which affects the
whole joint. Onset of deep aching pain is gradual and
early morning stiffness usually lasts for 15 to 30 min.

Inflammatory arthropathies

These include ankylosing spondylitis and psoriatic arthritis. Spondylitis is characterised by thinning or loss of
elasticity of the discs that cushion the vertebrae of the
spine, and is the most common cause of chronic low back
pain in the middle aged and elderly. Patients commonly have
marked stiffness on awakening and pain that alternates
from side to side of the lumbar spine. Exercise relieves
the pain but is made worse by bending, lifting and
prolonged sitting in one position (e.g. long car journeys).

 **TRIGGER POINTS indicative of referral: Low back
pain**

- Associated fever
- Back pain from structures above the lumbar region
- Bowel or bladder incontinence
- Failure to improve after 10 to 14 days since onset
- Numbness
- Patients under 20 and over 60
- Persistent and progressively worsening pain
- Referred pain into the lower leg
- Suspected fracture

Table 8.1
Specific questions to ask the patient: Back pain

Question	Relevance
Age	● *Children:* have a higher incidence of identifiable and potentially serious causes, e.g. spondylolysis, Scheuermann's disease (although pain is experienced in upper back and neck) and malignancy. All children should be referred unless backache is associated with recent participation in sport ● *Aged 15 to 30:* prolapsed disc, trauma, fractures, and pregnancy most likely ● *Aged 30 to 50:* degenerative joint disease (osteoarthritis), prolapsed disc and malignancy most likely ● *Older than 50:* patients are more likely to have serious underlying disorders such as osteoporosis, malignancy and metabolic bone disorders (Paget's disease)
Location	● Pain felt that radiates into the buttocks, thighs and legs implies nerve root compression. If pain is felt below the knee, this is highly suggestive of sciatica
Onset	● Low back pain that is acute and sudden in onset is likely to be muscle strain in the lumbosacral region and not serious. However, acute low back pain in the elderly should be referred as even slight trauma can result in compression fractures ● Low back pain that is insidious in onset should be viewed with caution
Restriction of movement	● People with disc herniation usually have difficulty in sitting down ● Mechanical causes of pain are exacerbated with physical activity and relieved by rest ● Systemic causes of back ache are usually worse with rest and disturb sleep
Weakness or numbness	● Progressive muscle weakness must be referred for further evaluation

Evidence base for over-the-counter medication

Pharmacists can appropriately treat patients with uncomplicated acute low back pain. The goal of treatment is to provide relief of symptoms and a return to normal mobility. The approach to managing low back pain should be a combination of rest and physical activity augmented by analgesic therapy.

Conservative treatment

Bed rest was once widely prescribed for patients with low back pain. However, a number of systematic reviews have now proven that prolonged bed rest is counter-productive. Patients might benefit from short-term rest, lasting no longer than 2 days, after which they should be encouraged to exercise. The level and length of exercise should be tailored to the individual and referral to a physiotherapist or the GP would be needed.

Analgesics (paracetamol, aspirin, ibuprofen and compound products)

All systemic analgesics when prescribed as monotherapy have proven efficacy in pain relief at standard doses. However, the use of NSAIDs for 7 to 10 days is widely advocated (naproxen, ketoprofen and diclofenac are available in other countries, for example New Zealand). This should produce a significant reduction in symptoms and patients must be advised to see their GP if symptoms fail to improve after this time.

Compound analgesics (paracetamol/codeine, aspirin/codeine or paracetamol/ dihydrocodeine)

Codeine and dihydrocodeine can be prescribed OTC provided their respective maximum strengths do not exceed 1.5% and the maximum dose does not exceed 20 or 10 mg, respectively. In practice, this equates to commercially available products with a maximum dose of 12.8 mg of codeine and 7.46 mg of dihydrocodeine.

At these doses their pain-killing effect has been called into question. A number of papers have concluded that OTC doses are too low to produce statistically significant reductions in pain compared to single agents. However, the opioid dose might be sufficient to cause side-effects such as constipation. Elderly patients are particularly susceptible to opioid side-effects and might, in rare circumstances, experience drowsiness even at OTC doses.

Caffeine

A number of proprietary products contain caffeine in doses ranging from 15 to 110 mg. It has been claimed that caffeine enhances analgesic efficacy but evidence is lacking to substantiate these claims. They may have a mild stimulant effect and should therefore be avoided before going to bed.

Topical therapy

NSAIDs
Topical NSAIDs have been available OTC since ibuprofen became available in topical form in 1988. Since then, a

number of other NSAIDs have been deregulated from prescription only control. They have proved popular with patients and are widely sold over the counter. Prior to 1998, publications such as *MeReC* and *The Drug and Therapeutics Bulletin* stated that although several trials had shown topical NSAIDs to be more effective than placebo, the quality of this evidence was poor. Subsequently, in 1998, Moore et al published a systematic review of the safety and effectiveness of topical NSAIDs in acute and chronic pain conditions involving over 10 000 patients from 86 trials. The review included all NSAIDs available OTC. Positive outcomes were defined as 50% pain relief after 1 week for acute conditions. The review concluded that topical NSAIDs were effective and had a lower incidence of side-effects than same drugs taken orally.

No trials appear to have been conducted comparing one NSAID against another and so it is not possible to say if one NSAID is more efficacious than the other.

Rubefacients

Rubefacients, also known as counterirritants, have been incorporated in topical formulations for decades. They cause vasodilation, producing a sensation of warmth that distracts the patient from experiencing pain. It has also been hypothesised that increased blood flow might help disperse chemical mediators of pain, although this is unsubstantiated. With the exception of capsaicin, there is no evidence to support their effect and they should not be routinely recommended as first-line treatment.

Capsaicin

Two POM products have been granted licences for post-herpetic neuralgia and painful diabetic neuropathy (Axsain, capsaicin 0.075%) and symptomatic relief in osteoarthritis (Zacin, capsaicin 0.025%). Although these are not available OTC, a number of OTC products do contain capsaicin (e.g. Balmosa, 0.035%; Ralgex cream, 0.12 and stick, 1.96% capsaicin) at concentrations equivalent or higher than those found in the POM products. Although no evidence exists for these products in relieving pain it would seem a reasonable supposition that they might show similar effects. Trials are therefore needed to determine if OTC products are effective.

Enzymes

Heparinoid and hyaluronidase are included in a number of products. Theoretically they are supposed to disperse fluids in swollen areas, reducing swelling and bruising but this is unproven.

Alternative remedies

Glucosamine

Although glucosamine is not used for acute low back pain it is widely advertised to the general public as a treatment for osteoarthritis. There appears to be a growing body of evidence to support the efficacy of glucosamine. However, one recent meta-analysis concluded that individual study conclusions had overestimated its effect and that if glucosamine is to be used then it should only be used for short periods, as there is no trial data to support long-term use.

Summary

Based on evidence, patients with acute low back pain should be encouraged to exercise and be given a short course of a systemic NSAID unless contraindicated. Topical NSAIDs could also be recommended for those patients in whom side-effects need to be minimised, for example elderly patients or patients who have experienced GI side-effects with previous NSAID use as plasma concentrations with topical therapy is substantially lower and the stomach is circumvented avoiding direct irritation.

Use of OTC compound analgesics should be avoided, although patients might perceive they are getting a stronger pain killer and the placebo response of such medicines should not be underestimated.

Practical prescribing and product selection

Prescribing information relating to systemic analgesics reviewed in the section 'Evidence base for over-the-counter medication' is discussed and systemic proprietary products summarised in Table 8.2; useful tips relating to systemic analgesics are given in Hints and Tips Box 8.1.

Paracetamol

Paracetamol is the safest analgesic. It can be given to all patient groups, has no significant drug interactions and side-effects are very rare. Patients with low back pain will benefit most from taking paracetamol regularly at its maximum dose of eight tablets per day.

Aspirin

Unlike paracetamol, aspirin is associated with problems in its use. Children under 16 should avoid any products containing aspirin (although children with low back pain should be referred). It can cause gastric irritation and is associated with gastric bleeds, especially in the elderly. For this reason, aspirin should not be given to elderly patients or to any patient with a history of peptic ulcer. In a small minority of asthmatic patients, aspirin can precipitate shortness of breath, therefore any asthmatic who has previously had a hypersensitivity reaction to aspirin should avoid aspirin. It should also be avoided in patients taking warfarin because bleeding time is increased. Aspirin is best avoided in pregnancy because adverse effects to the mother and fetus have been reported.

Table 8.2
Systemic proprietary analgesics available OTC

Product	Aspirin	Paracetamol	Ibuprofen	Codeine	Other	Children
Advil			200 mg			> 12 years
Alka-Seltzer XS	267 mg	133 mg			Caffeine 40 mg	> 16 years
Alka-Xs Go	300 mg	200 mg			Caffeine 45 mg	> 16 years
Anadin Extra Tablets/Soluble Tablets	300 mg	200 mg			Caffeine 45 mg	> 16 years
Anadin Ibuprofen			200 mg			> 12 years
Anadin Paracetamol		500 mg				> 6 years
Anadin	325 mg				Caffeine 15 mg	> 16 years
Anadin Ultra			200 mg			> 12 years
Askit Powders	530 mg				Aloxiprin 140 mg Caffeine 110 mg	> 16 years
Aspro Clear	300 mg					> 16 years
Aspro Clear Max	500 mg					> 16 years
Calpol products (see Chapter 9, page 217)						
Codis 500	500 mg			8 mg		> 16 years
Cuprofen			200 mg			> 12 years
Cuprofen maximum			400 mg			> 12 years
Disprin and Disprin Direct	300 mg					> 16 years
Disprin Extra	300 mg	200 mg				> 16 years
Disprol products (see Chapter 9, page 217)						
Hedex		500 mg				> 6 years
Hedex Extra		500 mg			Caffeine 65 mg	> 12 years
Hedex Ibuprofen			200 mg			> 12 years
Medinol products (see Chapter 9, page 217)						
Medised products (see Chapter 9, page 217)						
Nurofen Tabs, meltabs, liquid capsules and caplets			200 mg			> 12 years
Nurofen Long Lasting			300 mg			> 12 years
Nurofen Plus			200 mg	12.8 mg		> 12 years
Nurofen Recovery			200 mg			> 12 years
Nurse Sykes Powders	165 mg	120 mg			Caffeine 65 mg	> 16 years
Panadol Tablets and Actifast Tablets		500 mg				> 12 years
Panadol Extra Tablets and Soluble Tablets	500 mg				Caffeine 65 mg	> 12 years
Panadol Night Pain		500 mg			Diphenhydramine 25 mg	> 12 years
Panadol Ultra		500 mg		12.8 mg		> 12 years
Paracodol Tablets and Soluble Tablets		500 mg		8 mg		> 12 years
Paramol		521 mg			Dihydrocodeine 7.46 mg	> 12 years
Phensic	325 mg				Caffeine 22 mg	> 16 years
Propain		400 mg			Caffeine 50 mg Diphenhydramine 5 mg	> 16 years
Solpadeine Tablets/Capsules/ Soluble Tablets		500 mg		8 mg	Caffeine 30 mg	> 12 years
Solpadeine Max		500 mg		12.8 mg		> 12 years
Solpaflex			200 mg	12.8 mg		> 12 years
Syndol		450 mg		10 mg	Caffeine 30 mg Doxylamine 5 mg	> 12 years
Veganin		500 mg		8 mg	Caffeine 30 mg	

HINTS AND TIPS BOX 8.1:

Children and aspirin	Aspirin-taking in children has been linked to Reyes syndrome, a rare syndrome in which encephalopathy occurs and if not diagnosed early can lead to death. Until October 2002 advice from the CSM stated that no child under 12 should take aspirin. However, due to wide availability of aspirin and other safer treatment choices it was decided to simplify the advice in the interest of public health and raise the age to children under 16 should not take aspirin. Many parents might not be aware that the age restriction for aspirin has changed and it is important that pharmacists remind parents
Topical products	Gentle massage of the area on application can be beneficial in dissipating swelling and help reduce pain therefore products with no evidence base may still prove useful

Ibuprofen

Ibuprofen should be used as first-line therapy unless the patient is contraindicated from using an NSAID. Adults should take 200 to 400 mg (one or two tablets) three times a day, although most patients will need the higher dose of 400 mg three times a day. Ibuprofen is best avoided in certain patient groups, such as the elderly, because they are more prone to GI bleeds and have reduced renal function; patients with a history of peptic ulcers and those asthmatics who are hypersensitive to aspirin or any other NSAID. However, it appears to be safe in pregnancy.

For the majority of patients, ibuprofen is well tolerated, although gastric irritation is a well-recognised side-effect. It can interact with many medicines and although none of these interactions are truly significant, ibuprofen can alter lithium levels so that, where possible, an alternative should be recommended. If ibuprofen is given with lithium then the patient's serum lithium needs to be monitored more closely than normal.

Topical NSAIDs (e.g. ibuprofen, piroxicam, diclofenac, felbinac, ketoprofen)

Topical NSAIDs provide an alternative to those patients who should avoid systemic NSAID therapy. They have fewer side-effects than systemic therapy with the most commonly reported adverse events being skin reactions (maculopapular rash or itching) at the site of application. Gastrointestinal side effects have been reported but are rare.

Ibuprofen (e.g. Ibuleve range, Cuprofen, Deep Relief, Nurofen, Proflex)

Ibuprofen is the most well-known and bought topical NSAID. A range of formulations is available including cream, gel, spray and mousse. It is available as a standard 5% formulation or a maximum strength of 10% and should be applied no more than four times a day. Patients under 12 should not use any topical ibuprofen product, although some manufacturers state it should not be given to children under 14 (e.g. Nurofen products).

Piroxicam (Feldene P gel), diclofenac (Voltarol Emulgel P), ketoprofen (Oruvail), felbinac (Traxam Pain Relief), salicylic acid (Movelat) and benzydamine (Difflam) are all available commercially. Like ibuprofen, they are all applied three or four times a day and should not be given to children.

Rubefacients (e.g. Balmosa, Deep Heat, Radain B and Ralgex ranges)

Rubefacients can be used on all patients except young children; most manufacturers state they should not be used on children under 5 or 6 years of age. They can be used by all other patient groups, have no drug interactions and side-effects are localised to excessive irritation at the site of application. The majority of products contain two or more compounds, although most contain nicotinates and/or salicylates. Other compounds in rubefacients include menthol, camphor, capsaicin and turpentine oil.

Further reading

[Anonymous] 1993 Combination analgesics. MeReC Bulletin 4:45–47

[Anonymous] 1997 Topical NSAIDs: an update. MeReC Bulletin 8:29–32

[Anonymous] 1998 Managing acute low back pain. Drug and Therapeutics Bulletin 36:93–95

[Anonymous] 1999 Topical NSAIDs for joint disease. Drug and Therapeutics Bulletin 37:87–88

Bueff H U, Van Der Reis W 1996 Low back pain. Primary Care 23:345–364

Moore R A, Tramer M R, Carroll D et al 1998 Qualitative systematic review of topically applied NSAIDs. British Medical Journal 316:333–338

Towheed T E, Anastassiades T P 2000 Glucosamine and chondroitin for treating symptoms of osteoarthritis-evidence is widely touted but incomplete. Journal of the American Medical Association 283:1483–1484

Wood J 1999 Osteoarthritis and its management. Pharmaceutical Journal 262:744–746.

Activity-related/sports-related soft tissue injuries

This section will discuss common conditions affecting the shoulder, elbow, knee, ankle and foot.

Background

Muscle, tendons, ligaments, fascia and synovial capsules are all soft tissue structures. Damage to any of these structures will result in pain and/or inflammation. Historically, pharmacists see only a small proportion of acute soft tissue injuries; the majority of patients present to a GP, physiotherapist or casualty department. In a number of small studies, respondents did not consider the pharmacist as a source of advice or help, although the minority who consulted a pharmacist were satisfied with the advice received. This suggests that pharmacists could play a greater role in managing patients with activity-/sport-related problems.

Prevalence and epidemiology

Most injuries are as a direct result of physical activity or accident. Prevalence is therefore higher in people who actively participate in sports. In primary care the ankles and knees are the most common sites of injury.

Aetiology

The aetiology of soft tissue injury depends on the structures affected. Sprains are caused by forcing a joint in to an abnormal position that overstretches or twists ligaments, and can vary from damage of a few fibres to complete rupture. Strains involve tearing of muscle fibres, which can be partial or complete and is usually a result of over exertion when the muscle is stretched beyond its usual limits.

Arriving at a differential diagnosis

Patients will often state they have sprained or strained something. It is important to confirm their self-diagnosis as these terms are often used interchangeably. Sprains and strains can be graded according to the severity of the injury, but this is of little practical value. The major role of the pharmacist is to determine if the patient can manage the injury or whether referral is needed. This will be primarily based on questions asked (Table 8.3) of the patient but, even without an intimate knowledge of joint anatomy, limited physical examination can be performed to help decide if referral is necessary.

Clinical features of soft tissue injury

In general patients will present with pain, swelling and bruising. The extent and severity of symptoms will be determined by the severity of the injury.

Shoulder-specific conditions

The shoulder provides the greatest range of motion of any joint. It is a very mobile and complex interconnected structure (Fig. 8.3), consequently there are a number of commonly encountered shoulder injuries, such as frozen shoulder, impingement syndromes and rotator cuff syndrome. Within the confines of the community pharmacy, the patient can be asked to perform certain arm movements that will allow the range of motion of the shoulder to be determined (Fig. 8.4). Patients who show marked loss of motion should be referred.

Rotator cuff syndrome

The rotator cuff refers to the combined tendons of the scapula muscles that hold the head of the humerus in place. Rubbing of these tendons causes pain. It is most often seen in patients over the age of 40 and is associated with repetitive overhead activity. Pain tends to be worse at night and might disturb sleep. Reaching behind the back also tends to worsen pain. Also, the patient cannot normally initiate **abduction**.

Frozen shoulder

This term is used to describe the shoulder when it has marked restriction in all the major ranges of motion. It often occurs without warning or explanation and can vary in severity from day to day. NSAIDs could be offered but if symptoms fail to respond with treatment after 5 days then referral for alternative treatment and physiotherapy should be considered.

Elbow-specific conditions

In primary care pharmacists are only likely to see three elbow problems: tennis elbow (lateral **epicondylitis**); golfer's elbow (medial epicondylitis) and student's elbow (bursitis).

Tennis elbow is characterised by pain felt over the outer aspect of the elbow joint that might also spread up the upper arm. The patient should have a history of gradually increasing pain and tenderness. In comparison, the pain of golfer's elbow is noticed on the inner side of the elbow and can radiate down the forearm. Both names

Table 8.3
Specific questions to ask the patient: soft tissue injuries

	Relevance
When did it happen and when did the patient present	• The closer these two events are the more likely the patient will be suffering from a serious problem that is outside the remit of the pharmacist, unless the injury was sustained in close proximity to the pharmacy and the patient has asked for first aid
Presenting symptoms	• Marked swelling, bruising and pain occurring straight after injury is suggestive of more serious injury and referral to casualty for X-rays and further tests is needed
Nature of injury	• If the injury occurred in which impact forces were great then fracture becomes more likely • Sudden onset, associated with a single traumatic event suggests a mechanical problem such as tendon/ligament tearing • If the person has a foot injury and is unable to bear their full weight whilst walking then referral is needed
Range of motion	• If the affected joint shows marked reduction in normal range of motion this requires referral for fuller evaluation
Nature of pain	• Referred pain suggests nerve root compression involvement, for example a shoulder injury in which pain is also felt in the hand • Pain that is insidious in onset and progressive is more likely to be due to some form of degenerative disease and requires referral
Age of patient	• *Children:* Bones are softer in children and therefore more prone to greenstick fractures (fracture of the outer part of the bone) and should be referred to exclude such problems • *Elderly:* Risk factors for fracture, such as osteoarthritis and osteoporosis is higher in the elderly

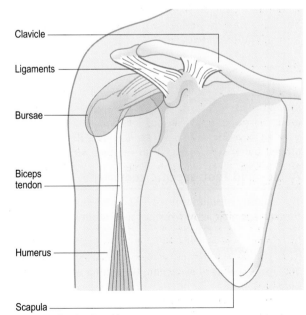

Clavicle

Ligaments

Bursae

Biceps
tendon

Humerus

Scapula

Fig. 8.3 Basic shoulder anatomy

are misleading as people other than tennis and golf players can suffer from the problems and, if not sports related, these conditions are usually related to a repetitive activity.

Knee-specific conditions

The knee is the largest joint in the body and is subject to extreme forces. Unsurprisingly, it is the most common site of sport injuries, especially among footballers. To help maintain stability the knee has three main pairs of ligaments: the medial collateral ligament, which connects the femur to the tibia; the lateral collateral ligament, which connects the femur to the fibula and the anterior cruciate ligament, which prevents the tibia from sliding forward on the femur (Fig. 8.5).

Ligament damage

Most often seen in footballers. Find out from the patient how the injury occurred. If the injury occurred when twisting this implies damage to medial meniscus (incomplete rings of cartilage that promote joint stability) as the medial collateral ligament is attached to the meniscus and forces applied to the ligament result in tears of the meniscus. This is less serious than damage to the anterior

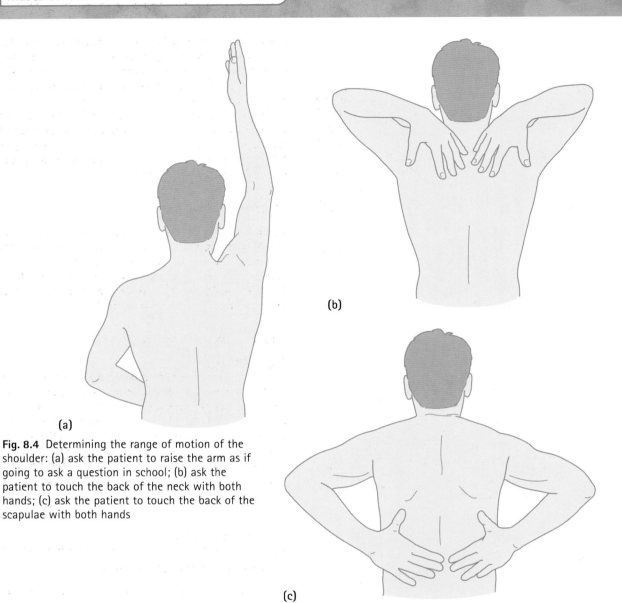

Fig. 8.4 Determining the range of motion of the shoulder: (a) ask the patient to raise the arm as if going to ask a question in school; (b) ask the patient to touch the back of the neck with both hands; (c) ask the patient to touch the back of the scapulae with both hands

cruciate ligament, which usually occurs when the person receives a blow to the back of the knee. The former can usually respond to NSAIDs and physiotherapy, whereas the latter can end careers.

Runner's knee (chondromalacia)

Most commonly noted in recreational joggers who are increasing their mileage, for example training to run a marathon. It develops insidiously with pain being the predominant symptom. Pain can be aggravated by prolonged periods of sitting down in the same position or climbing stairs. Treatment depends on the severity of pain but NSAIDs can be tried if the pain is mild to total rest and stopping running if severe.

Ankle- and foot-specific conditions

The majority of injuries involve sprained ankles, whether through sporting activity or just as a result of accidents.

Ankle sprains

The ankle acts as a hinge joint permitting up and down motion. Three sets of ligaments provide stability to the joint: the deltoid, lateral collateral and syndesmosis. The majority of ankle sprains involve the lateral ligamentous structures due to inversion of the joint leading to injury of (Fig. 8.6). Patients usually describe an accident when they 'went over their ankle'. Most patients will walk with a limp because the ankle cannot support their full weight.

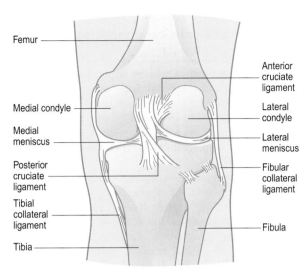

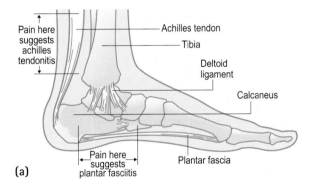

Fig. 8.5 Basic knee anatomy

Fig. 8.6 Basic anatomy of the ankle: (a) medial view; (b) lateral view

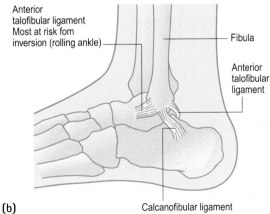

Achilles tendon injuries

Injuries to the structures associated with the Achilles tendon are usually seen in runners or athletes involved in jumping sports. Inflammation of bursae or the Achilles tendon itself will manifest with similar symptoms. Pain is felt behind the heel, just above the calcaneus, and progressively worsens the longer the injury lasts. It often occurs when runners increase their mileage or run over hilly terrain. Depending on the severity of the injury, treatment could be anything from NSAIDs, complete rest or having a cast fitted. If the injury is recent in onset and the pain not too severe, the pharmacist could suggest NSAID therapy and rest. If this fails to remedy the situation the person should be referred.

Plantar fasciitis

The plantar fascia extends from the calcaneus to the middle phalanges of the toes allowing toes to flex. Runners are most prone to plantar fasciitis. Patients will present with pain felt along the plantar surface of the foot and heel. Pain is insidious and progressively worsens until the person may alter their running style.

Common muscle strains

Thigh strains

Tears of the quadriceps (front of the thigh) and hamstring (back of the thigh) are very common. Patients will not always be able to recall a specific event that has caused the strain. Pain and discomfort is worsened when the patient tries to use the muscle but daily activities can usually be performed. RICE (see page 200) followed by NSAID treatment will usually resolve the problem, however, referral is needed if daily activities are compromised.

Conditions to eliminate

Delayed onset muscle soreness

This is a common problem and follows unaccustomed strenuous activity. For example, the patient might describe playing football for the first time in a long while or just started going to aerobic classes. Pain is felt in the muscles, which feel stiff and tight. Pain peaks within 72 h. Patients should be encouraged to properly stretch prior to exercising to minimise the problem. No treatment is necessary.

Shin splint syndrome

Recreational runners and people unaccustomed to regular running may experience pain along the front of the lower third of the tibia. Pressing gently on this area will cause considerable pain. It is caused by over-stretching the tibial muscle and is usually precipitated by running on hard surfaces. Pain is made worse by continued running or climbing stairs. Treatment involves running less frequently or for shorter distances and NSAID therapy for approximately one week.

Bursitis

Bursae can become inflamed that leads to accumulation of synovial fluid in the joint. Housemaid's knee and student's elbow are such examples. Clinically, joint swelling is the predominant feature with associated pain and local tenderness.

Stress fractures

Most commonly associated with the foot. Patients experience a dull ache along the affected metatarsal shaft that changes to a sharp ache behind the metatarsal head. It is often seen in those patients that have a history of increased activity or a change in footwear.

Gout

Acute attacks of gout are exquisitely painful, with patients reporting that even bedclothes cannot be tolerated. Approximately 80% of cases affect the big toe. Gout is more prevalent in men, especially over the age of 50.

Carpal tunnel syndrome

At the base of the palm is a 'tunnel' through which the median nerve passes; this narrow passage between the forearm and hand is called the carpal tunnel. If the median nerve becomes trapped, it can cause numbness and tingling in the hand. Often the patient will wake in the night with numbness and tingling pain that radiates to the forearm, and sometimes extends to the shoulder.

Repetitive strain injury

This condition, also termed chronic upper limb pain syndrome, often results after prolonged periods of steady hand movement involving repeated grasping, turning and twisting. The predominant symptom is pain in all or one part of one or both arms. Usually the person's job will involve repetitive tasks, such as keyboard operations.

TRIGGER POINTS indicative of referral: Soft tissue injury

- Acute injuries that show immediate swelling and severe pain
- Children under 12 and elderly patients
- Decreased range of motion in all directions involving the shoulder
- Excessive range of movement in any joint (can suggest major ligament disruption)
- Patients unable to bear any weight on an injured ankle/foot
- Suspected fracture
- Treatment failure

Evidence base for over-the-counter medication and practical prescribing and product selection

Prescribing information relating to medication for soft tissue injuries is the same as acute low back pain (see page 192). However, non-drug treatment plays a vital and major role in the treatment of soft tissue injuries. Standard advice follows the acronym RICE:

Rest: allows immobilisation, enhancing healing and reducing blood flow.

Ice: should be applied while the injury feels warm to the touch. Apply until the skin becomes numb and repeat at hourly intervals. Bags of frozen peas wrapped in a towel are ideal to use on the injury as they conform to body shape and provide even distribution of cold.

Compression: a crepe bandage provides a minimum level of compression. Tubular stockings (e.g. Tubigrip) are convenient and easy to apply but fail to give adequate compression.

Elevation: ideally the injured part should be elevated above the heart to help fluid drain away from the injury.

Further reading

Donnelly A E, Maughan R J, Whiting P H 190 Effects of ibuprofen in exercise induced muscle soreness and indices of muscle damage. British Journal of Sports Medicine 24:191–195

Kayne S, Reeves A 1994 Sports care and the pharmacist-an opportunity not to be missed. Pharmaceutical Journal 253:66–67

Knill-Jones R 1989 Survey of activity in Scottish sports medicine centres. Performance 1:4

Polisson R P 1986 Sports medicine for the internist. Medical Clinics of North America 70:469–489

Spiegel T M, Crues J V 1988 The painful shoulder: diagnosis and treatment. Primary Care 15:709–724

Stern S H 1988 Ankle and foot pain. Primary Care 15:809–826

West S G, Woodburn J 1995 Pain in the foot. British Medical Journal 310:860–864

Web sites

Society of Sports Therapists: www.society-of-sports-therapists.org

The Repetitive Strain Injury Association: rsi.websitehosting-services.co.uk/index.asp

Self-assessment questions

The following questions are intended to supplement the text. Two levels of questions are provided; multiple choice questions and case studies. The multiple choice questions are designed to test factual recall and the case studies allow knowledge to be applied to a practice setting.

Multiple choice questions

8.1. Which of the following is *not* used in topical formulations for musculoskeletal disorders?

a. nicotinates
b. hyaluronidase
c. choline
d. menthol
e. capsaicin

8.2. Which of the following statements is true of osteoarthritis?

a. Morning stiffness usually lasts less than 30 min
b. Pain is eased by movement
c. Pain is usually worst in the morning
d. Osteoarthritis commonly affects small joints
e. Inflammation is a key pathological finding

8.3. Which of the following patients would *not* be at increased risk of developing gastrointestinal problems when taking NSAIDs?

a. A patient taking Pariet
b. An elderly patient
c. A patient suffering from *H. pylori* infection
d. A patient with asthma
e. A patient with gastro-oesophageal reflux disease (GORD)

8.4. Vertebrae involved in sciatica are:

a. L1–L2
b. L2–L3
c. L3–L4
d. L4–L5
e. None of the above

8.5. Which ligament is most often damaged in a sprained ankle?

a. Cruciate ligament
b. Deltoid ligament
c. Medial collateral ligament
d. Posterior talofibular ligament
e. Anterior talofibular ligament

8.6. A strain is said to affect which structure?

a. Tendon
b. Ligament
c. Bursa
d. Muscle
e. Cartilage

8.7. From the following list, what common name is given to inflammation of the bursa?

a. Golfer's elbow
b. Student's elbow
c. Tennis elbow
d. Repetitive strain injury
e. Shin splints

8.8. In which of the following conditions does pain often wake the patient?

a. Rotator cuff syndrome
b. Frozen shoulder
c. Hamstring strain
d. Plantar fasciitis
e. Housemaid's knee

Questions 8.9 to 8.11 concern the following groups of people:

A. Runners/joggers
B. Footballers
C. Squash players
D. Occasional gardeners
E. Swimmers

Select, from A to E, which of the above groups of people are more prone to:

8.9 Anterior cruciate ligament damage

8.10. Plantar fasciitis

8.11. Tennis elbow

Questions 8.12 to 8.14 concern the following OTC medications:

A. Feldene P Gel
B. Codis tablets
C. Panadol tablets
D. Radian B cream
E. Voltarol emulgel

Select, from A to E, which of the above medicines

8.12. Can only be given to children older than 16

8.13. Has no evidence of efficacy

8.14. May cause constipation

Questions 8.15 to 8.17: for each of these questions *one* or *more* **of the responses is (are) correct. Decide which of the responses is (are) correct. Then choose:**

A. If a, b and c are correct
B. If a and b only are correct
C. If b and c only are correct
D. If a only is correct
E. If c only is correct

Directions summarised

A	B	C	D	E
a, b and c	a and b only	b and c only	a only	c only

8.15. Which of the following measures should be recommended to a patient who has just suffered an acute soft tissue injury?

   a. Heat and massage of the affected area
   b. Elevation of the affected area
   c. Compression of the affected area by means of an elastic bandage or support

8.16. Acute low back pain is characterised by:

   a. Insidious onset and progressively worsening pain
   b. Radiating pain toward the thoracic vertebrae
   c. Decreased mobility

8.17. Children under 12 with a soft tissue injury should be referred to the GP because:

   a. 'RICE' is only suitable for adults
   b. OTC medication is contraindicated
   c. More prone to greenstick fractures than adults

Questions 8.18 to 8.20: these questions consist of a statement in the left-hand column followed by a statement in the right-hand column. You need to:

● decide whether the first statement is true or false
● decide whether the second statement is true or false

Then choose:

A. If both statements are true and the second statement is a correct explanation of the first statement
B. If both statements are true but the second statement is *not* a correct explanation of the first statement
C. If the first statement is true but the second statement is false
D. If the first statement is false but the second statement is true
E. If both statements are false

Directions summarised

	First statement	Second statement	
A	True	True	Second explanation is a correct explanation of the first
B	True	True	Second statement is *not* a correct explanation of the first
C	True	False	
D	False	True	
E	False	False	

	First statement	*Second statement*
8.18.	Carpal tunnel syndrome causes hand numbness	Medial nerve impingement results in symptoms
8.19.	Low back pain with associated fever should be referred	Malignancy is the likely cause
8.20.	NSAIDs are the mainstay of systemic treatment for soft tissue injuries	They should be used for 7–10 days. If symptoms do not improve, referral is needed

Case study

CASE STUDY 8.1

Mrs AT is an overweight 65-year-old woman who comes to your community pharmacy to consult you regarding a musculoskeletal complaint.

a. Describe the signs and symptoms that can be associated with musculoskeletal conditions.

The following signs and symptoms can be associated with musculoskeletal pain:

- *Pain: need to know location, nature, severity and duration, whether it persists at rest, whether it restricts movement or prevents sleep.*
- *Stiffness: can occur in a joint as a result of inflammation or fluid accumulation or in muscles as a result of unaccustomed exercise or overuse.*
- *Inflammation: reaction of tissues to injury and results in redness, swelling, heat and pain, therefore can usually be seen as well as felt.*
- *Tenderness: soreness when affected part is touched or handled.*
- *Restricted movement: may be as a result of swelling (physical restriction) or limitation imposed by level of pain.*
- *Bruising: often develops later; might not be obvious in an acute presentation.*

You recommend a topical NSAID preparation to ease Mrs AT's symptoms until she is able to see her GP.

b. List the various NSAIDs available OTC to treat musculoskeletal conditions.

Ibuprofen, ketoprofen, piroxicam, felbinac, diclofenac.

c. What are the possible side-effects associated with their use and in what circumstances should you exercise caution when recommending them to patients.

Beware of GI disturbance. Dyspepsia, nausea and diarrhoea have been reported. Should be avoided in aspirin-sensitive asthmatics (reports of bronchospasm). Most manufacturers warn against use in pregnancy and breast-feeding.

Mrs AT's GP is concerned that she might have developed osteoarthritis in her knees and refers her to a hospital where the diagnosis is confirmed. Mrs AT is prescribed paracetamol to treat her pain. She asks you if there are any self-help measures she can employ, or OTC products she can buy, to reduce her discomfort and improve her mobility.

d. Detail the recommendations and counselling you would give her.

You would advise Mrs AT of the following:

- *Weight reduction: reduced strain on joints.*
- *Exercise: maintains muscle strength and increases joint stability. Also helpful in weight loss, combined with appropriate dietary restrictions. Swimming is very good as the weight of the body is supported by water, thus reducing strain on joints.*
- *Alternative remedies: glucosamine has been shown to be effective in reducing symptoms of osteoarthritis. However, many trials have involved small numbers, been poorly designed or failed to assess optimal dosing requirements.*
- *Physical aids: a variety of aids is available to use in the home, many via mail order. Her GP will be able to refer her to a physiotherapist or occupational therapist, if necessary.*

CASE STUDY 8.2

Mrs BB, a 69-year old woman, hobbles into your pharmacy, supported by her husband. She has just slipped off the pavement edge and believes she has sprained her ankle.

a. To ascertain if referral is necessary, describe the questions you would ask Mrs BB?

Find out exact nature of pain and its location. It is likely that the anterior talofibular ligament has been damaged. Symptoms that would warrant referral are severe pain in any bony prominence, if Mrs BB is unable to walk unsupported for at least four steps and marked swelling and bruising occurred straight after the fall. Mrs BB should be told

CASE STUDY 8.2

to go to casualty if these symptoms are present.

You decide that Mrs BB has indeed sprained her ankle but referral is unnecessary. You recommend RICE as the best course of action.

b. Explain the meaning of each of the letters in the mnemonic RICE and the rationale for each of its elements in the treatment of soft tissue injury.

RICE stands for the following:
R – Rest: allows immobilisation, which enhances healing and reduces blood flow to the affected tissue. Should ideally be for 24 to 48 h, but this is often difficult to achieve.
I – Ice: used to reduce blood flow to injured tissue and thus reduce bleeding and swelling. Cooling also has analgesic effect. The ice pack (a bag of frozen peas is ideal) should be separated from the skin by a thin towel or handkerchief to prevent skin damage. Should be continued for at least 30 min. Disadvantage is that it might encourage use of affected part too soon after injury.
C – Compression: allows haemostasis to occur, thereby reducing swelling. Supportive bandage can be applied. Elasticated supports also available.
E – Elevation: reduces blood flow and leakage of fluid into the extracellular spaces.

Mrs BB asks to purchase some OTC analgesia to alleviate her pain. Her regular medication is as follows:

● Bendroflumethiazide 2.5 mg od: used to treat hypertension. Taken for 5 years
● Fybogel sachets, 1 bd: taken for 4 years for constipation
● Lansoprazole 15mg od: maintenance therapy in treatment of GORD associated with hiatus hernia

c. Which OTC systemic analgesics would be most suitable for Mrs BB. Explain how you arrived at your choice and why you eliminated others.

Aspirin: can cause GI disturbance; Mrs BB has GORD, therefore aspirin is contraindicated.

Ibuprofen: NSAIDS can cause fluid retention and Mrs BB has hypertension. However, this is unlikely to be clinically significant, especially if only NSAIDs are recommended for only a few days. Like aspirin, ibuprofen can cause GI disturbances.
Codeine: Cannot be bought as a single agent. Combinations with aspirin need to be avoided. Paracetamol and codeine combinations could be offered but the codeine content is likely to cause constipation, which Mrs BB is already treated for. Therefore codeine is likely to worsen her already existing constipation. Finally, OTC analgesic combinations have been shown not to significantly reduce pain compared to monotherapy.
This leaves paracetamol as the medicine of choice for Mrs BB.

Mrs BB asks if she should also use a topical preparation on her ankle.

d. Describe the range of topical preparations available to treat soft tissue injuries and which would be suitable to recommend to Mrs BB, giving the reasons for your decision(s).

Rubefacients contain essential oils, salicylates, nicotinates, capsicum, camphor, terpentine and menthol. They provide warmth to the injury site, except menthol and camphor, which are cooling. These can be recommended to Mrs BB.
Ideally recommend a product with no salicylate because there is a low risk of systemic absorption and gastric irritation.
Topical NSAIDs: relatively low doses reach the bloodstream and there is therefore less risk of GI problems than with systemic NSAIDs. Use of topical NSAIDs are unlikely to cause side-effects if used for short periods of time (5 to 10 days) and could be given to Mrs BB even though she has GORD. However, she should be told that if she experiences any indigestion-type symptoms to stop using the product.

Answers to multiple choice questions

8.1 = c   8.2 = a   8.3 = d   8.4 = d   8.5 = e   8.6 = d   8.7 = b   8.8 = a   8.9 = b   8.10 = a,
8.11 = c   8.12 = b   8.13 = d   8.14 = b   8.15 = c   8.16 = e   8.17 = e   8.18 = a   8.19 = c   8.20 = b.

Paediatrics

Background

A number of conditions are encountered much more frequently in children than in the rest of the population. It is these conditions that this chapter focuses on. A small number of conditions that affect all age groups but are often associated with children are not included, for example middle ear infection. Such conditions are covered in other chapters and, where appropriate, will be cross-referenced to the relevant sections within the text.

History taking

In the majority of cases pharmacists will be heavily dependent on getting details about the child's problem from the parents or an adult responsible for the child's welfare. This presents both benefits and problems to the pharmacist. Parents will know when the child is not well and asking the parent about the child's general health will help to determine how poorly the child actually is. Additionally, a child who is running around and lively is unlikely to be acutely ill and referral to a GP is less likely. The major problem faced by all healthcare professionals is the difficulty in gaining an accurate history of the presenting complaint. This poses difficulties in assessing the quality and accuracy of the information, because children find it hard to articulate their symptoms. If a child can be asked questions, these often have to posed in either closed or leading formats to elicit information.

As a rule of thumb, any child who appears visibly ill should always be seen by the pharmacist and referral might well be needed, whereas children who are acting normally and appear generally well will normally not need to see the GP and can be managed by the pharmacist.

Head lice

Background

Humans act as hosts to three species of louse: *Pediculosis capitis* (head lice), *Pediculosis corporis* (body lice) and *Pediculosis pubis* (pubic lice). In this section only head lice are discussed.

Prevalence and epidemiology

Head lice rates are reported to be increasing. They affect all ages but are much more prevalent in children, especially girls (who tend to have longer hair). Head lice can occur at any time and do not show any seasonal variation. Most parents will have experienced a sibling who has had head lice, or received letters from school alerting parents to head lice infestation within the school.

Aetiology

Head lice can only be transmitted by head-to-head contact. Fleeting contact will be insufficient for lice to be transferred between heads. Once transmitted, lice begin to reproduce. The adult louse lives for approximately

1 month. Throughout this time the female louse lays several eggs at the base of hair shaft each night. Eggs hatch after 6–9 nine days, leaving the egg case attached to the hair shaft (known as a 'nit'). In the course of maturing to adulthood, the young louse – the nymph – undergoes three moults. Shortly after maturing, the female louse is sexually mature and able to mate.

Arriving at a differential diagnosis

Most parents will diagnose head lice themselves or be concerned that their child has head lice because of a recent local outbreak at school. Occasionally, parents will also want to buy products to prevent their child contracting head lice. It is the role of the pharmacist to confirm self-diagnosis and stop inappropriate sales of products. It should also be remembered that an itching scalp in children is not always due to head lice and other causes should be eliminated. Asking a number of symptom-specific questions should enable a diagnosis of head lice to be easily made (Table 9.1).

Clinical features of head lice

Unless live lice have been found, most patients will present with scalp itching. Itching is caused due to an allergic response of the scalp to the saliva of the lice and can take weeks to develop. However, only a third of patients experience itching.

Conditions to eliminate

Dandruff

Dandruff can cause irritation and itching of the scalp. However, the scalp should be dry and flaky. Skin debris might also be visible on the clothing.

Seborrhoeic dermatitis

Typically, seborrhoeic dermatitis will affect areas other than the scalp, most notably the face and napkin area. If only scalp involvement is present then the child might complain of severe and persistent dandruff. In infants the person will have large yellow scales and crusts of the scalp (cradle cap).

 TRIGGER POINTS indicative of referral: Head lice

- Parents who find cost of treatment prohibitive

Evidence base for over-the-counter medication

Insecticides are the mainstay of lice eradication. In the UK, malathion (organophosphate), permethrin and phenothrin (pyrethroids) are available OTC.

Many trials have investigated the efficacy of malathion and pyrethroids. However, poor trial design has made interpretation of their results difficult. In 1995 a review of 28 trials by Vander Stichele et al concluded that only permethrin has proven efficacy in a clinical setting, despite all three classes of insecticide demonstrating in vitro activity. However, the review was criticised and subsequently shown to be weak in certain areas of inclusion and exclusion criteria. A further review identified 70 trials, only three of which met the rigorous inclusion criteria. The authors concluded that malathion and permethrin were effective, with high cure rates, but there was insufficient evidence to demonstrate if one was more efficacious than the other.

Unfortunately, these trials were conducted in areas with no prior exposure to the insecticides and therefore

 Table 9.1
Specific questions to ask the patient: Head lice

Question	Relevance
Have live lice been seen	• The presence of live lice is diagnostic • Pharmacists can advise patients on how best to check for infection. The easiest detection method is to comb damp or wet hair forward using a fine metal-toothed comb over a pale or white piece of paper. If live lice are present then one or more will be visible on the paper • Proprietary products are available and will remove even the smallest of newly hatched nymphs
Empty egg shells (nits)	• This does not constitute evidence of current infection. This is a common misconception held by the general public and the pharmacist must ensure that parents seeking treatment have observed live lice • Egg shells are not removed by using insecticides. Patients need to be reassured that the presence of egg shells does not mean treatment failure
Presence of itching	• Itching is not always present with head lice. Inspection of the scalp should be made to check for signs of dandruff, psoriasis or seborrhoeic dermatitis

lice were fully susceptible to their effects. In the UK, evidence of developing resistance to insecticides is well recognised. To combat resistance, different strategies have been adopted. Until recently, most health authorities advocated a rotational policy on a biannual or triennial basis. This approach was abandoned as insecticides became more readily available and rotation became unenforceable. The current recommendation is a mosaic model whereby the same product is used for a course of treatment (two applications 7 days apart). If this fails, another product from a different class should be tried.

Because of the emerging problem of resistance, attention has focused on non-drug treatment options. The 'bug busting method' (wet combing) has received much attention although evidence of its effectiveness is only anecdotal. Even the Department of Health has supported the use of this method and in some areas the 'bug busting' programme is advocated rather than the use of insecticides.

Bug busting involves combing wet hair with a fine toothed comb every 3–4 days for 2 weeks. This removes all the lice as they hatch and ensures that none reach maturity and lay the next generation of eggs. A Cochrane review of insecticidal treatments published in 2000 called for this method to be evaluated to assess its effectiveness.

In August 2000 the results of such a study were published. The results showed that bug busting had a cure rate of 38% compared with 78% for malathion. Children were nearly three times as likely still to have head lice after bug busting than those who used malathion, even in a geographical location known to have intermediate insecticidal resistance. The authors concluded that bug busting was therefore not an appropriate first-line treatment for the eradication of head lice.

Other non-insecticidal methods of eradication are also promoted. These include herbal remedies such as tea tree oil. No evidence exists on the effectiveness of tea tree oil and it should not be recommended until such time that data supports its use.

Practical prescribing and product selection

Prescribing information relating to medicines for head lice reviewed in the section 'Evidence base for over-the-counter medication' is discussed and summarised in Table 9.2; useful tips relating to patients presenting with head lice are given in Hints and Tips Box 9.1.

All products can be used on children older than 6 months. When applying the products, particular attention should be paid to the areas behind the ears and at the

Table 9.2
Practical prescribing: Summary of head lice medicines

Medicine	Use in children	Likely side-effects	Drug interactions of note	Patients in whom care should be exercised	Pregnancy
Permethrin Phenothrin Malathion	> 6 months	Irritation of scalp (rare)	None	Asthmatics and patients with scalp conditions should avoid alcohol-based products	OK

HINTS AND TIPS BOX 9.1: HEAD LICE

Who to treat?	Different people advocate different solutions. Some say treat only those with live lice present, whereas others say that all close family contacts should be treated. In an ideal situation only patients with live lice would be treated and all close contacts, usually family members, would check regularly for lice. This requires high levels of motivation. A more pragmatic approach is to treat all family members if the pharmacist thinks that the above regime would not be followed
Products for prevention	Prevention of lice using insecticides is not advocated and the patient should be counselled on when treatment is required
Lotion, liquid or shampoo?	Do not recommend shampoos. The concentration of insecticide will be too low to ensure eradication because the shampoo is diluted by water. In addition, they have a much shorter contact time with the hair and scalp compared to lotions and liquids A liquid product is the most suitable formulation for very young children and asthmatics
Treatment failure	Although emergence of resistance is an established fact, it should be remembered that inappropriate usage and incorrect application would lead also to treatment failure. In theory, all lice and eggs are killed on a single application. However, studies suggest that some eggs survive, therefore a further application 7 days later is now recommended

nape of the neck, as these areas are where lice are most often found.

Permethrin (Lyclear Creme Rinse)

Before application the hair should be washed with a mild shampoo and towelled dry. Enough Lyclear should be applied to the hair to ensure the hair and scalp is thoroughly saturated. It should be left on the hair for 10 min before rinsing the hair thoroughly with water. One bottle is sufficient for shoulder length hair of average thickness. It might rarely cause scalp reddening and irritation.

Phenothrin (Full Marks)

Full Marks is available as liquid, lotion or mousse. Liquids and lotions are rubbed into the scalp until all the hair and scalp is thoroughly moistened and then allowed to dry naturally. They should be applied as close to the base of the hair and scalp as possible. Twelve hours later the hair should be shampooed in the normal way. Most parents find it easier and more convenient to apply the solution before bedtime and leave on overnight. The mousse is applied to dry hair at several points on the scalp and massaged into the scalp, ensuring no part of the scalp is left uncovered. After 30 minutes the hair can be washed with normal shampoo.

Malathion (e.g. Derbac-M, Prioderm, Quellada-M, Suleo-M)

Malathion is available as liquid, lotion or shampoo. Liquids and lotions are applied in exactly the same manner as Full Marks products.

Shampoos, if used, should be applied to wet hair and left on for 5 min before rinsing. After rinsing the process should be repeated. Two further treatment courses then have to be applied at 3-day intervals.

Two products (Prioderm lotion and Suleo-M) have an alcoholic base and should be avoided in asthmatics and small children because they might precipitate broncho-spasm. Like permethrin, skin irritation has been reported on application but is rare.

Further reading
[Anonymous] 1998 Treating head louse infections. Drug and Therapeutics Bulletin 36:45–46
Burgess I F 1998 Head lice-developing a practical approach. The Practitioner 242:126–129
Burgess I F, Brown C M, Peock S et al 1995 Head lice resistant to pyrethroid insecticides in Britain. British Medical Journal 311:752
Dodd C S 2000 Interventions for treating headlice (Cochrane Review). In: The Cochrane Library, Issue 4. Update Software, Oxford
Ibarra J 1994 Coping with head lice in the 1990s. Primary Health Care 4:19–21

Roberts R J, Casey D, Morgan D A, Petrovic M 2000 Comparison of wet combing with malathion for treatment of head lice in the UK: a pragmatic randomised controlled trial. Lancet 356:540–544
Vander Stichele R H, Dezeure E M, Bogaert M G 1995 Systematic review of clinical efficacy of topical treatments for head lice. British Medical Journal 311:604–608
Vermaak Z 1996 Model for the control of pediculus humanus capitis. Public Health 110:283–288

Web sites
Community Hygiene Concern: www.chc.org/bugbusting/
Pediculosis.com: www.pediculosis.com/products.html

Threadworm (*Enterobius vermicularis*)

Background

Worm infections are extremely common both in the developed and developing world. In the UK the most common worm infection is threadworm, which is a cause of inconvenience and embarrassment rather than morbidity. However, a social stigma surrounds the diagnosis of threadworm, with many patients believing that infection implies a lack of hygiene. This belief is unfounded and infection occurs in all social strata. The patient might benefit from reassurance from the pharmacist, explaining that the condition is very common and is nothing to be ashamed or embarrassed about.

Prevalence and epidemiology

Threadworm is the most common helminth infection throughout temperate and developed countries. This is primarily due to threadworm transmission not being waterborne, unlike other helminth infections. Threadworm prevalence is difficult to establish due to the high number of people who self medicate or are asymptomatic. However, UK prevalence rates have been estimated at 20% in the community, rising to 65% in institutionalised settings. Higher prevalence rates have been observed in developing countries, with some authors suggesting prevalence can reach 100% in certain populations.

Aetiology

Eggs are transmitted to the human host primarily by the faecal–oral route (autoinfection) but also by retroinfection and inhalation. Faecal–oral transmission involves eggs lodging under fingernails, which are then ingested by finger sucking after anal contact. Retroinfection occurs when larvae hatch on the anal mucosa and migrate back into the sigmoid colon. Finally, threadworm eggs are highly resistant to environmental factors and can easily be transferred to clothing, bed linen and inanimate objects (e.g. toys), resulting in dust-borne infections. Once eggs are ingested, duodenal fluid breaks them down and releases larvae, which migrate into the small and large intestines. After mating, the female migrates to the anus, usually at night, where eggs are laid on the perianal skin folds, after which the female dies. Once laid, the eggs are infective almost immediately. Transmission back into the gut can then take place again via one of three mechanisms outlined above and so the cycle is perpetuated.

Arriving at a differential diagnosis

Threadworm diagnosis should be one of the more simple conditions to diagnose. Patients who are not asymptomatic generally present with very specific symptoms.

Clinical features of threadworm

Night-time perianal itching is the classic presentation. However, patients might experience symptoms ranging from a local 'tickling' sensation to acute pain. Any child with night-time perianal itching is almost certain to have threadworm. Itching can lead to sleep disturbances resulting in irritability and tiredness the next day. Diagnosis can be confirmed by observing threadworm on the stool, although they are not always visible.

Complicating factors such as excoriation and secondary bacterial infection of the perianal skin can occur due to persistent scratching. The parent should be asked if the perianal skin is broken or weeping.

Conditions to eliminate

Other worm infections

Roundworm and tapeworm infections are encountered occasionally. However, these infections are usually contracted by adults when visiting poor and developing countries.

Contact irritant dermatitis

Occasionally, dermatitis can cause perianal itching especially in adults. If there is no recent family history of threadworm or there is no visible sign of threadworm on the faeces then dermatitis is possible.

TRIGGER POINTS indicative of referral:
Threadworm

- Medication failure
- Secondary infection of perianal skin due to scratching

Evidence base for over-the-counter medication

Mebendazole and piperazine are available OTC for the treatment of threadworm. There is a large body of evidence to support the effectiveness of mebendazole in roundworm infections but for other worm infections, including threadworm, there is less evidence to show consistently high cure rates. For threadworm, cure rates between 60 and 82% for single-dose treatment of mebendazole have been reported.

Piperazine appears to have less evidence supporting its effectiveness than mebendazole. One study has compared piperazine against mebendazole and found mebendazole to have a higher cure rate than piperazine; although the number of patients in the trial was low.

The difference in cure rates might be, in part, due to their respective mechanism of action. Mebendazole inhibits the worm's uptake of glucose, thus killing them, whereas piperazine paralyses the worm. To optimise worm clearance from the gut one piperazine formulation also contains senna. However, if paralysis wears off the worm might be able to migrate back into the colon and thus treatment would fail.

Practical prescribing and product selection

Prescribing information relating to medicines for threadworm reviewed in the section 'Evidence base for over-the-counter medication' is discussed and summarised in Table 9.3; useful tips relating to patients presenting with threadworm are given in Hints and Tips Box 9.2.

Treatment should ideally be given to all family members and not only the patient with symptoms, as it is likely that other family members will have been infected even though they might not show signs of clinical infection. A repeated dose 14 days later is often recommended to ensure worms maturing from ova at the time of the first dose are also eradicated.

It is also worth mentioning at this time that mebendazole and piperazine should be avoided in pregnancy because fetal malformations have been reported. Patients should be advised to practise hygiene measures. If treatment is absolutely essential, piperazine has been used, although this should not be in the first trimester.

Mebendazole (e.g. Ovex, Pripsen Mebendazole)

The dose for adults and children over 2 is a single tablet. Young children might prefer to chew the tablet and it has been formulated to taste of orange. It has been reported to cause abdominal pain, diarrhoea and rash. It does interact with cimetidine, increasing mebendazole plasma levels but this is of little clinical consequence. However, phenytoin and carbamazepine decrease mebendazole plasma levels and the dose of mebendazole may need to be increased.

Table 9.3
Practical Prescribing: Summary of Medicines for Threadworm

Medicine	Use in children	Likely side-effects	Drug interactions of note	Patients in whom care should be exercised	Pregnancy
Mebendazole	> 2 years	Abdominal pain, rash	Phenytoin and carbamazepine	None	Avoid
Piperazine	> 3 months	Diarrhoea, rash	None	None	

HINTS AND TIPS BOX 9.2: THREADWORM

Hygiene measures	Complementary to drug treatment is the need for strict personal hygiene
	Nails should be kept short and clean
	Careful washing and nail scrubbing prior to meals and after each visit to the toilet is essential to prevent autoinfection
	Bed linen should be washed frequently, ideally every day, although this might not be practical
	Underwear should be worn underneath night clothes to prevent scratching

Piperazine (e.g. Pripsen Piperazine Phosphate Powder or citrate elixir)

Piperazine is available as either sachets or elixir, with the sachets also containing senna. Both can be given to children from 1 year of age. Children over 6 should take the contents of one full sachet whereas children aged between 1 and 6 should be given one level 5 mL spoonful of the sachet contents. Children over 3 months old should take half a level 5 mL spoonful. The dose should be given in the morning (for adults the dose is recommended to be taken at night).

The elixir is much less convenient for patients to take as the manufacturers recommend that the dose has to be given for seven consecutive days.

A number of side-effects have been reported with piperazine but all are rare and generally are of GI origin such as diarrhoea or allergic reactions, for example rash.

Further reading

Albonico M, Smith P G, Hall A et al 1994 A randomized controlled trial comparing mebendazole and albendazole against ascaris, trichuris and hookworm Infections. Transactions of the Royal Society of Tropical Medicine and Hygiene 88:585–589

Cook G C 1990 Threadworm infection and its treatment. Pharmaceutical Journal 254:765–767

Rafi S, Memon A, Billo A G 1997 Efficacy and safety of mebendazole in children with worm infestation. Journal of the Pakistan Medical Association 47:140–141

Russell L J 1991 The pinworm, Enterobius vermicularis. Primary Care 18:13–24

Sorensen E, Ismail M, Amarasinghe D K et al 1996 The efficacy of three anthelmintic drugs given in a single dose. Ceylon Medical Journal 41:42–45

Zaman V 1987 Other gut nematodes. In: Weatherall D J, Ledingham J G G, Warrell D A, eds Oxford textbook of medicine. Oxford University Press, Oxford

Web sites

Division of parasitic diseases: www.cdc.gov/ncidod/dpd/parasites/pinworm/default.htm

Colic

Background

There is no universally agreed definition of colic. A widely used definition is that proposed by Wessel et al (1954) that has come to be known as the 'rule of threes'. Wessel proposed that an infant could be considered to have colic if it cries for more than 3 hours a day for more than 3 days a week for more than 3 weeks.

Prevalence and epidemiology

The prevalence of colic is unknown, although clinical practice and sales of products for colic would suggest that colic-like symptoms are common.

Aetiology

The cause of colic is poorly understood. A number of theories have been put forward, from an immature digestive system to problems in under- or overfeeding. Pain and crying in an infant might be due to excessive wind caused by air swallowing during crying or feeding. If the infant is bottle fed this is almost always due to the teat hole being too small. If the infant is breast fed then air swallowing can be due to sucking too long on the breast or sucking on an empty breast.

Arriving at a differential diagnosis

It is difficult to determine if the baby is considered to have colic or is just crying excessively, as the diagnosis of the condition depends on qualitative descriptions. However, the term 'colic' is often wrongly applied to any infant who cries more than usual. The definition by Wessel has its limitations because it is arbitrary and few parents are willing to wait 3 weeks to see if the infant meets the criteria for colic. As a result, the third criterion is usually dropped in the clinical setting. Asking a number of symptom-specific questions should enable a diagnosis of colic to be made Table 9.4.

Clinical features of colic

Besides obvious crying, the infant might show signs of abdominal pain, having a rigid abdomen with the legs drawn up towards the chest. Fists may be clenched and the infant resists acts of comfort and cuddling. Pain might be mild, merely causing the child to be restless in the evenings or severe, resulting in rhythmical screaming attacks lasting a few minutes at a time, alternating with equally long quiet periods in which the child almost goes to sleep, before another attack starts. Attacks appear to be more common in the early evening, giving rise to the name 6.00 p.m. colic.

Conditions to eliminate

Acute infection

Colic and acute infections of the ear or urinary tract can present with almost identical symptoms. However, in acute infection the child should have no previous history of excessive crying and have signs of systemic infection such as fever.

Intolerance to cow's milk protein

Colicky pain in infants is sometimes due to intolerance to cow's milk protein. This is far less common than generally believed but should be considered if the infant is failing to thrive.

TRIGGER POINTS indicative of referral: Colic

- Infants that are failing to put on weight
- Medication failure
- Overanxious parents

Evidence base for over-the-counter medication

Dimethicone (simethicone) is reported to have anti-foaming properties, reducing surface tension and allowing easier elimination of gas from the gut by passing flatus or belching. It is widely used yet no evidence of its efficacy exists. It might be a useful placebo for anxious and often tired and irritable parents who want to give their baby some form of medication.

Practical prescribing and product selection

Prescribing information relating to dimethicone is discussed and summarised in Table 9.5: useful tips relating to colic are given in Hints and Tips Box 9.3.

Dimethicone (e.g. Infacol, Dentinox, Woodward's Colic Drops)

Dimethicone is pharmacologically inert, it has no side-effects, drug interactions or precautions in its use and can therefore be safely prescribed to all children. It is administered with or just after each feed. All products

Table 9.4
Specific questions to ask the patient: Colic

Question	Relevance
Duration of crying	● If colic is suspected the baby will usually cry for more than 3 h day for more than 3 days per week
History of crying	● Excessive crying is not isolated and will have been present for some time. Acute infections are normally sudden in onset and the baby will not exhibit a long-standing history of excessive crying

Table 9.5
Practical prescribing: Summary of medicines for colic

Medicine	Use in children	Likely side-effects	Drug interactions of note	Patients in whom care should be exercised	Pregnancy
Dimethicone	Infant upwards	None	None	None	Not applicable

HINTS AND TIPS BOX 9.3: COLIC

Review feeding technique	Before recommending a product it is worth checking feeding technique. Underfeeding the baby can result in excessive sucking resulting in air being swallowed leading to colic-like symptoms. Additionally, the teat size of the bottle should be checked. When the bottle is turned upside down the milk should drop slowly from the bottle

contain different strengths of dimethicone, however the dose administered to the child is almost equivalent, for example Infacol 0.5 to 1 mL (20 to 40 mg), Dentinox 2.5 mL (21 mg) and Woodward's Colic Drops 0.3 to 0.6 mL (20 to 40 mg).

Further reading
Barr R G, Lessard J 2001 Excessive crying. In: Bergman A B, ed. 20 common problems in paediatrics. McGraw-Hill, New York

Wessel M A, Cobb J C, Jackson E B et al 1954 Paroxysmal fussing in infancy, sometimes called 'colic'. Pediatrics 14:421–434

Web sites
General site on colic: www.colichelp.com/

Atopic dermatitis

Background

Atopic dermatitis is an allergic skin condition that mainly affects infants and young children. The vast majority of patients will 'grow out' of the condition by their early teens. However in a small number of patients in whom atopic dermatitis persists into adulthood the condition becomes chronic. Generalised dry skin with **lichenification** at the elbow and knee is common and patients have a predispositon to irritant contact dermatitis.

Prevalence and epidemiology

The prevalence of atopic dermatitis is unclear. It has been reported to affect anything between 1 and 15% of people at some time during their lifetime. The condition usually presents in infants aged between 2 and 6 months but it can also occur in older children. Upwards of 60% of children will have onset within the first year, rising to 80% within the first 5 years. Although the prevalence is unclear, it has been shown that the incidence of atopic dermatitis is rising.

Aetiology

Atopic dermatitis has a strong genetic component, with most patients having a positive family history of one or more parents suffering from asthma, eczema or hayfever. The chance of a sibling having atopic dermatitis if one parent has the condition is 20%, rising to 50% if both parents are affected. In addition a number of environmental factors have been implicated in the development or worsening of the condition and include certain foods (e.g. diary products), stress and heat or cold.

Arriving at a differential diagnosis

To help with diagnosis, criteria-based protocols are available, for example those produced by the *British Journal of Dermatology*, which state that atopic dermatitis can be diagnosed as an itchy skin (Fig. 9.1) plus three or more of the following:

- onset before age of 2 years (Fig. 9.2)
- history of dry skin
- history of eczema in the skin creases (and also the cheeks in children under 10 years)
- visible flexural eczema (inside elbows, behind knees or involvement of the cheeks/forehead and outer limbs in children under 4 years; Fig. 9.3)
- personal history of other atopic disease.

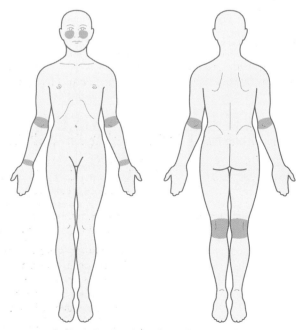

Fig. 9.1 Typical distribution of atopic dermatitis

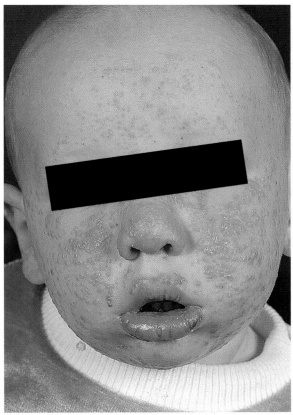

Fig. 9.2 Atopic dermatitis in an infant. Reproduced from *Dermatology: An Illustrated Colour Text* by D Gawkrodger, 2002, Mosby, with permission

Asking a number of symptom-specific questions should enable a diagnosis of atopic dermatitis to be made (Table 9.6).

Clinical features of atopic dermatitis

A typical presentation of a child with atopic dermatitis is an irritable, scratching child with dermatitis of varying

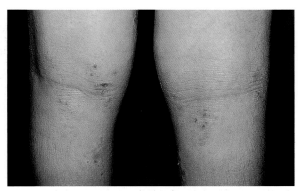

Fig. 9.3 Atopic dermatitis in the popliteal fossa (bend of the knee). Reproduced from *Dermatology: An Illustrated Colour Text* by D Gawkrodger, 2002, Mosby, with permission

severity. The child might have had the symptoms for some time and the parent has often already tried some form of cream to help control the itch and rash. Scratching can lead to broken skin, which then can become infected.

Conditions to eliminate

Seborrhoeic dermatitis

Seborrhoeic dermatitis in infants typically occurs in the first 6 months. Itching is generally not present and the condition usually spontaneously resolves after a few weeks and seldom recurs. It usually affects the scalp, face and napkin area. Large yellow scales and crusts often appear on the scalp and are often referred to as 'cradle cap'.

Psoriasis

Psoriasis can be mistaken for atopic dermatitis because the rash is **erythematous** and can occur on parts of the body such as the scalp, elbows and knees, which is a

Table 9.6
Specific questions to ask the patient: Atopic dermatitis

Question	Relevance
Is itching present	● Atopic dermatitis is classically associated with intense itching ● Psoriasis and seborrhoeic dermatitis are not usually associated with itching
Distribution of rash	● Varies according to age (Fig. 9.1) but in infants the nappy area is not involved; this is a useful distinction between atopic dermatitis and seborrhoeic dermatitis
Age of child	● Presentation varies with age ● *Babies:* facial involvement (the cheeks) is common along with patchy red scaly lesions on the wrists and hands (Fig. 9.2) ● *Toddlers and older children:* the antecubital (in front or at the bend of the elbow), popliteal fossae (behind the knee) and ankles are more commonly involved (Fig. 9.3)
Family history of atopy	● If a parent has eczema, hayfever or asthma then the likelihood of atopic dermatitis rises

common location for atopic dermatitis in older children. However, the rash is raised, has well defined boundaries with a silvery-white scaly appearance; it rarely itches.

Herpes simplex complications

Sufferers from atopic dermatitis are susceptible to the herpes simplex virus. If herpes is suspected the patient should be referred quickly for aciclovir. For further information on herpes simplex the reader is referred to page 177.

TRIGGER POINTS indicative of referral: Atopic dermatitis

- Children with widespread or severe dermatitis
- Medication failure
- Presence of secondary infection (weeping and crusting lesions)

Evidence base for over-the-counter medication

The mainstay of treatment for atopic dermatitis consists of avoiding potential irritants, managing dry skin, controlling itching using systemic antihistamines and topical corticosteroids to treat flare ups. The latter option is not available OTC because license restrictions mean that children only over the age of 10 can be given OTC corticosteroids.

The approach to the management of atopic dermatitis does not appear to be based on evidence of efficacy drawn from clinical trials but on clinical experience and common sense.

Avoiding irritants

The use of highly perfumed soaps and detergents should be discouraged and replaced with soap substitutes (e.g.

Alpha Keri, Neutrogena, Dove). Patients should be told to have luke warm not hot baths because in some patients hot water can aggravate the problem. In addition, a bath additive should be used (e.g. Balneum, Oilatum, Emulsiderm) to help hydration of the skin.

Emollients

No published literature appears to have addressed whether one emollient is superior to another in treating atopic dermatitis. Patients might have to try several emollients before finding one that is most effective for their skin.

Antihistamines

There appears to be no clinical trial data on the use of sedative antihistamine for reducing pruritus in atopic dermatitis, however they are often prescribed to children to help with itching. Additionally, they can also help prevent night-time scratching.

Corticosteroids

A substantial body of evidence exists for corticosteroids in controlling all types of dermatitis, including atopic dermatitis. If the symptoms warrant corticosteroid therapy then the patient needs to be referred to the GP. Usually mild steroids such as hydrocortisone (1% to 2.5%), preferably in an ointment base should be prescribed for twice daily administration.

Practical prescribing and product selection

Prescribing information relating to medicines for atopic dermatitis reviewed in the section 'Evidence base for over-the-counter medication' is discussed and summarised in Table 9.7; useful information regarding emollients containing lanolin is given in Hints and Tips Box 9.4.

Table 9.7
Practical prescribing: Summary of medicines for atopic dermatitis

Medicine	Use in children	Likely side-effects	Drug interactions of note	Patients in whom care should be exercised	Pregnancy
Emollients	Birth onwards	None	None	None	Not applicable
Antihistamines					
Brompheniramine	mg/kg doses for children up to the age of 3	Sedation	Increased sedation with opioid analgesics, anxiolytics, hypnotics and antidepressants. However, it is unlikely a child will be taking such medicines	None	Not applicable
Chlorphenamine	> 1 year				
Clemastine	> 1 year				
Cyproheptadine	> 2 years				
Hydroxyzine	> 6 months				
Promethazine	> 2 years				

HINTS AND TIPS BOX 9.4: DERMATITIS

Lanolin-containing emollients	Emollients that contain lanolin, e.g. Keri Lotion and E45, should be avoided or patch tested first because they are known to cause sensitisation

Emollients

There is a plethora of emollient products on the market and which one a patient uses will be dictated by patient response and acceptability. All emollients should be regularly and liberally applied, with no upper limit on how often they can be used. All are chemically inert and therefore can be safely used from birth upwards. For a summary of emollient products see Table 7.25 (page 184).

Sedating antihistamines

Although no sedating antihistamine products, except hydroxyzine, have a specific product licence for the treatment of pruritus, they are frequently prescribed by GPs and could be given OTC. However, it must be remembered that if recommended then the person concerned is acting outside the product licence and will be therefore liable for any clinical consequence associated with the use of the product. The doses that can be given for the various sedating antihistamines are listed below.

Brompheniramine (Dimotane)

For children up to the age of 3 the dose should be based on a milligram per kilogram basis (0.4 to 1.0 mg/kg) in four divided doses. For older children, aged between 3 and 6 years, the dose is 5 mL (2 mg) and for those over 6 years it is 5 to 10 mL (2 to 4 mg) three or four times a day.

Chlorphenamine (Piriton)

Chlorphenamine can be given from the age of 1 year. Children up to the age 2 should take 2.5 mL of syrup (1 mg) twice a day. For children aged between 2 and 5 the dose is 2.5 mL (1 mg) three or four times a day and those over the age of 6 should take 5 mL (2 mg) three or four times a day.

Clemastine (Tavegil)

Clemastine is taken twice a day by children of all ages. Those aged between 1 and 3 should take 2.5–5 mL (250 to 500 µg), children aged between 3 and 6 should take 5 mL (500 µg) and for those aged over 6 the dose is 5 to 10 mL (500 µg to 1 mg).

Cyproheptadine (Periactin)

Children between 2 and 6 should take 2 mg (half a tablet) and for children over 7 the dose is 4 mg (one tablet) two or three times a day.

Hydroxyzine (Atarax, Ucerax)

Hydroxyzine is the medicine most commonly prescribed by GPs, probably because it has a license for pruritus and can be given from 6 months of age. Children up to the age of 6 should take 5 to 15 mg (2.5 to 7.5 mL of Ucerax liquid, or one to one-and-a-half Atarax 10 mg tablets) daily. For children over the age of 6 the dose is 15 to 25 mg daily.

Promethazine (Phenergan)

Children between 2 and 5 years should take 5 to 15 mg (5 to 15 mL) daily in one to two divided doses. For those aged over 5 the dose is 10 to 25 mg daily in one to two divided doses.

Further reading

Agarwal A, Berth-Jones J 1999 Guide to the treatment of atopic eczema 1999. The Prescriber 10:31–45
Clark C, Hoare C 2001 Making the most of emollients. Pharmaceutical Journal 266:227–229
Hanifin J M 1991 Atopic dermatitis in infants and children. Pediatric Clinics of North America 38:763–789

Web sites

National Eczema Society: www.eczema.org/
General dermatology site: www.dermatologist.co.uk/index.html

Fever

Background

Normal oral temperature is 37°C (98.6°F), plus or minus 1°C, although rectal temperature is about 0.5°C higher and underarm temperature 0.5°C lower than oral temperature. Ideally, rectal temperature should be taken because it gives the most reliable results, but this method is probably the least convenient and acceptable. Using forehead strip thermometers is popular because it is easy, but it should be discouraged because it is not very precise. Therefore, for pragmatic purposes, an oral or underarm temperature should be conducted.

Prevalence and epidemiology

Fever is a common symptom of many conditions and in children viral and bacterial causes are most commonly implicated. Therefore fever is extremely common and its prevalence and epidemiology within the population are determined by those conditions.

Aetiology

Body temperature is regulated closely because temperature changes can significantly alter cellular functions and, in extreme cases, lead to death. Thermoregulation is a balance between heat production and heat loss. Cellular metabolism produces heat and this means that energy – in the form of heat – is produced continually by the body. This heat production is lost through the skin by radiation, evaporation, conduction and convection. The thermoregulation centre located in the hypothalamus controls the whole process. When body temperature reaches its 'set point' (approximately 37°C), mechanisms to lose or conserve heat are activated. When a person suffers from a fever this suggests that there is some defect in the temperature regulating control system. In fact, the system is functioning normally but with an adjusted higher 'set point'. This process is complex and involves the production of pyrogens (fever-causing substances) that alter the set point.

Arriving at a differential diagnosis

The parent, in nearly every instance, will diagnose fever in the child. This is usually a subjective perception by the parent that the child feels warm or is off colour. The importance of the parent's perception should not be underestimated or dismissed if the child's temperature has not been taken. Many healthcare professionals often place too much value on an empirical figure when in many instances the look of the child is more important than the height of the fever. Nearly all cases of fever will be a result of either a bacterial or viral infection. Asking a number of symptom-specific questions should enable the pharmacist to treat or refer the child with fever (Table 9.8).

Clinical features of fever

A child with fever will generally be irritable, off his or her food and seek greater parental attention than usual. Depending on the cause of fever, the child might exhibit other symptoms such as cold, cough, sore throat and earache.

Conditions to eliminate

Upper respiratory tract infections

It is rare for upper respiratory tract infections to present with fever alone. Cough, cold or sore throat is usually present. Treatment can be offered and referral is generally not needed unless secondary bacterial infection is suspected; earache symptoms might suggest this.

Roseola infantum (sixth disease)

Roseola infantum is probably caused by a neurodermotropic virus and is most prevalent in children under 1 year of age. Onset is with a sudden high fever (40°C) that usually subsides by the third or fourth day once the rash, which blanches when pressed, appears on the trunk and limbs. The condition is self-limiting and referral is not usually necessary.

Glandular fever

Most commonly seen in young adults rather than children but any patient who has a long-standing history of fatigue and a low fever (< 38.5°C) should be referred for further evaluation.

Urinary tract infection

One of the most common causes of fever in children is urinary tract infection. Often the child will present only with fever and no other symptoms will be present. Referral is needed.

Table 9.8
Specific questions to ask the patient: Fever

Question	Relevance
How old is the child	● Children under 3 months should be referred automatically because diagnosis can be very difficult and serious complications can arise
How poorly is the child	● The parent will know how poorly the child is relative to normal behaviour. A child might have a high temperature but be relatively normal whereas a child with a mild temperature might be quite poorly
Associated symptoms	● Viral upper respiratory tract infections are usually accompanied by one or more symptoms including cough, cold or sore throat ● Glandular fever is usually accompanied by fatigue and lymph node enlargement (usually teenagers) ● If no other symptoms are present fever suggests a bacterial infection, often a urinary tract infection

Medicine-induced fever

A number of medicines can elevate body temperature and should be considered if no other cause can be determined. Penicillins, cephalosporins, macrolides, tricyclic antidepressants, anticonvulsants and anti-inflammatory medicines, when associated with hypersensitivity, have all been associated with increasing temperature.

Meningitis

Meningitis can present with fever. However, there will be other symptoms present such as severe headache, photophobia, lethargy, drowsiness and neck stiffness. A non-blanching petechial rash might also be present as the condition progresses.

 TRIGGER POINTS indicative of referral: Fever

- Any feverish child under 3 months old
- Fever accompanied with no other symptoms
- If the patient has suffered any febrile convulsion
- Purpuric rash
- Stiff neck

Evidence base for over-the-counter medication

Paracetamol and ibuprofen have proven efficacy as antipyretics and either can be used to reduce temperature. However, there is a lack of evidence to show that combinations of both or alternating paracetamol and ibuprofen are better than using a single agent.

Practical prescribing and product selection

Prescribing information relating to medicines for fever reviewed in the section 'Evidence base for over-the-counter medication' is discussed and summarised in Table 9.9; useful tips relating to patients presenting with fever are given in Hints and Tips Box 9.5.

Paracetamol (e.g. Calpol, Disprol, Medinol)

Paracetamol is the most widely used antipyretic. It is available as liquid, soluble tablets, sachets and melt tabs, although the most frequently purchased formulation is liquid. In addition, paracetamol antihistamine combination (Medised Infant, Tixyplus (diphenhydramine) and Medised Suspension (promethazine)) is available. Children should be given paracetamol every 4 to 6 h, with a maximum of four doses in 24 h. Children between 3 months and 1 year of age should take 60 to 120 mg (2.5 to 5 mL of the paediatric version), in those aged between 1 and 5 years the dose is 120 to 250 mg (5 mL of a paediatric version or 5 mL of Calpol 6 Plus or Medinol Over 6). For children over the age of 6 the dose is 250 to 500 mg (5 to 10 mL of Calpol 6 Plus or Medinol Over 6). Paracetamol has no commonly occurring side-effects and does not interact with any medicines and so can be safely taken by all children.

Ibuprofen

Ibuprofen can be given to children over 6 months old. The dose can be given three or four times a day for children of all ages. Infants 6 to 12 months should take 2.5 mL (50 mg), those aged between 1 and 3 should take

Table 9.9
Practical prescribing: Summary of medicines for fever

Medicine	Use in children	Likely side-effects	Drug interactions of note	Patients in whom care should be exercised	Pregnancy
Paracetamol	> 3 months	None	None	None	Not applicable
Ibuprofen	> 6 months	GI disturbances		Children with known hypersensitivity to NSAIDs	

HINTS AND TIPS BOX 9.5: FEVER

Taking a temperature	If using a mercury thermometer, make sure the thermometer is shaken before use. When taking an oral temperature the thermometer should be placed under the tongue for 2 or 3 min. Before the temperature is taken it is important to wait at least 10 min after eating anything hot or cold
Drinking fluids	Children should be told to drink additional fluid to prevent dehydration because a fever will make them sweat more than usual

5 mL, children 4 to 6 years should take 7.5 mL, children 7 to 9 should take 10 mL and children 10 to 12 should take 15 mL.

Ibuprofen can cause gastrointestinal side-effects such as nausea and diarrhoea and also interacts with many other medicines, although those medicines that interact with ibuprofen are very unlikely to be taken by children. Any child who has previously taken an NSAID and had an allergic reaction to it should avoid ibuprofen.

Further reading

Nowak T J, Handford A G 2000 Essentials of pathophysiology. McGraw-Hill, New York

Web sites

The Joanna Briggs Institute for Evidence Based Nursing & Midwifery: www.nottingham.ac.uk/nursing/jbi
General site on fever: www.nlm.nih.gov/medlineplus/fever.html

Infectious childhood conditions

Background

A number of infectious diseases are more prevalent in children than the rest of the population. Many of these diseases are now vaccine preventable and the provision of immunisation programmes has almost eradicated them from developed countries. However, some conditions have no vaccine or incomplete vaccine cover is provided, which means that contraction of the disease is still possible. This usually results in the child suffering from mild symptoms from which a full and speedy recovery is made but in some circumstances, for example meningitis, infection can result in death. In addition, recent controversy over the safety of the triple vaccine for measles, mumps and rubella has seen UK vaccination rates fall. This raises the possibility of children contracting these diseases and outbreaks in other Western countries have been reported. Mention of measles, mumps and rubella is therefore made at the end of this section for completeness.

Meningitis

Meningitis is usually caused by bacterial or viral infection. Viral meningitis is much more common than bacterial meningitis but – thankfully – viral infections are much less serious than bacterial causes.

Signs and symptoms are non-specific in the early stages of the disease and range from fever, nausea, vomiting and headache to irritability. Symptoms can develop quickly and be unpredictable, especially in infants and young children. Symptoms of fever, lethargy, vomiting and irritability are common in children aged between 3 months and 2 years; severe headache, stiff neck and photophobia are more common in older children and adults. In the latter stages of the disease a petechial or purpuric non-blanching rash characteristically develops in meningococcal infection.

The number of cases in the UK is now at their lowest ever levels due to the introduction of two vaccines into the UK vaccination schedule. The Hib vaccine was introduced in 1992 (active against *Haemophilus influenzae*) and the meningococcal C conjugate vaccine introduced in 1999 (active against serogroup C *Meningococcus*).

Glandular fever

Glandular fever is caused by the Epstein–Barr virus and is most commonly seen in patients aged between 15 and 24. It is rare in children under 5 and less frequent in those aged between 5 and 14.

It is transmitted from close salivary contact and is also known as the kissing disease. It has an incubation period of 4 to 7 weeks. Symptoms are vague but characterised by fatigue, headache, sore throat and swollen and tender lymph glands. The symptoms tend to be mild but can linger for many months.

Chicken pox

Chicken pox is very common and is probably the most likely infectious childhood rash to be seen in community pharmacy. It is the primary infection observed when the patient contracts the varicella zoster virus and is transmitted either by droplet infection or with contact with vesicular exudates. The incubation period ranges from 10 to 20 days and prior to the rash developing the patient will experience up to 3 days of prodromal symptoms that could include fever, headache and sore throat. Small red lumps appear that rapidly develop into vesicles, which crust over after 3 to 5 days. New lesions tend to occur in crops of three to five for the first 4 days and begin on the head and neck before moving onto the trunk (Fig. 9.4). The vesicles are often extremely itchy and secondary bacterial infection due to the vesicles being scratched is not unusual. A person is contagious until all lesions have crusted over. A vaccination has been available in America since 1995 and has shown to be 70 to 90% effective. In the UK a vaccine was launched in July 2002 but currently it is only being given to selected patients and is not part of the standard vaccination schedule.

Molluscum contagiosum

This is caused by a pox virus and is usually transmitted by indirect contact for example sharing towels, although it is not very contagious. The face and axillae are common sites of infection. They generally appear in crops and appear as pink pearl-like spots usually less than 0.5 cm

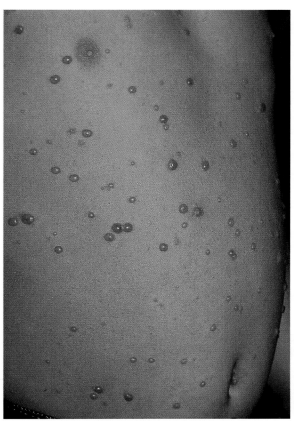

Fig. 9.4 Chicken pox. Reproduced from *Color Atlas of Dermatology* by G White, 2004, Churchill Livingstone, with permission

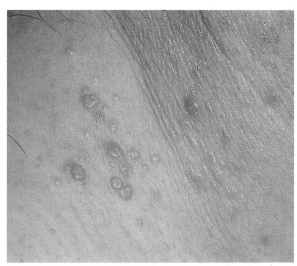

Fig. 9.5 Molluscum contagiosum. Reproduced from *Dermatology: An Illustrated Colour Text* by D Gawkrodger, 2002, Mosby, with permission

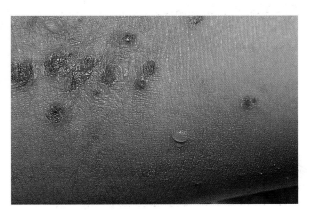

Fig. 9.6 Impetigo. Reproduced from *Color Atlas of Dermatology* by G White, 2004, Churchill Livingstone, with permission

in diameter. All lesions have a central punctum that is a diagnostic feature (Fig. 9.5). Confusion should not arise with other conditions other than viral warts (for further information on warts see page 165). The condition will resolve spontaneously but if the parent or child is anxious then referral to the GP should be made because liquid nitrogen can be used to remove the lesions.

Impetigo

Impetigo is caused by a bacterial infection, most notably *Staphylococcus aureus* or *Streptococcus pyogenes*. It presents mainly on the face, around the nose and mouth. It usually starts as a small red itchy patch of inflamed skin that quickly develops into vesicles that rupture and weep. The exudate dries to a brown, yellow sticky crust (Fig. 9.6). It is contagious and children should be kept off school until the rash clears. General hygiene measures should include not sharing towels, which will help to stop household contacts contracting the infection. The child's nails should be kept short to stop him or her scratching the lesions. Currently, referral is needed for either topical (e.g. fusidic acid) or systemic (flucloxacillin) therapy.

Measles

Since 1968 all infants in the UK have routinely been offered vaccination against measles. It is caused by the paramyxo virus and spread by droplet inhalation. It is the most dangerous of childhood diseases because of the complications that can occur. Approximately 7% of patients develop respiratory complications such as otitis media and pneumonia but encephalitis is seen in about one in every 600 to 1000 cases of measles.

Measles has an incubation period of between 7 to 14 days, which is then followed by 3 or 4 days of prodromal symptoms where the child will have a fever, head cold, cough and conjunctivitis. On the inner cheek and gums small white spots are visible, like grains of salt and are known as Koplik's spots; these are diagnostic for measles. A blotchy red rash appears around the ears before moving on to the trunk and limbs. Immediate referral to the GP is needed.

German measles (rubella)

Rubella is caused by an RNA virus and spread by either close personal contact or airborne droplets. It is less contagious than measles and if contracted many people suffer from mild symptoms and the infection passes undiagnosed. After the incubation period of 14 to 21 days the child experiences up to 5 days of prodromal symptoms, which include cold-like symptoms and swollen glands in the neck before a rash appears on the face that quickly moves on to the trunk and extremities. The rash tends to be pinpoint and macular. The biggest problem posed by rubella is to women in early pregnancy, as fetal damage is possible.

Mumps

Mumps is caused by a paramyxo virus and is transmitted by airborne droplets from the nose and throat. It is the least contagious of the childhood diseases and requires close personal contact before infection can occur. The virus causes an increase in temperature followed by swelling of one or both parotid glands and the child will experience pain when the mouth is opened.

Mumps is much more unpleasant if contracted as an adult and in 20 to 30% of men the disease affects the testicles, with a serious infection possibly causing sterility. The most serious complication from mumps is meningitis.

To aid in differential diagnosis of childhood conditions see Table 9.10.

Table 9.10
Differential diagnosis of childhood conditions

	Measles	German measles	Meningitis	Glandular fever	Chicken pox	Molluscum contagiosum	Mumps	Impetigo
Prodromal stage								
Fever	Yes	No	Yes	Yes	Yes, in older individuals	No	Yes	No
Swollen glands	No	Yes	No	Yes	No	No	Yes	No
Cold-like symptoms	Yes	Yes	No	No	No	No	No	No
Other signs	Koplik's spots*	Malaise	Lethargy, stiff neck, vomiting, photophobia	Malaise and headache	Malaise and headache	None	None	None
Rash								
Location	Ears and face progressing to trunk and limbs	Face moving quickly to trunk	Trunk and limbs	Trunk	On trunk and face, rarely on extremities	Face and axillae	Not Applicable	Facial area especially around nose and mouth
Character	Maculo-papular	Macules, often pinpoint by second day	Purplish blotches Do not blanch	Maculo-papular About 10% have rash	Lesions discrete and appear in crops	Pink pearl-like spots with central punctum*		Vesicles that exude forming yellow crusts
Epidemiology								
Age group most affected	Children and adolescents	Children under 12	Childhood to adulthood	15- to 24-year-olds most at risk	Very common in children	Young children	Children under 12	School-aged children

* Diagnostic.

Self-assessment questions

The following questions are intended to supplement the text. Two levels of questions are provided; multiple choice questions and case studies. The multiple choice questions are designed to test factual recall and case studies allow knowledge to be applied to a practice setting.

Multiple choice questions

9.1 The common name of 'nits' refers to:

  a. An adult head louse
  b. An immature head louse
  c. Live eggs
  d. Egg cases
  e. None of the above

9.2. Which antihistamine has a license for pruritus?

  a. Chlorphenamine
  b. Clemastine
  c. Cyproheptadine
  d. Hydroxyzine
  e. Azatadine

9.3. A low grade fever is defined as a temperature of?

  a. Less than 36.5°C
  b. Less than 37.5°C
  c. Less than 38.5°C
  d. Less than 39.5°C
  e. Less than 40.5°C

9.4. Which patient group should avoid using alcoholic insecticides?

  a. Asthmatics
  b. Patients with coeliac's disease
  c. Those with hypertension
  d. Patients with peptic ulcer
  e. Epileptics

9.5. Fever in children with no associated symptoms or signs is usually due to:

  a. Gastroenteritis
  b. Urinary tract infection
  c. Upper respiratory tract infection
  d. Bacterial tonsillitis
  e. Impetigo

9.6. What are the usual age children present with atopic dermatitis?

  a. In the first month of life
  b. Before 6 months
  c. Before 1 year
  d. Before 2 years
  e. Before 5 years

9.7. Mebendazole can be given to patients from what age?

  a. 1
  b. 2
  c. 3
  d. 4
  e. 5

9.8. How many days after initial treatment should a second application of insecticide be used to eradicate head lice?

  a. 3
  b. 5
  c. 7
  d. 10
  e. 14

Questions 9.9 to 9.11 concern the following conditions:

A. Chicken pox
B. Measles
C. German measles
D. Glandular fever
E. Impetigo

Select, from A to E, which of the above conditions:

9.9. Is often caused by *Staphylococcus*

9.10. Is characterised by a vesicular rash

9.11. Is transmitted by close salivary contact

Questions 9.12 to 9.14 concern the following medicines:

A. Piperazine
B. Mebendazole
C. Permethrin
D. Dimethicone
E. Brompheniramine

Select, from A to E, which of the above medicines:

9.12. Is associated with sedation

9.13. Is contraindicated in pregnancy

9.14. Causes abdominal pain

Questions 9.15 to 9.17: for each of these questions *one* or *more* of the responses is (are) correct. Decide which of the responses is (are) correct. Then choose:

A. If a, b and c are correct
B. If a and b only are correct
C. If b and c only are correct
D. If a only is correct
E. If c only is correct

Directions summarised

A	B	C	D	E
a, b and c	a and b only	b and c only	a only	c only

9.15. Colic is generally due to:

    a. The teat hole being too large
    b. Swallowing air when being breast fed
    c. Being given too much food

9.16. Atopic dermatitis can be defined as itchy skin plus:

    a. History of dry skin
    b. Flexural eczema
    c. A personal history of other atopic disease

9.17. Which statement(s) about head lice treatment is/are true:

    a. Shampoos are not as effective as lotions
    b. Alcoholic lotions are suitable for all patients
    c. They can be used prophylactically

Questions 9.18 to 9.20: these questions consist of a statement in the left-hand column followed by a statement in the right-hand column. You need to:

● decide whether the first statement is true or false
● decide whether the second statement is true or false

Then choose:

A. If both statements are true and the second statement is a correct explanation of the first statement
B. If both statements are true but the second statement is *not* a correct explanation of the first statement
C. If the first statement is true but the second statement is false
D. If the first statement is false but the second statement is true
E. If both statements are false

Directions summarised

	First statement	Second statement	
A	True	True	Second explanation is a correct explanation of the first
B	True	True	Second statement is *not* a correct explanation of the first
C	True	False	
D	False	True	
E	False	False	

	First statement	Second statement
9.18.	Emollients are the mainstay of treatment of atopic dermatitis	Products with lanolin should be avoided
9.19.	Oral temperature is the most accurate measure of temperature	Normal body temperature is 37°C
9.20.	Measles is vaccine preventable	It is usually given as a triple vaccine

Case study

CASE STUDY 9.1

Ms JP, a young mother of two children comes in to the pharmacy one afternoon clutching a letter from the children's primary school. The letter says that there is a head lice outbreak and instructs parents to treat their children for head lice.

a. How do you respond?

You need to find out if her children actually have head lice or if she is trying to buy a product to stop them getting head lice. She should be told that products cannot be bought to prevent her children contracting head lice and she should inspect their heads regularly, and only when live lice are found should a product be bought. Ms JP should be told how to inspect her children's hair for signs of head lice.

Ms JP returns to the pharmacy 4 days later and says her youngest daughter does now have head lice. She is 5 and suffers from no medical problems.

b. What product are you going to recommend?

Malathion or a pyrethroid would be acceptable treatment options. Patient acceptability will primarily drive choice of product.

c. What patient factors will influence your recommendation?

If the child has broken scalp skin then an alcoholic product should be avoided because irritation and stinging could occur. Additionally, very long hair might require more than one bottle of product.

Ms JP says she is not very keen on using chemicals on her daughter's hair. She has heard that you can use conditioner and that will get rid of the problem.

d. How do you respond?

Mrs JP is probably referring to the 'bug busting' technique. She should be told that the effectiveness of bug busting is lower than using chemicals but can be tried if she really does not want to use insecticides. You should stress that it is very important to adhere to the regimen as poor compliance with the bug busting method is probably why it has been shown to be less effective.

Ms JP then asks you whether her older daughter, Samantha, should also be treated even though she has not got head lice.

e. What do you say?

There is no definitive answer. Some authorities say treat all people whereas others say treat only the person with head lice. Your primary care trust might issue local guidelines and it would be worth finding out if any guidance is available.

CASE STUDY 9.2

Mr PB is looking after his grandson for the weekend. He asks for some advice because he has noticed a rash on his grandson's body and wants something to help get rid of it.

a. What do you need to know?

You need to know:

- *The location of rash*
- *What the rash looks like*
- *When the rash appeared*
- *Associated symptoms, such as itch*
- *General health of the child*
- *If the child has a temperature*
- *What, if any, symptoms the child had before the rash appeared*
- *The age of his grandson.*

All Mr PB is able to tell you is that his grandson has been with him for the last day and he only noticed the rash this morning when he was dressing him. The boy is 4 years old and the rash is on his chest and back; Mr PB describes them as spots. He thinks it is probably itchy because he saw his grandson scratching this morning.

b. What do you think could be the problem?

Without seeing the child and the rash it is always difficult to make a differential diagnosis from information from a third party, but it appears the child might have chicken pox.

c. Are there any further questions you could ask the man to confirm your diagnosis?

Further questions you could ask are:

- *Are the spots coming out in groups?*
- *Have any of the spots turned into little blisters?*
- *Has he been exposed to other children with chicken pox?*

Mr PB is unsure and concerned that his grandson is OK.

d. What could you do?

It appears that his grandson is not poorly and unless he deteriorates there is probably no need to call out the GP. You could recommend an antihistamine to help with the itching and reassure him that his grandson will be OK, but that if he becomes poorly the GP should be called out. You also tell him that the rash fits the description of chicken pox but without seeing the rash you cannot be sure. It would therefore be useful if you could see the child or if the child could be seen by someone over the next couple of days to confirm your suspicions.

Answers to multiple choice questions

9.1 = c   9.2 = d   9.3 = c   9.4 = a   9.5 = b   9.6 = b   9.7 = b   9.8 = c   9.9 = e   9.10 = a,
9.11= d   9.12 = e   9.13 = b   9.14 = b   9.15 = b   9.16 = a   9.17 = d   9.18 = b   9.19 = d   9.20 = b.

Specific product requests

Background

Many patients will present in the pharmacy requesting a specific product rather than wanting advice on symptoms. They might have seen a product advertised on the television or been told to purchase it by their doctor. Regardless of the reason why they are asking for the product, it is the responsibility of the pharmacist to ensure that patients receive the most appropriate therapy. This chapter therefore deals with situations where patients ask for a particular product or class of product but the pharmacist needs to elicit more information from the patient before complying with the request.

Motion sickness

Background

Motion sickness is characterised by nausea, pallor and occasionally vomiting. Pharmacists are frequently asked to recommend a travel-sickness remedy, especially by anxious parents. Motion sickness can affect any individual in any form of moving vehicle.

Prevalence and epidemiology

The exact prevalence of motion sickness is unknown. Children between the ages of 2 and 12 are most commonly affected. However, certain sectors of the population, for example naval crew and pilots, also show a higher prevalence rate than the normal population. This

is obviously due to the greater exposure they have to potential motion sickness.

Aetiology

It is widely believed that motion sickness results from the inability of the brain to process conflicting information received from sensory nerve terminals concerning movement and position, the eyes and the vestibular system of the ear.

Evidence base for over-the-counter medication

First-generation antihistamines (cyclizine, cinnarizine, meclozine and promethazine) and the anticholinergic hyoscine are routinely recommended to prevent motion sickness. All have shown various degrees of effectiveness, with hyoscine consistently proving the most effective.

Non-pharmacological approaches to the prevention of motion sickness using acupressure are also available OTC. Bruce et al (1990) investigated the use of Sea Band acupressure bands versus hyoscine and placebo. Eighteen healthy volunteers were subjected to simulated conditions to induce motion sickness. The findings showed that whereas hyoscine exerted a preventative effect, Sea Bands were no more effective than placebo. Further trials have confirmed these findings, although a small trial by Stern et al (2001) reported positive findings. Further trials are needed because acupressure has shown positive effects for the nausea and vomiting associated with pregnancy.

Practical prescribing and product selection

Prescribing information relating to medicines for motion sickness reviewed in the section 'Evidence base for over-the-counter medication' is discussed and summarised in Table 10.1.

Product selection should be based on matching the length of the journey with the duration of action of each medicine (see Hints and Tips box 10.1).

Antihistamines

Antihistamines in products for motion sickness are associated with sedation. They therefore have the same side-effects, interactions and precautions in use as other first-generation antihistamines used in cough and cold remedies. For further information on these, see page 21.

Cyclizine (Valoid)

Cyclizine is prescribed very rarely. It is subject to abuse by drug misusers and many pharmacies do not stock it. If taken, adults and children over 12 should take one tablet (50 mg) three times a day. The dose for children over the age of 6 is half the adult dose.

Cinnarizine (Stugeron)

Adults and children over 12 should take two tablets 2 h before travel. The dose can be repeated every 8 h (one tablet) if needed. For children aged between 5 and 12 the dose is half the adult dose.

Meclozine (Sea-Legs)

Adults and children over 12 years should take two tablets (25 mg) 1 h before travel, however, as activity lasts 24 h, the dose can be taken the night before travel. Children aged between 6 and 12 years should take half the adult dose (one tablet, 12.5 mg) and for children over 2, half a tablet (6.25 mg) should be taken.

Promethazine (Avomine)

Adults and children over the age of 10 should take one tablet 1–2 h before travel; for children over 5 the dose should be half that of the adult dose.

Hyoscine hydrobromide (e.g. Joy-Rides, Kwells)

Products containing hyoscine should be taken 20 to 30 min before the time of travel; because they have a short half life they have a short duration of action and the dose might therefore have to be repeated on journeys longer than 4 h.

Although hyoscine hydrobromide appears to be safe in pregnancy, the manufacturers state that it should be avoided. It interacts with other medicines that have anticholinergic side-effects and should therefore not be co-prescribed, if possible. Because hyoscine hydromide crosses the blood–brain barrier, it can cause sedation.

Joy-Rides

Joy rides can be given from age 3 upwards. Children aged between 3 and 4 years should take half a tablet

Table 10.1
Practical prescribing: Summary of medicines for travel sickness

Medicine	Use in children	Likely side-effects	Drug interactions of note	Patients in whom care should be exercised	Pregnancy
Cyclizine (Valoid)	> 6 years	Dry mouth, sedation	Increased sedation with alcohol, opioid analgesics, analgesics, anxiolytics, hypnotics and antidepressants	Angle-closure glaucoma, prostate enlargement	OK, but manufacturers state avoid
Cinnarizine (Sturgeron 15)	> 5 years				
Meclozine (Sea-Legs)	> 2 years				
Promethazine (Avomine)	> 5 years				
Hyoscine					
Joy-Rides	> 3 years	Dry mouth, sedation	Increased anticholinergic side-effects with TCAs and neuroleptics	Angle-closure glaucoma, prostate enlargement	OK, but manufacturers state avoid
Kwells	> 10 years				
Junior Kwells	> 4 years				

HINTS AND TIPS BOX 10.1: TRAVEL SICKNESS

Dry mouth problems	Many people complain of a dry mouth with travel sickness medicines. This is easily overcome by sucking a sweet, which will stimulate saliva production and get rid of a dry mouth
Matching up length of journey with product	Hyoscine should be recommended for journeys up to 4 h; cinnarizine for journeys over 4 h but less than 8 h and promethazine and meclozine for journeys longer than 8 h

(75 µg) and no more than one tablet (150 µg) in 24 h. Children between the ages of 4 and 7 should take one tablet (150 µg) to a maximum of two tablets (300 µg) in 24 h, and children aged between 7 and 12 should take one to two tablets.

Kwells

Kwells can only be given to children aged 10 and over. Children over 10 should take half to one tablet. For adults the dose is one tablet. The dose can be repeated every 6 h when needed.

Junior Kwells

Junior Kwells contain half the amount of hyoscine hydrobromide (150 µg) than Kwells and are marketed at children under the age of 10, although older children can take them. Children aged between 4 and 10 should take half to one tablet. The dose should be taken 30 min before the start of the journey.

Further reading

Bruce D G, Golding J F, Hockenhull N et al 1990 Acupressure and motion sickness. Aviation, Space and Environmental Medicine 61:361–365

Dahl E, Offer-Ohlsen D, Lillevold P E et al 1984 Transdermal scopolamine, oral meclizine and placebo in motion sickness. Clinical Pharmacology and Therapeutics 36:116–120

Klocker N, Hanschke W, Toussaint S et al 2001 Scopolamine nasal spray in motion sickness: a randomised, controlled and crossover study for the comparison of two scopolamine nasal sprays with oral dimenhydrinate and placebo. European Journal of Pharmaceutical Science 13:227–232

Noy S, Shapira S, Zilbiger A et al 1984 Transdermal therapeutic system scopolamine (TTSS), dimenhydrinate and placebo-a comparative study at sea. Aviation, Space and Environmental Medicine 55:1051–1054

Pingree B J, Pethybridge R J 1994 A comparison of the efficacy of cinnarizine with scopolamine in the treatment of seasickness. Aviation, Space and Environmental Medicine 65:597–605

Stern R M, Jokerst M D, Muth E R, Hollis C 2001 Acupressure relieves the symptoms of motion sickness and reduces abnormal gastric activity. Alternative Therapy and Health Medicine 7:91–94

Emergency hormonal contraception

Background

Emergency hormonal contraception (EHC) became available to the public, through community pharmacies and without the need for a prescription, in January 2001. Greater access to emergency contraception fits in with the government policy of trying to reduce the number of unwanted pregnancies (see Hints and Tips Box 10.2). It is expected that pharmacy supply will provide a welcome additional route for patients requiring EHC at times when other providers might be closed, for example at weekends and in the evenings. The product contains progestogen in the form of two levonorgestrel 0.75 mg tablets and is marketed under the name of Levonelle.

Aetiology

The exact mechanism of action for levonorgestrel is not clear and, indeed, it appears to have more than one mode of action at more than one site. It is thought to work mainly by preventing ovulation and fertilisation if intercourse has taken place in the preovulatory phase, when the likelihood of fertilisation is the highest. It is also thought to cause endometrial changes that discourage egg implantation.

Evidence base for over-the-counter medication

The exact effectiveness of Levonelle is hard to establish, as many people who have been treated with emergency contraception will not have become pregnant even without treatment. However, when Levonelle was compared against the Yuzpe regimen (Schering PC4) the progestogen-only regime was found to prevent 86% of expected pregnancies, when treatment was initiated within 72 h, compared with 57% with PC4. Levonorgestrel is more effective the earlier it is taken after unprotected sex; it prevents 95% of pregnancies if taken within 24 h of unprotected sex, 85% between 24 and 48 h, and 58% if used within 48 to 72 h.

In addition to being more effective than the **Yuzpe method**, trials have shown Levonelle to have a more

---

HINTS AND TIPS BOX 10.2: EMERGENCY HORMONAL CONTRACEPTION

Who is eligible?	Only patients over the age of 16 can be supplied with Levonelle, although family planning services, GPs and pharmacists acting under a patient group direction can supply EHC to patients under 16
Do you have to supply EHC?	The supply of EHC is at the discretion of the individual pharmacist and some, for religious beliefs, might choose not to supply EHC. However, the patient should be advised on other local sources of supply so that she can access the service

Table 10.2
Practical prescribing: Summary of medicines for emergency hormonal contraception

Medicine	Use in children	Likely side-effects	Drug interactions of note	Patients in whom care should be exercised	Pregnancy
Levonelle	> 16 years	Nausea	Anticonvulsants, rifampicin, griseofulvin, St John's Wort and ciclosporin	Conditions in which Levonelle absorption might be impaired, for example Crohn's disease	Not applicable

favourable side-effect profile, with lower incidences of nausea and vomiting.

Practical prescribing and product selection

Prescribing information relating to Levonelle is discussed and summarised in Table 10.2.

Assessing patient suitability

Prior to any sale or supply of Levonelle the pharmacist has to be in a position to determine if the patient is suitable to take the medicine. To do this, an assessment has to be made on the likelihood that the patient is pregnant:

- First, has the patient had unprotected sex, contraceptive failure or missed taking contraceptive pills in the last 72 h? EHC can only be given to patients who present within 72 h. If more than 72 h have elapsed but less than 120 h (5 days) then the patient will need to have an intrauterine device fitted.
- Is the patient already pregnant? Details about the patient's last period should be sought. Is the period late, and if so how many days late? Was the nature of the period different or unusual. If pregnancy is suspected, a pregnancy test could be offered.
- What method of contraception is normally used? Patients who take combined oral contraceptives might not need EHC, depending on which part of the cycle the pill was forgotten. The Royal College of Obstetricians and Gynaecologists guidelines on missed pills are:
  - if two or more pills are missed from the first seven pills in a packet or four or more pills are missed mid-packet then EHC should be given
  - if two or more pills are missed from the last seven pills in a packet, EHC is not needed providing the pill-free break is omitted
  - if the patient uses a progestogen-only form of contraception then EHC should always be given if the tablet is taken more than 3 h late.

A number of useful checklists have been produced and are used in practice, an example of one such form is

shown in Fig. 10.1. Many pharmacists ask patients to complete one of these forms, instead of asking potentially embarrassing questions in the pharmacy. When the form has been completed, the pharmacist can decide whether EHC should be supplied to the patient.

Levonelle

Levonelle should be taken as soon as possible after unprotected sex or contraceptive failure. The dose consists of two tablets taken as a single dose. About 1 in 5 patients experience nausea but only 1 in 20 go on to be sick. If the patient vomits within 3 h of taking the dose she should be advised to take another two tablets immediately. Taking EHC can affect the timing of the next menstrual period and patients should be told that the period might be earlier or later than usual. However, if the period is different than normal or more than 5 days late then she should be advised to have a pregnancy test.

A number of medicines do, theoretically, interact with Levonelle, most notably enzyme inducers, including anticonvulsants, rifampicin, griseofulvin and St John's wort, although the clinical significance of the interactions appear low as only a handful of drug interaction reports have been received by the manufacturers. It seems prudent, until such time that more substantial evidence is available, that patients taking these medicines are referred to the GP. In such circumstances, doubling the dose of Levonelle is commonly practised (although not licensed). If this is not the preferred option then an alternative form of EHC can be given, for example an intrauterine device.

Further reading

[Anonymous] 1998 Randomised controlled trial of levonorgestrel versus the Yuzpe regimen of combined oral contraceptives for emergency contraception. Task Force on Postovulatory Methods of Fertility Regulation. Lancet 352:428–433

Centre for Pharmacy Postgraduate Education (CPPE) 2003 Emergency hormonal contraception e-learning material. CPPE, University of Manchester. Available online to qualified pharmacists: www.cppe.man.ac.uk

Emergency Hormonal Contraception (Levonelle)

Before the pharmacist can supply you with emergency contraception you are asked to answer the questions below. Your answers will allow the pharmacist to decide if it is safe for you to have these pills. Any information you give will be treated confidentially and you will be given this sheet of paper to take home with you. If you have any difficulty with any of the questions the pharmacist will be happy to help you.

You will be charged £19.99 for a box of Levonelle. Levonelle is free from a family planning clinic or your GP. Information about these services is on the other side of this sheet or ask the pharmacist for help.

1. What was the date of your last period?

2. Was your last period unusually light or unusually heavy?   Yes ☐   No ☐   Don't know ☐

3. Is your cycle between 24 and 32 days
   (i.e. from the start of one period and the start of another)   Yes ☐   No ☐

4. If you answered NO to the above question, how many days are there usually between the start of one period and the start of the next?   _____ days

5. How many hours is it since you had unprotected sex?   _____ hours

6. Is this the only time you have had unprotected sex since your last period   Yes ☐   No ☐

7. Have you used emergency contraception since your last period or within the last 4 weeks?   Yes ☐   No ☐

8. What form of contraception do you normally use?

9. Have you been jaundiced or had any sort of liver disease within the last six months?   Yes ☐   No ☐

10. Are you taking any other medicines or tablets – either prescribed or bought over the counter (e.g. St John's Wort)? **If YES please tell the pharmacist**   Yes ☐   No ☐

11. Are you completing this form to get emergency contraception for yourself?   Yes ☐   No ☐

12. What is your date of birth?

Fig. 10.1a) An emergency hormonal contraception request form supplied by Portsmouth and the Isle of Wight Health Authority for Community Pharmacists (part (b) overleaf). Reproduced with permission

After you have obtained the emergency pills

- Read the booklet inside the box of Levonelle
- Take the first pill as soon as possible
- Take the second pill 12 hours later (the booklet advises what to do if you are late taking the second pill or if you are sick taking either of the 2 pills)
- Carry on using your normal contraception until your next period
- If you have missed pills use condoms as well for at least 7 days
- Your next period will come at about the normal time. Sometimes it occurs a little earlier or a little later
- If you have not had a period within 3 weeks of taking the emergency pills, you should have a pregnancy test
- If you need to take the emergency pill again in this cycle, before your next period has come, then return to the pharmacist or see your GP or go to a family planning clinic

IMPORTANT
The pharmacist is not able to sell Levonelle to people under the age of 16, but they will be able to tell you where you can obtain it. This information is also given below.

If you have had unprotected sex you may also be at risk of a sexually transmitted or shared infection, for example Chlamydia. For further advice or help, ring the local genito-urinary clinic on 023 92866792 or go to a family planning clinic or see your GP.

For further information or advice regarding where you can obtain emergency contraception or get help about a sexually transmitted infection contact:

Portsmouth Family Planning Helpline - 023 866301

Or any of the following -   NHS Direct 0845 4647
Portsmouth Genito-urinary Clinic 023 92866792
Your own GP

Emergency contraception can also be obtained at the following places in the evenings and weekends:

Accident and Emergency, QA Hospital, Cosham. **Tel: 023 92286000**

Accident Treatment Centre, Haslar Hospital, Gosport. **Tel: 023 92584255**

Havant War Memorial Hospital. **Tel: 023 92484256**

Petersfield Hospital. **Tel: 01730 263221**

Emsworth Cottage Hospital. **Tel: 01243 376041**

Fig. 10.1b) Emergency hormonal contraception request, cont'd.

Piaggio G, von Hertzen H, Grimes D A et al 1999 Timing of emergency contraception with levonorgestrel or the Yuzpe regimen. Task Force on Postovulatory Methods of Fertility Regulation. Lancet 353:721

Web sites
British Pregnancy Advisory Service: www.bpas.org
Brook Advisory Centres: www.thebabyregistry.co.uk/advice/b/bac.htm
Family Planning Association: www.fpa.org.uk
Marie Stopes Clinics: www.mariestopes.org.uk

Nicotine replacement therapy

Background

Smoking represents the single greatest cause of preventable illness and premature death worldwide. It is responsible or contributes to a myriad of conditions including lung cancer, ischaemic heart disease and chronic obstructive pulmonary disease. Of these, ischaemic heart disease is the most important smoking-related disease with more deaths attributable to this than any other, including lung cancer. Smoking kills over 120 000 people each year. Successive UK governments have placed great importance on reducing the number of smokers. The current Government White Paper *Smoking kills* outlines targets to decrease smoking rates and can be accessed at www.archive.official-documents.co.uk/document/cm41/4177/4177.htm

Prevalence and epidemiology

According to UK government figures published for 1998, 27% of the adult population smokes – a staggering 12 million people. Encouragingly, this figure is lower than it was 20 years ago, when almost 1 in 2 of the population smoked. However, worrying recent trends show that the number of new young smokers is increasing, especially teenage girls. There are also large differences in the number of smokers between socioeconomic groups. For example, unskilled male workers are three to four times more likely to smoke than professional males.

Globally, the incidence of smoking is mixed, with some Western countries seeing a decrease in smoking rates whereas in other countries it is on the increase. As legislation governing tobacco sales and advertising becomes stricter in developed countries, the tobacco industry is seeking easier markets in developing countries, where intensive marketing is still permitted and it can gain new customers.

Aetiology

Hundreds of compounds have been identified in tobacco smoke, however only three are of real clinical importance:

- tar-based products, which have carcinogenic properties
- carbon monoxide, which reduces the oxygen-carrying capacity of the red blood cells
- nicotine, which produces dependence by activating dopaminergic systems.

Tolerance to the effects of nicotine is rapid. Once plasma nicotine levels fall below a threshold, patients begin to suffer nicotine withdrawal symptoms and will crave another cigarette. Treatment is therefore based on maintaining plasma nicotine just above this threshold.

Evidence base for over-the-counter medication

Nicotine replacement therapy (NRT) has established itself as an effective treatment option. Numerous well-designed clinical trials have shown that NRT doubles the success rate of those attempting to stop smoking when compared with placebo. There are a number of drug delivery systems, all of which have been shown to be more effective than placebo, although it is not possible to say if one delivery system is better than another because comparative trials between them do not appear to have been conducted. The patient's personal choice of delivery system will therefore be the determining factor.

In 1998, evidence-based smoking cessation guidelines were produced by the Health Education Authority and published in the journal *Thorax*. These guidelines recommended the use of NRT and advocated that healthcare professionals should give smokers accurate information on NRT products; pharmacists are ideally placed to do this.

Practical prescribing and product selection

Prescribing information relating to the medicines for NRT reviewed in the section 'Evidence base for over-the-counter medication' is discussed and summarised in Table 10.3.

Before instigating any treatment, it is important that the patient does *want* to stop smoking. Work has shown that motivation is a major determinant for successful smoking cessation and interventions based on the trans-theoretical model of change have proved effective (Fig. 10.2). The model identifies six stages; progress through these is cyclical and patients need different types of support and advice at each stage.

Table 10.3
Practical prescribing: Summary of medicines used as nicotine replacement therapy

Medicine	Use in children	Likely side-effects	Drug interactions of note	Patients in whom care should be exercised	Pregnancy
Nicorette Nicotinell NiQuitinCQ	> 18 years	GI disturbances	None	Patients with heart disease	Not recommended

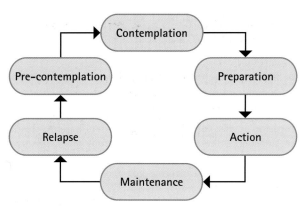

Fig. 10.2 Stages of change

Most patients who ask directly for NRT will be at the preparation stage of the model and ready to enter the action stage. However, a small number of patients might well be buying NRT to please others and are actually in the precontemplation stage and do not want to stop smoking.

NRT is formulated as gum, lozenges, patches, nasal spray, inhalator and sublingual tablets, therefore there should be a treatment option to suit all patients (see Hints and Tips Box 10.3). All patients can use them, except in pregnancy. Patients with pre-existing heart disease are not contraindicated from using NRT and research has shown that NRT can be safely given in this patient group, although product licences for OTC products state they should not be given. In practice it would seem unreasonable not to allow these patients to use NRT, although it might be prudent to speak first with the patient's GP.

Side-effects with NRT are rare and are normally limited to gastrointestinal problems associated with accidental ingestion of nicotine when chewing gum or to local skin irritation and vivid dreams associated with patches. Headache, nausea and diarrhoea have also been reported. NRT also appears not to have any significant interactions with other medicines.

Nicorette

Nicorette is available as gum (2 and 4 mg), inhalation cartridge (10 mg), microtab (2 mg) and patch (5, 10 and 15 mg).

Gum

Nicorette gum is available as either citrus or mint flavour (unflavoured gum leaves a bitter taste in the mouth). The gum should be chewed slowly until the taste becomes strong, it should then be rested between the cheek and gum until the taste fades. The gum can then be re-chewed. Each piece of gum lasts approximately 30 min. A maximum of 15 pieces of gum can be chewed in any 24-h period.

Inhalation cartridge

The inhalator can be particularly helpful to those smokers who still feel they need to continue the hand-to-mouth movement. Each cartridge is inserted into the inhalator and air is drawn into the mouth through the mouthpiece. Deep drawing or short sucking can be used as required by the individual. Each cartridge lasts about 20 min. Cessation of smoking is planned to take 3 months. For the first 2 months patients should use between 6 and 12 cartridges a day. During weeks 8 to 10 the aim is to reduce the number of cartridges used by half and after the final 2 weeks the number of cartridges used should be zero.

Microtabs

Microtabs are delivered sublingually and patients who smoke less than 20 cigarettes a day should use one tablet per hour (doubled for heavy smokers), increased to two tablets per hour if the patient fails to stop smoking with the one tablet per hour regimen or for those whose nicotine withdrawal symptoms remain so strong they believe they will relapse. Most patients require between 8 to 24 tablets a day, although the maximum is 40 tablets in 24 h. Treatment should be stopped when daily consumption is down to 1 or 2 tablets a day.

Patches

Nicorette patches are usually applied at bedtime and left on for 16 h. Patients who smoke more than 20 cigarettes a day should start on the highest strength patch (15 mg) for 8 weeks before stepping down to the 10 mg patch for a further 2 weeks. The lowest-strength patch (5 mg) should be finally worn for another 2 weeks.

HINTS AND TIPS BOX 10.3: NICOTINE REPLACEMENT THERAPY

Application of patches	Patches should be applied to non-hairy skin on the hip, chest or upper arm. The next patch should be placed on a different site to avoid skin irritation
16- or 24-h patches?	A 16-h patch will be suitable for most patients, however, if a patient requires a cigarette within the first 20 to 30 min of waking then a 24-h patch should be given. If sleep disturbances are experienced with the 24-h patches the patient can switch to a 16-h patch or alternatively remove the 24-h patch at bed time

Nicotinell

Nicotinell is available as gum (2 or 4 mg), patches (7, 14 and 21 mg) and lozenge (1 mg).

Gum

Nicotinell gum is flavoured and available as fruit or mint gum. The dosage and administration of Nicotinell gum is the same as that for Nicorette gum.

Patches

Nicotinell patches are suitable for those smokers who must have a cigarette as soon as they wake up. The patches are worn continuously and changed every 24 h, thus when the patient awakes nicotine levels will be above the threshold of nicotine withdrawal. People who smoke more than 20 cigarettes a day should use the highest strength patch (TTS 30 patch, 21 mg) for 3 to 4 weeks, after which the strength of the patch should be reduced to the middle strength (TTS 20 patch, 14 mg) for a further 3 to 4 weeks before finally using the lowest patch (TTS 10 patch, 7 mg). If the patient smokes less than 20 cigarettes a day then they should start on the middle strength patch.

Lozenges

Patients should be instructed to suck one lozenge every 1–2 h when they have the urge to smoke. The usual dosage is 8 to 12 lozenges per day, with a maximum of 25 lozenges in 24 h. Lozenges are mint flavoured and should be sucked until the taste becomes strong, and then placed between gum and cheek (similar to the gum) until the taste fades, when sucking can recommence. Each lozenge takes approximately 30 min to dissolve completely.

NiQuitinCQ

NiQuitinCQ is only available as patches (7, 14 and 21 mg) and the manufacturer recommends an 8- or 10-week treatment course, depending on the number of cigarettes smoked each day. Patients who smoke more than 10 cigarettes a day should use the 21 mg patch for 6 weeks, followed by the 14 mg patch for 2 weeks and finally the 7 mg for the last 2 weeks. Patients who smoke less than 10 cigarettes a day should start on the middle-strength patch (14 mg) for 6 weeks followed by the 7 mg for a final 2 weeks.

Further reading

Callum C 1998 The UK smoking epidemic: deaths in 1995. Health Education Authority (now called the Health Development Agency), London

Hajek P 1994 Treatments for smokers. Addiction 89:1543–1549

Raw N, McNeill A D, West R 1998 Smoking cessation guidelines for health professionals. A guide to effective smoking cessation interventions for the health care system. Thorax 53; suppl 5(1):S1–S9

Web sites

Action on Smoking and Health (ASH): www.ash.org/
Department of Health information site: www.givingupsmoking.co.uk
Novartis company site giving general advice on smoking cessation: www.nicotinell.com/intl/firstmoment.php

Malaria prophylaxis

Background

Malaria is a parasitic disease spread by the female anopheles mosquito. Four species of the protozoan *Plasmodium* produce malaria in humans: *P. vivax, P. ovale, P. malariae* and *P. falciparum. P. falciparum* is the most virulent form of malaria and is responsible for the majority of deaths associated with malaria infection. It acts by altering the surface of red blood cells, making them adhere to blood vessel walls and resulting in **sequestration**. Clinically, patients suffer from chills, nausea, vomiting and headache. This is followed by fever, which concludes with sweating. This cycle repeats every 2 to 3 days.

Prevalence and epidemiology

Malaria is a leading cause of death in areas of the world where the infection is endemic, with an estimated 300 million cases each year resulting in over 1 million deaths. However, malaria is not only confined to endemic malarial areas and the number of cases reported in Western countries, for example the UK, is on the increase as more and more people travel to countries where malaria is common. More than 2000 cases of malaria are reported in England and Wales each year, resulting in around 12 deaths a year. The majority of cases contracted are the *P. vivax* found in the Indian subcontinent.

The risk of contracting malaria varies greatly and depends on the area visited, the time of year and altitude. In general, the risk tends to be greater in more remote areas than in urban/tourist areas, after rainy or monsoon seasons and at low altitude. It is therefore possible to have a different risk of contracting malaria within the same country, for example visiting the Southern lowlands of Ethiopia after the rainy season would pose a very high risk whereas trekking in the Simien mountains in the north of the country during the dry season would pose minimal risk.

Aetiology

Malarial parasites are transmitted to humans when an infected female anopheles mosquito bites its host. Once in the human host, the parasites (which at this stage of their life-cycle are known as 'sporozoites') are transported via the bloodstream to the liver. In the liver they divide and multiply (they are now known as 'merozoites'). After 5 to 16 days the liver cells rupture, to release up to 400 000 merozoites, which invade the human host's **erythrocytes**. The merozoites reproduce asexually in the erythrocytes before causing them to rupture and release yet more merozoites into the blood to invade yet more erythrocytes. Any mosquito that bites an infected person at this stage will ingest the parasites and the cycle will begin again. It is worth noting that *P. vivax* and *P. ovale* parasites can remain dormant in the liver, which explains why malarial symptoms can manifest months after return from an infected region.

Evidence base for over-the-counter medication

Not being bitten is the only guaranteed way of not contracting malaria. Although this is almost impossible to ensure, protective measures should always be taken. General advice includes:

- using insect repellents, particularly those containing diethyl toluamide (DEET), which are the most effective and best studied insect repellents on the market
- wearing long-sleeved shirts and trousers, especially at dawn and dusk
- checking hotel windows to make sure they have adequate screening
- sleeping in a bed with a mosquito net
- keeping doors and windows closed during the evening and night
- using mosquito coils or plug-in dispensers.

People travelling to more remote areas should buy their own mosquito net that has been impregnated with an insecticide. A number of travel centres and specialist outdoor shops sell such products.

Chemoprophylaxis

In addition to taking precautions to avoid being bitten, travellers should take antimalarial medication. Chloroquine and proguanil are licensed for pharmacy sale when used for prophylaxis of malaria and have proven efficacy. However, there is now widespread drug resistance to these two medicines and their use is limited. It is therefore important to check the current guidelines for the destination the client is travelling to or through. Two easily available reference sources in which UK recommendations can be found are the *British National Formulary* and *MIMS*. In addition, a number of organisations produce reference material on current recommendations. In most instances, *MIMS* is the first-line reference source because the guidelines are updated monthly (the *British National Formulary* is produced every 6 months) and are more likely to be up to date. For travellers who are travelling to very high-risk areas (usually sub-Saharan Africa or South East Asia) or travelling for extended periods, it might be better to refer the client to a specialist centre.

Practical prescribing and product selection

Prescribing information relating to medicines for malaria reviewed in the section 'Evidence base for over-the-counter medication' is discussed and summarised in Table 10.4; useful tips relating to patients travelling to regions where malaria is endemic are given in Hints and Tips Box 10.4.

Medicine regimens

Antimalarials need to be taken at least 1 week before departure, during the stay in the malaria endemic region and for 4 weeks on leaving the area. Taking the medication prior to departure allows the patient to know whether they are going to experience side-effects and, if they do, still have enough time to obtain a different antimalarial before departure. It also helps to establish a medicine-taking routine that will – hopefully – help with compliance. Medicine-taking for a further 4 weeks after leaving the region is to ensure that any possible infection that could have been contracted during the final days of the stay does not develop into malaria.

Chloroquine (e.g. Avloclor, Nivaquine)

Chloroquine can be given alone or in combination with proguanil and is restricted to areas in which the risk

Table 10.4
Practical prescribing: Summary of medicines for malaria prophylaxis

Medicine	Use in children	Likely side-effects	Drug interactions of note	Patients in whom care should be exercised	Pregnancy
Chloroquine	All ages	GI disturbances and visual problems	Amiodarone, flecainide, sotalol, astemizole and terfenadine	Avoid in epilepsy	OK
Paludrine		Diarrhoea	None	Renal impairment	

HINTS AND TIPS BOX 10.4: MALARIA

Application of DEET	The concentration of DEET in commercial products varies widely. Products with concentrations in excess of 50% can cause skin irritation and occasionally skin blistering. It is advisable that these are patch tested first before widespread application DEET should be re-applied every 3–4 h to ensure adequate protection DEET can damage certain plastics, e.g. sunglasses. It is important to emphasise to clients that they must wash their hands after applying DEET
Illness on return from malarial region	Patients should be told to report cold or flu-like symptoms to their GP for 3 months after returning from holiday. However, symptoms of malaria can take up to a year to manifest themselves because the liver can harbour a reservoir of parasites

of chloroquine-resistant falciparum malaria is still low. Adults and children over 13 should take 300 mg of chloroquine base each week; this is equivalent to two tablets. Chloroquine can be given to children of all ages and is calculated on a milligram per kilogram basis. A syrup formulation of Nivaquine is available (50 mg of base/5 mL) and should be recommended for children because an accurate dose can be given according to their weight.

Chloroquine is associated with a number of side-effects including nausea, vomiting, headaches and visual disturbances. Most patient groups, including pregnant women, can take chloroquine, although it is contra-indicated in epilepsy because it might lower the seizure threshold and tonic–clonic seizures have been reported with prophylactic doses. Patients with psoriasis might notice a worsening of their condition. Chloroquine should be avoided in patients taking amiodarone, flecainide, sotalol, astemizole and terfenadine because there is a risk of QT prolongation and ventricular arrhythmia.

Proguanil (Paludrine)

Proguanil is always used in combination with chloroquine unless the patient is contraindicated from taking chloroquine. Adults and children over the age of 13 should take 200 mg (two tablets) daily. Like chloroquine, proguanil can be given to children of all ages and the dose should be on a milligram per kilogram basis. A problem with dosing regimens involving proguanil is that it has to be taken daily in addition to weekly taking of chloroquine. To aid this, a travel pack suitable for adults on a 2-week holiday is available. This combines 14 chloroquine tablets with 28 proguanil tablets. Side-effects associated with proguanil are usually mild and include diarrhoea. Patients with known mild renal impairment should take 100 mg daily and the dose should be further reduced if renal impairment is moderate or severe.

Further reading

[Anonymous] 2001 Giving advice on malaria prevention. Pharmaceutical Journal 267: 92–97

Goodyear L 2000 Malaria. Pharmaceutical Journal 264: 405–410

Web sites

NHS advice for travellers: www.fitfortravel.scot.nhs.uk

WHO advice on international travel and health: www.who.int/ith

Sunburn

Background

Rays from the ultraviolet region of the light spectrum are responsible for suntan and sunburn. The ultraviolet spectrum is subdivided in to three regions:

- UVA (320–400 nm)
- UVB (290–320 nm)
- UVC (200–290 nm).

Although UVC light is effectively filtered out by the ozone layer, light from the UVA spectrum is responsible for causing skin tanning and UVB light causes sunburn.

Prevalence and epidemiology

The prevalence and epidemiology of sunburn is unknown but the incidence of cancers related to long-term skin damage has dramatically increased since the 1980s. The incidence of sun-related cancers are greatest in white-skinned people living in equatorial regions.

Aetiology

The body's response to the effects of UVA and UVB light is protective. On exposure to ultraviolet light, melanocytes in the skin increase their production of the compound melanin, causing a darkening of the skin – the all important suntan! Melanin absorbs both UVA and UVB and effectively protects the skin from damage, unfortunately melanin synthesis is slow and skin damage might well have occurred already (sunburn). In addition to melanin production, epidermal hyperplasia occurs, causing the skin to thicken; this provides further protection against the skin.

Sunburn is an inflammatory response to excessive exposure to ultraviolet light whereby an increase in inflammatory mediators results in capillary vasodilatation and increased capillary permeability. Long-term problems of sun-induced skin damage are premature skin ageing and, more importantly, acute exposure to ultraviolet light is associated with increased incidence of basal cell carcinoma and malignant melanoma. Skin surfaces (e.g. face and hands) that are exposed to a lifetime accumulation of UV radiation are also associated with squamous cell carcinoma.

Evidence base for over-the-counter medication

Very few medicines offer a specific treatment for sunburn; prevention is truly better than cure. Sunscreens allow UVA and UVB to be filtered, preventing burning and premature ageing of skin. The sun protection factor (SPF) gives a rough estimate of the efficiency of the product to block UVB:

> for example, if a person normally shows signs of burning in 30 min without protection, a product with an SPF of 6 would extend the period of time until burning begins to 3 hours (i.e. it extends the time taken to burn by six times).

A controversial star rating also exists to indicate the level of protection offered against UVA relative to protection against UVB. A four-star rating indicates the product has a balanced amount of UVA and UVB protection. The lower the star rating, the greater the protection offered against UVB compared to UVA.

Practical prescribing and product selection

Prescribing information relating to sunscreen products reviewed in the section 'Evidence base for over-the-counter medication' is discussed and summarised in Table 10.5; useful tips relating to patients asking for advice about protection from the sun are given in Hints and Tips Box 10.5.

A plethora of sunscreen products are marketed. All products should be reapplied every 2 to 3 h and after swimming to ensure maximum protection. Standard practice until recently was to match skin type with the level of SPF protection the person should seek. However, although preventing sunburn, this approach does not prevent long-term skin damage. Rather than selecting a specific sunscreen for skin type it is advocated that all white-skinned people should use a sunscreen with an SPF of 15. This level of protection is effectively a sun block because it absorbs more than 90% of UV radiation and, provided it is applied in sufficient quantity and regularly (every 2 to 3 h), then higher SPF sunscreens are not needed.

Chemical sunscreens

Chemical sunscreens work by absorbing UV energy and give protection against either UVA or UVB, although they tend to be more effective against UVB radiation. The majority of marketed products contain a combination of agents including benzophenones, cinnamates, dibenzoylmethanes and para-aminobenzoic acid. The latter is infrequently used now because it has been associated with contact sensitivity.

Physical sunscreens

Physical sunscreens are opaque reflective agents and offer protection against UVA and UVB radiation. Examples of physical sunscreens include zinc and titanium oxide.

Table 10.5
Practical prescribing: Summary of sun protection products

Medicine	Use in children	Likely side-effects	Drug interactions of note	Patients in whom care should be exercised	Pregnancy
Chemical sunscreens	Infant upwards	Allergic reactions, but might be linked to the vehicle and not the active ingredients	None	None	OK
Physical sunscreens		None, but can be cosmetically unacceptable			

HINTS AND TIPS BOX 10.5: SUNBURN

How to avoid sunburn	People can develop sunburn even on cloudy days because ultraviolet light is not effectively filtered; therefore patients should be told to still apply sunscreen Avoid the hottest parts of the day (between 10.00 a.m. and 2.00 p.m.) as the chances of being burnt are greatest Wear a hat with a brim and also long-sleeved shirts and trousers during the hottest parts of the day
Water-resistant sunscreens	These are claimed to be effective after immersion in water. However, studies have shown that sunscreen effectiveness decreases after water exposure. It would therefore be prudent to reapply sunscreens after swimming
Eye protection	Prolonged (over years) sun exposure can contribute to age-related macular degeneration. Therefore wrap around sunglasses and lenses that effectively filter UV light should be worn
But what if the person has got sunburn?	Mild sunburn can be managed with a combination of topical cooling preparations, such as calamine and systemic analgesia
Medicine-induced photosensitivity	Piroxicam, tetracyclines, chlorpromazine, phenothiazines and amiodarone can cause pruritus and skin rash when the skin is exposed to natural sunlight

Further reading

Goodyear L 2001 Skin conditions associated with the sun and heat. Pharmaceutical Journal 266: 892–897

Kricker A, Armstrong B K, English D R et al 1995 Does intermittent sun exposure cause basal cell carcinoma? a case-control study in Western Australia. International Journal of Cancer 60:489–494

Wong J G, Feussner J R 1994 Screening for melanoma. 'Here's looking at you, kid'. North Carolina Medical Journal 55:142–145

Web sites

Article on sunscreens and cancer: www.com/healthnews/sunscreens.html

Electronic textbook of dermatology: www.telemedicine.org/stamford.htm

The Skin Cancer Foundation: www.skincancer.org/

Self-assessment questions

The following questions are intended to supplement the text. Two levels of questions are provided; multiple choice questions and case studies. The multiple choice questions are designed to test factual recall and case studies allow knowledge to be applied to a practice setting.

Multiple choice questions

10.1. Which antihistamine used for motion sickness is subject to abuse?

a. Cinnarizine
b. Cyclizine
c. Promethazine
d. Meclozine
e. Hyoscine

10.2. What is the main side-effect of Levonelle?

a. Vomiting
b. Headache
c. Diarrhoea
d. Nausea
e. Dizziness

10.3. In which group of the population is smoking on the increase?

a. Middle-aged males
b. Middle-aged females
c. Teenage females
d. Teenage males
e. None of the above

10.4. Which patients should use 24-h patches?

a. People who smoke more than 20 cigarettes a day
b. People who smoke more than 40 cigarettes a day
c. People who need a cigarette within 20 min of waking up
d. People who need a cigarette before they go to sleep
e. People who smoke cigars

10.5. Which dermatological condition can be worsened by taking chloroquine?

a. Psoriasis
b. Acne vulgaris
c. Eczema
d. Rosacea
e. Atopic dermatitis

10.6. How long after unprotected sex can emergency hormonal contraception be given?

a. 24 h
b. 48 h
c. 72 h
d. 96 h
e. 120 h

10.7. What is regarded as the most important smoking-related disease?

a. Lung cancer
b. Chronic obstructive pulmonary disease
c. Throat cancer
d. Motor neurone disease
e. Ischaemic heart disease

10.8. With which patient group should care be taken when recommending promethazine for motion sickness?

a. Glaucoma
b. Hypertension
c. Peptic ulceration
d. Diabetes mellitus
e. Parkinson's disease

Questions 10.9 to 10.11 concern the following NRT products:

A. Patch
B. Gum
C. Inhalator
D. Lozenge
E. Microtab

Select, from A to E, which of the above products:

10.9. Is most suitable for patients in whom compliance might be an issue

10.10. Delivers constant levels of plasma nicotine

10.11. Is useful for those people who need to have their hands occupied

Questions 10.12 to 10.14 concern the following medicines:

A. Chloroquine
B. Proguanil
C. Hyoscine
D. Nicotine replacement therapy
E. Levonorgestrel

Select, from A to E, which of the above medicines:

10.12. Causes diarrhoea

10.13. Causes visual disturbances

10.14. Causes dry mouth

Questions 10.15 to 10.17: for each of these questions *one* or *more* of the responses is (are) correct. Decide which of the responses is (are) correct. Then choose:

A. If a, b and c are correct
B. If a and b only are correct
C. If b and c only are correct
D. If a only is correct
E. If c only is correct

Directions summarised

A	B	C	D	E
a, b and c	a and b only	b and c only	a only	c only

10.15. When using DEET, the following rule(s) should be followed:

   a. It should be applied regularly
   b. It should be kept away from plastic
   c. It should never be applied to the face

10.16. *Plasmodium falciparum* is associated with:

   a. High levels of drug resistance
   b. The highest incidence of death compared to other forms of malaria
   c. Widespread distribution on the African continent

10.17. What side-effects are commonly associated with chewing nicotine gum?

   a. Hypotension
   b. Taste disturbance
   c. GI disturbances

Questions 10.18 to 10.20: these questions consist of a statement in the left-hand column followed by a statement in the right-hand column. You need to:

● decide whether the first statement is true or false
● decide whether the second statement is true or false

Then choose:

A. If both statements are true and the second statement is a correct explanation of the first statement
B. If both statements are true but the second statement is *not* a correct explanation of the first statement
C. If the first statement is true but the second statement is false
D. If the first statement is false but the second statement is true
E. If both statements are false

Directions summarised

	First statement	Second statement	
A	True	True	Second explanation is a correct explanation of the first
B	True	True	Second statement is *not* a correct explanation of the first
C	True	False	
D	False	True	
E	False	False	

	First statement	*Second statement*
10.18.	Antimalarials have to be taken before travel	Side-effects may preclude patient from taking antimalarials
10.19.	Malaria can be contracted months after return from endemic area	The liver holds a reservoir of parasites that are hard to eradicate
10.20.	Pregnancy is a contraindication for malaria prophylaxis	Infants cannot take antimalarials

Case study

CASE STUDY 10.1

Mr and Mrs J and their two children, Sammy aged 5 and Jessica aged 12 are going on their summer holidays. They want to know what travel sickness tablets they should take.

a. What information do you need to know before recommending a suitable product? For each question state your rationale

You need to know:

- *Who is affected by travel sickness: this will influence recommendation, especially if it affects one of the parents who might be driving.*
- *The length of the trip: this will influence which product will be the most appropriate. It is sensible to match up the length of journey with a medicine that has the same duration of action as the trip.*
- *Medication history: patients who are taking medication for glaucoma or prostate enlargement should avoid taking OTC medicines. Additionally, medicines with anticholinergic side-effects will potentiate the side-effects of OTC medication.*
- *Past medication for similar journeys: it is likely that the family has bought such products in the past. It is worth finding out what they were and how well tolerated they were before potentially recommending the same product.*

You find out they are going to northern France by ferry. This is a 2-hour boat journey followed by a further 2-hour drive. Mr Jones gets seasick and neither of the children likes boats or car journeys. Jessica also suffers from narcolepsy.

b. What would be the best drug regimen for the family? State your rationale.

It appears that the total journey time is relatively short and a hyoscine-based product would be the most suitable product for the two children and their father. Junior Kwells could be used by everyone; Mr Jones would have to take two tablets, Jessica one tablets and Sammy half a tablet. As Jessica has narcolepsy it is necessary to see if she takes any medication to help with the condition. If she does then checks would have to be made to ensure that she could still take hyoscine.

c. What practical advice would you also offer the Jones family?

Hyoscine will cause dry mouth and potential sedation. Sucking sweets can compensate dry mouth. Sedation might be a problem for Mr Jones because he has to drive after the ferry crossing. He should be told about the possible effects of hyoscine. He might choose not to take the medication, although no alternative is available that does not cause possible sedation.

The two children might experience less nausea if they are kept occupied by playing games.

CASE STUDY 10.2

Ms HS walks in to the pharmacy on Saturday morning and asks to buy Levonelle.

a. What questions do you need to ask?

You need to discover:

- *Her age*
- *How long ago she had unprotected sex*
- *Whether she used a form of contraception. If so, what form*
- *The date of her last period and whether it was different to normal.*

You find out she is 18 and had sex last night. She normally takes Microgynon. Her period was about 3 weeks ago and was the same as previous periods.

b. What else do you need to know?

You also need to know about her pill taking compliance.

She says that she has not taken her pill for the last 2 days (Thursday and Friday) and doesn't know whether she should take today's tablet. She has three tablets left before the end of the packet.

c. What advice are you going to give her?

There is no need for EHC because she has forgotten to take her tablets at the end of the cycle. She should be told to continue taking the rest of her tablets but that when the last tablet is taken she should not have a 7-day pill-free period but go straight on to the next packet.

She is very anxious and doesn't feel confident in the advice you have given.

d. Could you supply EHC even though it is not necessary?

There is no reason why you could not supply Levonelle. If this would relieve her anxiety then supply would not be unreasonable.

Answers to multiple choice questions

10.1 = b 10.2 = d 10.3 = c 10.4 = c 10.5 = a 10.6 = c 10.7 = e 10.8 = a 10.9 = a 10.10 = a,
10.11= c 10.12 = b 10.13 = a 10.14 = c 10.15 = b 10.16 = a 10.17 = c 10.18 = a 10.19 = a 10.20 = c.

Abbreviations

µg:	microgram	L:	litre
ACE:	angiotension converting enzyme	MAOI:	monoamine oxidase inhibitor
ADR:	adverse drug reaction	MAU:	minor aphthous ulcers
CB:	chronic bronchitis	mEq:	milliequivalent
CSM:	Committee for Safety of Medicines	mg:	milligram
DEET:	diethyl toluamide	MI:	myocardial infarction
DPH:	diphenhydramine	mL:	millilitre
EHC:	Emergency hormonal contraception	mmol:	millimole
FDA:	Food and Drug Administration (equivalent to the Medicines Control Authority in the UK)	NRT:	Nicotine replacement therapy
		NSAID:	non-steroidal anti-inflammatory drug
GORD:	gastro-oesophageal reflux disease	ORT:	oral rehydration therapy
GP:	general practitioner	OTC:	over-the-counter
GSL:	general sales list	P:	pharmacy
h:	hour	PD:	primary dysmenorrhoea
IHS:	International Headache Society	PID:	pelvic inflammatory disease
HMG-CoA:	beta-hydroxy beta-methyl glutaryl coenzyme A	PMS:	premenstrual syndrome
		POM:	prescription-only-medicine
HPV:	human papilloma virus	PV:	per vagina
HSV:	herpes simplex virus	SSRI:	selective serotonin reuptake inhibitor
IBS:	irritable bowel syndrome	STD:	sexually transmitted disease
IgE:	immunoglobulin E	TB:	tuberculosis
INR:	international normalised ratio	TCA:	tricyclic antidepressant
IUCD	intrauterine contraceptive device	UTI:	urinary tract infection
KCS:	keratoconjunctivitis sicca	WHO:	World Health Organization

Glossary of terms

Chapter 1

Atopy: A form of hypersensitivity characterised by a familial tendency.

Cervical lymphadenopathy: Enlargement of the cervical lymph nodes.

Agranulocytosis: Acute deficiency of neutrophil white blood cells leading to neutropenia.

Auroscopical examination: Examination of the ear drum by means of an apparatus that shines light on to the ear drum.

Haemoptysis: Coughing up blood.

Dyspnoea: Difficulty in breathing.

Malaise: General feeling of being unwell.

Gastro-oesophageal reflux: The back flow of gastric contents in to the oesophagus.

Pleurisy: Inflammation of the pleural membranes caused by the two pleural membranes adhering to one another.

Purulent: Term used to describe a material containing pus.

Rhinorrhoea: Watery nasal discharge.

Vascular engorgement: An area of tissue that has been excessively perfused with blood.

Vasodilatation: Increase in the diameter of the blood vessels.

Chapter 2

Chalazion: Also referred to as meibomian cyst.

Glands of Zeiss and Moll: Both are located within the eyelid. The gland of Zeiss secretes sebum; the gland of Moll secretes sweat.

Hordeola: Commonly known as styes.

Limbal area: Area where the cornea meets the sclera.

Meibomianitis: Inflammation of the meibomian gland caused by increased production of sebum from the sebaceous glands located at the base of the eyelids

Photophobia: A dislike of bright lights.

Visual acuity: The ability to read text. For example, distance visual acuity is the person's ability to read letters across the room and near visual acuity is the person's ability to read letters close to.

Chapter 3

Conductive deafness: Sound waves are hindered from reaching the inner ear (e.g. by ear wax) resulting in distortion of sounds that impairs the understanding of words.

Effusion: Escape of fluid, e.g. exudate from the ear.

Laceration: A tear in the skin causing a wound.

Oedamatous: Abnormal accumulation in intercellular spaces of the body.

Tinnitus: A noise in the ears likened to ringing or buzzing.

Chapter 4

Haematoma: A localised collection of blood, usually clotted, in an organ, space or tissue.

Myalgia: Muscular pain.

Paraesthesia: An abnormal sensation, for example, a burning or prickling sensation.

Pericranial: Area relating to around the skull.

Purpuric rash: Rash with a distinctive red–purple colouration caused by haemorrhage of small blood vessels in the skin.

Chapter 5

Amenorrhoea: Absence or the stoppage of menstruation.

Anovulatory: Term used to describe women that do not ovulate.

Bacteriuria: Bacteria in the urine.

Dyspareunia: Difficult or painful sexual intercourse.

Dysuria: Painful or difficult urination.

Haematuria: Blood in the urine.

Menarche: Onset of menstruation.

Nocturia: Excessive urination at night.

Perianal: The area around the anus.

Perineal: The area around the perineum, i.e. that area between the vulva and anus.

Postmenopausal women: Women that have finished menstruating. The average age for women to become postmenopausal in the UK is 51.

Prostate gland: The gland that surrounds the neck of the bladder and urethra in men.

Pyelonephritis: Inflammation of the kidney due to bacterial infection.

Suprapubic: Area above the pubic region.

Chapter 6

Annular lesions: Skin lesions that are circular.

Diverticulitis: Inflammation of a diverticulum, which is a pouch or sac. It occurs normally after herniation.

Halitosis: Bad breath.

Suprapubic: Area above the pubic area of the abdomen.

Tenesmus: Cessation of incomplete bowel evacuation.

Ureter: Tube connecting the kidney to the bladder.

Chapter 7

Atopy: Literally means 'strange disease'. The triad of atopic dermatitis, asthma and allergic rhinitis.

Comedone: A plug of oxidised sebaceous material obstructing the surface opening of pilosebaceous follicle, commonly referred to as a 'blackhead'.

Crust: The term given to dried exudate.

Erythema: Redness of the skin.

Intertrigo: Dermatitis on apposing areas of skin in flexural body sites, e.g. groin, axillae.

Papules: Raised palpable spots.

Pustule: A pus-filled lesion.

Vesicles: Small, raised, fluid-filled lesions or blisters.

Chapter 8

Abduction: Describes movement of a part away from the median plane of the body, e.g. moving the leg straight out to the side.

Articular cartilage: Cartilage occurring in the joint.

Disc herniation: Abnormal protrusion of the nucleus pulposus of the disc that might impinge on a nerve root.

Epicondylitis: Inflammation of the epicondyle, the protuberance above the condyle (the rounded part at the end of the bone used for articulation with another bone).

Chapter 9

Erythematous: Redness of the skin due to capillary vasodilation.

Lichenification: Thickenening and hardening of the skin.

Chapter 10

Erythrocytes: Red blood cells.

Melanocytes: Cells in the skin epidermis responsible for producing the pigment melanin.

Sequestration: An increased amount of blood within a limited vascular region.

Yuzpe method: The name given to the combined oestrogen and progestogen method of emergency contraception.

Index